Oral Rehabilitation

A Case-Based Approach

Oral Rehabilitation
A Case-Based Approach

Edited by

Professor Iven Klineberg

Chair, Nobel Biocare Centre of Oral Rehabilitation
Professor of Oral Rehabilitation
Faculty of Dentistry
The University of Sydney
Westmead Centre for Oral Health, Westmead Hospital
Sydney, Australia

Dr Diana Kingston

Information Consultant
Faculty of Dentistry
The University of Sydney
Sydney, Australia

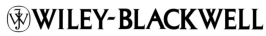

WILEY-BLACKWELL

A John Wiley & Sons, Ltd., Publication

Library of Congress Cataloging-in-Publication Data

Oral rehabilitation : a case-based approach / edited by Iven Klineberg, Diana Kingston.
    p. ; cm.
  Includes bibliographical references and index.
  ISBN 978-1-4051-9781-6 (hard cover : alk. paper)
  I. Klineberg, Iven. II. Kingston, Diana.
  [DNLM: 1. Oral Surgical Procedures, Preprosthetic–methods–Case Reports.   2. Prosthodontics–methods–Case Reports.   WU 500]
  617.6'9–dc23
                                                                 2011038021

A catalogue record for this book is available from the British Library.

Wiley also publishes its books in a variety of electronic formats. Some content that appears in print may not be available in electronic books.

Set in 10/12 pt Univers Light by Toppan Best-set Premedia Limited
Printed and bound in Singapore by Markono Print Media Pte Ltd

1   2012

Contents

Contributors

Dr Johnson P.Y. Chou
BDS *Otago*, DClinDent *Sydney*, FRACDS, MRACDS
Prosthodontist, Private Practice, Department of Oral
Restorative Sciences, Westmead Centre for Oral
Health, Westmead, NSW 2145, Australia

Dr Tuan Dao
BDS (Hons), MDSc (Pros) *Sydney*
Prosthodontist, Private Practice, Maroubra, NSW 2035,
Australia

Associate Professor Max Guazzato
DDS (Hons) *Milan*, PhD, DClinDent (Pros) *Sydney*,
MRACDS, FRACDS, DT
Associate Professor in Oral Rehabilitation,
Prosthodontist, Private Practice, Faculty of Dentistry,
University of Sydney, Westmead Centre of Oral Health,
Westmead, NSW 2145, Australia

Adjunct Associate Professor Robin Hawthorn
OAM, BDS (Hons), MDS *Sydney*, FICD
Prosthodontist, Private Practice, Tutor and Mentor,
Sydney, NSW 2000, Australia

Dr Ken Hooi
BDS, GradDipClinDent (Oral Implants), MDSc *Sydney*
Prosthodontist, Private Practice, The Dental Specialists,
Sydney, NSW 2000, Australia

Dr Diana Kingston
BA *Sydney*, MLib, PhD *UNSW*
Information Consultant (Dentistry & Medicine), Oatley,
NSW 2223, Australia

Professor Iven Klineberg
AM, RFD, BSc, MDS *Sydney*, PhD *London*, MRACDS,
FRACDS, FDSRCS *Eng and Edin*, FICD
Chair, Nobel Biocare Centre of Oral Rehabilitation,
Prosthodontist, Faculty of Dentistry, University of
Sydney, Westmead Centre of Oral Health, Westmead,
NSW 2145, Australia

Dr Agnes T.C. Lai
BDS, DClinDent *Sydney*, MRACDS
Lecturer in Oral Rehabilitation, Prosthodontist, Faculty
of Dentistry, University of Sydney, Westmead Centre of
Oral Health, Westmead, NSW 2145, Australia

Dr Michael Lewis
BDS (Hons), DClinDent (Pros) *Sydney*, MRACDS
Prosthodontist, Private Practice, Bondi, NSW 2026,
Australia

Dr Glen Liddelow
BDSc, MScD *WA*, DClinDent *Sydney*, MRACDS,
FRACDS
Prosthodontist, Private Practice, The Branemark Center,
West Perth, WA 6005, Australia

Professor Chris Peck
BDS, MSc (Dent), GradDipScMed (Pain) *Sydney*, PhD
UBC
Professor and Dean, Faculty of Dentistry, University of
Sydney, NSW 2006, Australia

Dr Robert Santosa
BDS *Adelaide*, MDSc *Sydney*
Prosthodontist, Private Practice, Sydney, NSW 2000,
Australia

Dr Christine Wallace
BDS, MDSc *Sydney*, CertMaxFacPros (*Iowa*),
GradCertSocSc (HEd) *Sydney*, MRACDS, FRACDS
Head, Department of Oral Restorative Sciences, Clinical
Senior Lecturer, Lane Cove, NSW 1595, Australia

Clinical Professor Terry Walton
AM, BDS, MDSc *Sydney*, MS *Michigan*, FRACDS, FICD
Prosthodontist, Private Practice, Sydney, NSW 2000,
Australia

Dr Alan Yap
BDS, MDSc (Pros) *Sydney*, MRACDS
Lecturer, Prosthodontist, Private Practice, Killara, NSW
2071, Australia

Foreword

Dental education has routinely sought to initiate and nurture the special relationship that should exist between dentist and patient. Hence our profession's ethical code and commitment to behave according to the highest standards. Yet current dental practice has never seemed as vulnerable as it is today to commercial pressures to sell restorative interventions. This is probably because so much of today's continuing education culture seems to encourage a professional health-care approach that is more responsive to consumer choice. Far too many meetings, commercial initiatives and web-based information seem to convey the message that dental care is no different from a commercial transaction, such as buying a suit or an expensive household appliance.

The resultant and increasingly blurred demarcation line between patient care and consumerism remains a pervasive challenge in prosthodontic practice – an even more serious one keeping in mind the biotechnological breakthrough of osseointegrated implants and the inflated promise of cosmetic solutions. It is therefore reassuring to find a book of this calibre. It underscores old principles and values as it seeks to reconcile erudition with prudence, scrupulous analysis with much wisdom. It is clearly the coherent result of over three decades of clinical scholarship that went into its conception, with the authors providing sensible understanding and context for assessing patients' oral rehabilitative needs in a manner that marries common sense with best available clinical evidence.

In the book's first half, review chapters cover essential determinants of diagnosis, treatment planning and patient management – strong reminders that even traditional basic principles need to be refined as better understanding of form and function yield clearer treatment considerations, as well as acknowledging more unanswered questions. The second half offers a spectrum of well-argued and described case histories that may be regarded as reflecting the broad range of prosthodontic expertise. This is the contributors' impressive and successful way of reaching across the dental disciplines that underpin so much of the oral rehabilitative effort. These case histories are an exemplary collection of teachable information within a methodological framework that connects them to the real clinical world. The result is a reliable and necessary blend of best available evidence and the sort of theory and empiricism that clinical expertise continues to depend on. This is a particularly insightful way to teach dentists how to approach the challenge of oral rehabilitation, always having, as an integral part, a patient-centred approach.

The authors and contributors have done the profession, and the discipline of prosthodontics in particular, an outstanding service by writing this book. It certainly deserves the widest possible readership.

George A. Zarb, CM, BChD, MS, DDS, MS, FRCD(C), PhD, DSc, MD, LLD (HC)
Emeritus Professor University of Toronto,
Editor-in-Chief International Journal of Prosthodontics

Acknowledgements

The Prosthodontics Specialty programme

This work would not have been contemplated without the important contributions from many colleagues, some of whom assisted in the early development of the programme some 30 years ago. Of these colleagues, some have continued to contribute and support the academic and/or clinical aspects of the coursework. Not surprisingly, the programme has required ongoing revisions, restructuring and upgrading of seminars and lectures, embracing new developments and contemporary technologies. The refocusing of patient care as patient centred and evidence based has been crucially important with the evolution and availability of electronic information and the internet. This is transforming every aspect of communication, community awareness, health management and education – all of which lead to a more informed community and one that is often prepared to challenge the knowledge base of the generalist as well as the specialist clinician.

The initial core group of clinical prosthodontists who assisted the academic and clinical programme include Robin Hawthorn and Terry Walton, who are to be especially acknowledged, as well as the first graduate from the programme Keith Baetz, who joined the teaching team after completing the programme. This core group was joined by other colleagues, including sequentially: Cyril Thomas, Christine Wallace, Dan Brener, Catherine Collins, Geoff Cook, Greg Charlesworth, David Sykes, Geoff Borlase, Chris Peck, Matthew McLaughlin, Suhas Deshpande, Norton Duckmanton, Peter Hell, Anthony Au, Sunny Hong and Neil Peppitt.

The programme was built around a principle of shared decision-making through a Planning Committee, which has in general met every 3 months to discuss and plan new developments and review all aspects of the programme. This has proven to be especially valuable and is a model that can be recommended for developing a new initiative. Those members of the Planning Committee must be recognised, as meetings take place early evening, requiring members to travel to the meeting and contribute to a planned agenda after a busy clinical day. Meetings are informal, but are built around a specific agenda, and are minuted with action items being progressed to ensure continuity of input and engagement of members. The development of electronic communication has greatly facilitated this. Those who have contributed to Planning Committee meetings since 1983 include: Bruce Burns, Roland Bryant, Robin Hawthorn,* Peter Howell, Michael Kafalias, Cyril Thomas, Terry Walton,* Keith Baetz, George Hewitt, Jim Ironside, Christine Wallace,* Catherine Collins, Melissa Kah, Sybille Lechner, Greg Murray, Neil Peppitt, Brian Roberts, David Roessler, Stephen Travis, Dan Brener,* Greg Charlesworth,* Geoff Cook,* David Sykes,*Geoff Borlase,* Norton Duckmanton,* Chris Peck, Suhas Deshpande,* Matthew McLaughlin,* Stefan Scholz and Max Guazzato.*

The present publication

This book would also not have been possible without the specific material prepared for the chapters and cases.

Section 1 to Section 3

We acknowledge the contributors to the first three sections of the book who were selected to prepare material of special importance to prosthodontic education, clinical assessment, diagnosis and treatment planning. These chapters cover a small aspect of clinical prosthodontics but are included to emphasise their relevance: literature searching as a key element of evidence-based practice; consent and clinician–patient relationship as a crucial aspect of patient management and gaining pretreatment agreement; treatment decision-making that underpins each case progression; orofacial pain and temporomandibular disorders as an important aspect of pretreatment for oral rehabilitation; diagnostic planning for a biological approach to tooth preparation; provisionalisation as an important aspect of management of dental, periodontal and patient needs; and maintenance and long-term outcomes. We are indebted to the chapter authors who are recognised for their special contribution to this work including: Chris Peck, Robin Hawthorn, Max Guazzato, Robert Santosa, Johnson Chou, Terry Walton, in addition to the editors. Special appreciation is acknowledged of

* Denotes current members.

the assistance of Daniel Klineberg for his critical and helpful comments for Chapter 3.

Section 4

The cases and case presentations are the core element of this text, as those selected are a representation of the case types managed by candidates in the specialty programme. They showcase the work of the programme and the level of clinical expertise expected at the conclusion of each candidature. Although only a small number of clinicians were selected, and often with more than one case each, their work reflects the standard approach to treatment planning and delivery that has been developed and followed. The authors – Ken Hooi, Johnson Chou, Max Guazzato, Agnes Lai, Glen Liddelow, Michael Lewis, Alan Yap and Tuan Dao – are to be congratulated for having completed the programme and for agreeing to provide the material for the case chapters. Others from the programme had also provided cases, but the word size and continual interaction required in preparation limited the author contributions.

In addition, each chapter has an introduction to define the case material to follow. Those colleagues who prepared these introductions, in addition to the editor, are Christine Wallace and Alan Yap who are to be acknowledged for their expertise in the specific clinical area.

Preparation for publication

The oversight provided throughout the project by our publisher Wiley-Blackwell has been constructive and supportive. We wish to thank Sophia Joyce, our Senior Commissioning Editor, and also Project Managers James Benefield and Catriona Cooper. Our sincere thanks go to members of other teams involved in the book's production including: Nick Morgan (production editor), Lucy Nash (editorial assistant), Ruth Swan (project manager), Maggie Beveridge (copyeditor), the typesetters at Toppan, the proofreaders and the indexer Allison McKechnie. Finally, the assistance with preparation provided by our local administrative group led by Natasha Pavic, and assisted initially by Alison Reid and Catherine Sperling, has been meticulous. Special acknowledgement is made of the ongoing support of Natasha, which has been indispensable and without which this work would not have been possible.

Iven Klineberg and Diana Kingston
Sydney, August 2011

Abbreviations

A	point A (anatomical landmark)	iCAT	imaging technique
ACC	all-ceramic crown	ICP	intercuspal contact position (of teeth)
adj	adjustment	INR	international normalised ratio
Ag	silver	L	left
ANB	anatomical landmarks for lateral cephalometric measurement (point A nasion point B)	lat ceph	lateral cephalometry
		LHS	left hand side
		LR	lower right
AP	antero-posterior	Lt	left
B	point B (anatomical landmark)	µm	micron, micrometre
B	buccal (restoration)	M	mesial (restoration)
BL	buccal lingual	MB	mesio-buccal
BOP	bleeding on probing	MCC	metal-ceramic crown
BWs	bite wing radiographs	MI	maximum intercuspation
CAD/CAM	computer-aided design/computer-aided manufacture	MIDB	mesial, incisal, distal, buccal (restoration)
		MIDBP	mesial incisal disto-buccal and palatal
CMC	ceramo-metal crown	MIDP	mesial incisal disto-palatal
CEJ	cemento-enamel junction	ML	mesio-lingual
CMC	ceramo-metal crown	MM	maxillo-mandibular
CO	centric occlusion	MMR	maxillo-mandibular relationship
CoCr	cobalt chrome (alloy for partial denture castings)	Mni	mandibular incisal
		MO	mesio-occlusal
CPITN	Community Periodontal Index of Treatment Needs	mod	modification
		MOD	mesio-occlusal distal
CR	centric relation	MODL	mesio-occluso-disto-lingual
CT	computed tomography	MODB	mesio-occluso-disto-buccal
D	distal (restoration)	MODP	mesio-occluso-disto-palatal
DB	disto-buccal	MOL	mesio-lingual
DO	disto-occlusal	MP	mesio-palatal or maximum protrusion
DP	disto-palatal	MPD	myofacial pain dysfunction
DPI	disto-palatal incisal	Mxi	maxillary incisal
Dx	diagnosis	N	nasion (anterior point on the frontonasal suture)
F	complete denture		
FDI	Federation Dentaire International	N/A	not apparent/not applicable
F/F	complete maxillary/complete mandibular dentures	NAD	no appreciable disease/no abnormalities detected
FDP	fixed dental prosthesis	Nil	no entry required
FGC	full gold crown	NKA	no known allergies
FGM	full gold margin	O	occlusal
FWS	free way space	OB	occluso-buccal
GIC	tooth coloured restorative material	OD	occluso-distal
GORD	gastro-oesophageal reflux disease	OHI	oral health instruction
GP	general medical practitioner/family physician	OHRQL	oral health related quality of life
I	implant	OJ	orange juice

OMFS	oral and maxillofacial surgery	ref	reference
OP	occluso-palatal	RFA	resonance frequency analysis
OPG	orthopantomogram	RHS	right hand side
OVD	occlusal vertical dimension	RP	retruded position
P	posterior	S	sella (centre of sella turcica)
PA	posterio-anterior	SC	single crown
pal	palate	SCC	squamous cell carcinoma
PAL	palatal	SDA	shortened dental arch
PDL	periodontal ligament	SI	anatomical landmark for lateral
perp	perpendicular		cephalometric imaging
PFM	porcelain fused to metal (crown)	SNA	sella nasion point A
pit	pit on occlusal surface of tooth	SNB	sella nasion point B
Po (or Pog)	pogonion	TMD	temporomandibular disorder
PPD	partial denture	TMJ	temporomandibular joint
R	right	TSL	tooth surface loss
R/L	right/left	UL	upper left
RBB	resin-bonded bridge	UR	upper right
RCP	retruded contact position (of teeth)	V	vertical
RCT	root canal treatment	VD	vertical dimension
RDP	removable dental prosthesis	VDO	vertical dimension of occlusion

Section 1

Introduction and Literature Searching

1

Introduction

Iven Klineberg and Diana Kingston

During the past decade in particular, dental education and clinical practice in contemporary prosthodontics have progressively embraced biological principles and evidence-based decision-making. They have distanced themselves from prosthodontics' mechanical beginnings. This emphasis on the biological basis of case assessment, including an empathetic history, a patient-centred treatment plan and emphasis on explicit and judicious patient consent to support clinical decision-making, allows the careful and meticulous delivery of treatment as a confident and predictable process. Each patient is entitled to, expects and depends on such an approach.

These fundamental changes in philosophy arose as a function of interprofessional dialogue and were influenced significantly by a comprehensive review of dental education presented in *Dental Education at the Crossroads – Challenges and Change* (Field 1995). There has also been a recognition of the importance of evidence-based dentistry. These factors have stimulated a review of core values in education and practice, as has been the case in medical education and practice (Sackett *et al.* 2000).

In recognition of these changes, the authors aim to provide the reader with a contemporary approach based on available evidence to define prosthodontic treatment planning and clinical application. The authors recognise that this is a requirement of educational programmes and are mindful of the need for applying this knowledge in clinical practice.

Restorative dentistry and prosthodontics involve tooth restoration and recognition of the importance of occlusal form to provide improved aesthetics as well as stable tooth contacts at an appropriate occlusal vertical dimension for optimising jaw function. This has a significant bearing on tooth mobility, is relevant for orthodontic treatment and is an important consideration in treatment planning for maxillofacial reconstruction. Enhancing jaw function, defining lower face height and satisfying aesthetic needs, are key issues in optimising oral health. This needs to be appreciated as a global construct, where crucial elements of psychosocial well-being and self-confidence are facial appearance and orofacial integrity as a patient-specific need.

Clinical studies in dentistry are now addressing long-term outcomes which represent major advances in evidence to support clinical decision-making. It is recognised that in the past there was no uniformity in clinical study design to allow meaningful data comparison. Study design has not consistently addressed issues of patient numbers, long-term follow-up, blinding of clinical treatment options, bias and critical assessment of outcome measures. In the absence of appropriate clinical trials and long-term studies on outcomes, clinical practice continues to be primarily based on clinical experience and may be tempered by clinical convenience (operator bias). However, more carefully designed clinical trials of an expected standardised and validated design are now emerging, which are beginning to provide treatment guidelines based on biological research and long-term outcomes of treatment.

An Oral Health Group has been established within the Cochrane Collaboration to coordinate the production of systematic reviews of the literature on interventions in dental and oral health care. The Cochrane Collaboration website provides access to training and resources for authors, such as a glossary and the *Cochrane Handbook for Systematic Reviews of Interventions*. It is possible to browse and search online for completed systematic reviews, reviews in progress (known as *Protocols*) and clinical trials in the *Cochrane Library*. The website of the Centre for Evidence-Based Medicine provides documents on levels of evidence and other training tools. Within the dental literature we find periodical articles on the topic (e.g. see in the serial publications *Evidence-based Dentistry* and the *Journal of Evidence-based Dental Practice*). For monographs on evidence-based dentistry, see Clarkson *et al.* (2002), Hackshaw *et al.* (2006), Chiappelli (2007), Richards *et al.* (2007) and Forrest *et al.* (2009).

Oral Rehabilitation: A Case-Based Approach, First Edition. Edited by Iven Klineberg, Diana Kingston.
© 2012 Blackwell Publishing Ltd. Published 2012 by Blackwell Publishing Ltd.

Evidence-based practice is important for medicine and dentistry to provide a standardised approach to optimise treatment outcomes as the cornerstone of best practice. Although it may sometimes appear to be conceptually difficult to implement, it is important to recognise that evidence-based practice includes several components:

- high-quality scientific and long-term clinical trials that provide objective evidence to support a particular clinical decision;
- clinical experience to ensure a full understanding of each patient's needs and to meet those expectations in the care delivered;
- the ability to ask specific questions in searching for the information required in the assessment and preparation of each case;
- the ability to search for and interpret the information so that it may be applied to each patient's particular clinical situation and explicit needs.

In the past, clinical experience exclusively directed the path of clinical treatment. The acknowledgement of a patient-centred and evidence-based approach is a welcome development for advancing both the clinical science and psychosocial foundation of successful clinical management.

This book arose from a desire to share the philosophy of case assessment, treatment planning and case delivery for a range of patient treatments offered by representative postgraduate students in the specialty programme in prosthodontics at the University of Sydney. It is written to provide a structured approach to decision-making for treatment planning and restoration in oral rehabilitation as an evidence-based process; there is a focus on interdisciplinary interaction to support prosthodontics.

This approach is targeted at those students wishing to advance their learning through a formal approach to clinical decision-making, whether they are beginning their learning or are at an advanced level.

The programme has matured progressively since its commencement by the Faculty of Dentistry at the University of Sydney in 1980. It includes formal coursework and supervised clinical practice in removable, fixed and maxillofacial prosthodontics, involving the use of implants as an integral part of prosthodontic care. It also includes diagnosis and management of orofacial pain and temporomandibular disorders.

The programme is offered as a 3-year full-time coursework programme with the academic and clinical component representing 60–70% and the research component 30–40%. Clinical coursework is primarily based at the Westmead Hospital Centre for Oral Health, a teaching hospital of the University of Sydney and the majority of the postgraduates are full-time in the hospital as Prosthodontic Registrars. Since 2005, provision has been made for selected candidates with extended clinical practice experience and an additional qualification to complete aspects of the clinical requirements in practice with clinical mentor guidance.

The programme is accredited by the Australian Dental Council. Since 2008, the qualification of Doctor of Clinical Dentistry (Prosthodontics), formerly Master of Dental Science (Prosthodontics), has been recognised for specialist description of Prosthodontist by the Australian State Dental Registration Boards and by the Australian Registration Board since 2010. The programme is designed for international equivalence. Postgraduates undertake teaching of undergraduate (predoctoral) students as an educational requirement, and many prosthodontic graduates contribute to the undergraduate and sometimes the postgraduate programme as clinical tutors. They make uniquely important contributions to prosthodontic education and gain significant personal benefits in the process. The strength of the undergraduate programme depends on there being a well-structured postgraduate programme to provide the necessary teaching support.

This book presents cases varying from less complex to more advanced and is designed for undergraduate and postgraduate students and prosthodontic educators. The cases represent the range of complexity presented to a tertiary referral centre as a specialist clinic of a teaching hospital. This demographic may be different from that of a specialist prosthodontic practice but the varied degree of complexity of cases managed ensures that graduates are well prepared for the requirements of specialist practice. Undergraduates will appreciate what is possible in oral rehabilitation and may be encouraged to consider postgraduate education, while postgraduates will become more aware of management options.

Case reports have a regular format and, although each presentation is not identical, they follow an approach that has been developed from evidence-based data to guide clinical decisions: they have a patient-centred focus. The latter defines the uniquely individual nature of each case and recognises that there is a range of treatment options that needs to be considered for each patient's specific needs.

The cases selected are from more recent graduates but are representative of the types of cases that have characterised the programme since its beginning. The cases are from those graduates who wished to contribute and their willingness to share this information is gratefully acknowledged.

Websites

Centre for Evidenced-Based Medicine. EBM tools (http://www.cebm.net, accessed 18 August 2010).

Cochrane Collaboration. Homepage (http://www.cochrane.org, accessed 24 August 2010).

Cochrane Library. Homepage (http://www.thecochranelibrary.com or http://www.cochrane.org, accessed 18 August 2010).

Cochrane Oral Health Group. Homepage (http://www.ohg.cochrane.org, accessed 18 August 2010).

References

Chiappelli, F. (ed.) (2007) *Manual of Evidence-based Research for the Health Sciences: Implication for Clinical Dentistry.* Nova Science, Hauppauge, NY.

Clarkson, J., Harrison, J., Ismail, A. *et al.* (eds) (2002) *Evidence Based Dentistry for Effective Practice.* Martin Dunitz, New York.

Cochrane Handbook for Systematic Reviews of Interventions (http://www.cochrane-handbook.org, accessed 24 August 2010).

Evidence-based Dentistry (1998–) British Dental Journal, London.

Field, M.J. (ed.) (1995) *Dental Education at the Crossroads: Challenges and Change.* Committee on the Future of Dental Education, Division of Health and Services, Institute of Medicine; Marilyn J. Field (ed.) National Academy Press, Washington, DC.

Forrest, J.L., Miller, S.A., Overman, P.R. *et al.* (2009) *Evidence-based Decision Making: A Translational Guide for Dental Professionals.* Wolters Kluwer Health, Philadelphia.

Hackshaw, A.K., Paul, E.A. & Davenport, E. (2006) *Evidence-based Dentistry: an Introduction.* Blackwell Munksgaard, Oxford.

Journal of Evidence-based Dental Practice (2001-) Mosby, St Louis.

Richards, D., Clarkson, J., Matthews, D. *et al.* (2007) *Evidence-based Dentistry: Managing Information for Better Practice.* Quintessence, London.

Sackett, D.L., Straus, S.L. & Richardson, W.S. *et al.* (2000) *Evidence-based Medicine: How to Practice and Teach EBM,* 2nd edn. Churchill Livingstone, Edinburgh.

2

Searching the Literature: An Evidence-Based Approach

Diana Kingston

This chapter considers principles and processes of literature search design with a focus on literary sources of information for subjects (topics). Similar principles may also be relevant to searches for authors and titles. Although the context is the clinical situation, information for researchers is also included.

The following aspects of search design are emphasised:

- needs identification;
- selection of information sources;
- concepts and their relationships;
- terminology for concepts and relationships;
- search design elements and launch points;
- refinement and choice of search designs.

These aspects may be thought of as subprocesses or design stages that tend to overlap. Work back and forth between the different stages of design, using feedback from progress to build (construct) an efficient and effective search strategy. A search design should be logical and complete. It should withstand peer review. Usually, a series of search designs for a topic is required (see Section 6). Each search design must be an appropriate three-way fit for a particular:

- research purpose;
- aspect of topic;
- chosen information source (database features, etc.).

Within the confines of a single chapter, an apparently simple sample topic best illustrates the issues that dentists as search designers need to address.

Sample topic: Longevity of single tooth implants

At this point some readers may prefer to proceed to Section 6 of this chapter and work through the accompanying examples, then return to follow the explanation of

search design preparation that starts here. Good preparation is vital to good search design and efficient, effective literature searching.

1. Needs identification

Needs identification is a very important first stage in the search design process. Aspects of a subject that are necessary inclusions are identified and recorded in a tabular fashion as search requirements (Table 2.1). Careful consideration of purpose and aims is required as is exploration in the field of interest to inform the search design process. It is very useful to record and consider any relevant citations or references found during this process, including terminology recorded as subject descriptors (see Section 4).

Specified inclusions and exclusions define and limit final literature search design and thus retrieval (results). However, some limitations should not be used too soon, otherwise they may limit the potential of the literature search. Refine the search requirements table from feedback with progress. The needs identification stage of search design overlaps with the next few stages of search design.

2. Selection of information sources

Information sources are of two (overlapping) groups. First, some resources are primarily used to explore, define and refine the direction and area of interest. Second, some resources are particularly relevant to evidence-based approaches for literature searching. In this chapter, for both the exploratory and main search stages, we concentrate on high-quality resources as our information sources of choice, in particular the *Cochrane Library* provided by the Cochrane Collaboration and *PubMed* (including the *MEDLINE* database) provided by the National Library of Medicine/National Institutes of Health in the USA (Table 2.2). It is suggested that the reader opens these online information sources and tries out the options.

Oral Rehabilitation: A Case-Based Approach, First Edition. Edited by Iven Klineberg, Diana Kingston.
© 2012 Blackwell Publishing Ltd. Published 2012 by Blackwell Publishing Ltd.

2.1 Exploratory sources

It is important to seek out definitions of ideas, concepts and terms, so that one can accurately pinpoint one's area of interest within the literature and gain an insight into the variations of terminology used by authors and indexers. Exploration of the boundaries and scope of a subject for our current purpose/s is very important. Various authoritative sources are available: library catalogues, dictionaries, thesauri, textbooks, articles and even internet sources. However, the latter should always be used with care and discrimination because general search engines do not filter for evidence-based material. In any case, at least look for the endorsement of a website by the Health on the Net Foundation (HON) logo. Of course, there are other sources of information in addition to these, such as clinical records and expert advice from colleagues. One aims to ascertain how much literature there may be on a topic, trends and the dates of the publications involved.

2.1.1 MeSH Browser

The *MeSH* thesaurus at the *MeSH Browser* website is designed for use with the *MEDLINE* database. It is a very important tool that may be used both as a dictionary and a guide to appropriate search terminology (primarily but not only) for the *MEDLINE* database and also the *Cochrane Database of Systematic Reviews* in the *Cochrane Library*. This tool may be approached in one of two ways:

- Type in term or beginning of any root fragments, then scroll down and click on an option [Find Term/s . . .]. For examples, see Table 2.3 and Table 2.4.
- Search by tree category – use [Navigate from tree top].

Table 2.1 Search requirements

Parameters and concepts	Priority
Description of topic (short paragraph): Longevity of single tooth implants	
Results required (e.g. comprehensive search or just a few references)	
Primary concept (e.g. Patient/Population/ Condition/Disease): single tooth implants	1
Secondary publication type/Type of article: meta-analyses	2.1
Secondary publication type/Type of article: systematic reviews	2.2
Primary publication (research study) type: randomised controlled trials	2.3
Second concept (continued): longevity	2.4
Controlled clinical trials (*CCTR – Cochrane*)	2.5
Prognosis clinical queries	2.6
Intervention/therapy clinical queries/Broad	2.7
Aetiology/causation/harm clinical queries	2.8
Diagnosis/diagnostic tests clinical queries	2.9
Publication form/s (e.g. books/articles/full-text/ abstract only)	

Notes:
1. Add rows to table for additional concept pools as required (e.g. Journal sets, Dates of publication, Dates of entry into database, Human/animal/species, Age group/s, Gender, Language/s of publication, Geographical area/s, Specific exclusions).
2. List citations (useful references already used): Torabinejad et al. (2007); Pjetursson et al. (2007); Jung et al. (2008).
3. List likely information sources (e.g. e-databases): *Cochrane Library* and *PubMed* (including *MEDLINE*).
4. Expect retrieval from priority 2 concept pools to overlap.

Table 2.3 Primary concept – *MeSH Browser*

Aim: to find *MeSH* term/s for primary concept via http://www.nlm.nih.gov/mesh/MBrowser.html

Enter the term 'single tooth' and click below on the option button labelled [Find Terms with ALL fragments] and retrieve the preferred *MeSH* term for our topic: **Dental Implants, Single-Tooth**. If we click on the link provided from this point we step into further details about this term including the:

- *Scope Note* (for the definition)
- *Previous Indexing* term was *Dental Implants* (used 1990–1996; this is relevant to a comprehensive search for older material)
- *History Note* (date given is 1997 when *MEDLINE* indexers started using this term officially – see above point)
- *MeSH Tree Structures* – the list indicates that our subject is indexed both as part of topic tree *Dentistry/ Prosthodontics* (in class E06) and topic tree *Equipment and supplies/Prostheses and implants* (in class E07). The subject hierarchy is expressed in both the subject class numbers and also the indenting or layout. From the visible patterns in these two lists (E06 and E07) we can see that *Dental Implants, Single-Tooth* is currently the most specific suitable term available in *MeSH* for the first concept in our topic

Table 2.2 Sources of information (this chapter)

Resource	Internet address
MeSH Browser	http://www.nlm.nih.gov/mesh/MBrowser.html
NLM Gateway	http://gateway.nlm.nih.gov/gw/Cmd
Cochrane Library	http://www.thecochranelibrary.com or link via http://www.cochrane.org
PubMed (including *MEDLINE*)	http://www.pubmed.gov or http://www.ncbi.nlm.nih.gov/sites/entrez?db=pubmed

Table 2.4 Secondary concept – MeSH Browser

<table>
<tr><td>

Aim: to find *MeSH* term/s for secondary concept via http://www.nlm.nih.gov/mesh/MBrowser.html

Through a similar process to Table 2.3, the *Scope Note* for 'longevity' makes it clear that this is an unsuitable *MeSH* term for the current research topic. This term is used in *MeSH* to refer to the lifespan of an organism. What do we mean by 'longevity' in the context of single tooth implants? Approach this question in various ways, including:

- Investigate (as above) *MeSH* terms attached to known citations noted during progress (e.g. **Dental Restoration Failure**, **Treatment Outcome**, **Dental Health Surveys**, **Survival Analysis**, **Longitudinal studies**)
- Use the root of terms (e.g. 'long' from 'longevity') to search the *MeSH Browser*. We find **Longitudinal Studies** listed in the results.
- Consult the *MeSH Trees* using the class numbers around a term such as *Longitudinal Studies* to find broader and narrower terms located on the same branch nearby topic branches
- Keep in mind an evidence-based perspective and use the saved search filters at *PubMed/Advanced Search/More Resources/Clinical Queries/*
- Remember that we may use other facilities listed in *MeSH Tree* class V03 (e.g. **Meta-Analysis [Publication Type]** to retrieve high quality reviews of the literature and **Clinical Trial [Publication Type]**, see Table 2.7)

Clearly we need to unpack and expand what we mean by 'longevity' and how to approach it in our present context. We know that this area will require further consideration in an evidence-based context as discussed in the text

</td></tr>
</table>

In summary, one should read the *Scope* and other notes attached to relevant *MeSH* terms. Also explore the relationships between relevant concepts. These are set out in the *MeSH Trees,* which is the subject classification system integrated into the *MeSH* database. The management and organisation of information in the light of new knowledge is an ongoing process for the *MeSH* database team.

2.1.2 NLM Gateway

The *NLM Gateway* is also a useful exploration point because its search software accesses simultaneously several National Library of Medicine database resources. However, simultaneous database searching has serious limitations (not being highly integrated with some specific features of each resource searched). However, at the exploratory phase of one's search design work a search at the *NLM Gateway* is useful to increase awareness of the scope of a subject in the literature. It may

provide some useful references and lead in unanticipated directions.

2.1.3 Other sources

When relevant, the dentist as searcher should consider exploration of major information sources based in related disciplines such as biology, chemistry, materials engineering and psychology. In addition, other information resources such as *ISI Web of Knowledge* provided by Thomson Reuters through licences to institutions and libraries should be investigated at some stage. The mention of various sources raises issues related to access (conditions may apply) and training for use of multiple sources of information. This broad area is outside the scope of a single chapter. Consult affiliated library personnel regarding information access and retrieval, indexing guidelines, data formats, search functions and user interface screen options. As usual, readers are advised to ask a librarian and to take classes.

2.2 Evidence-based sources

There are various primary and secondary evidence-based sources of information as discussed at the Centre for Evidence-Based Medicine website (e.g. see under their *EBM Tools* tab). The *Cochrane Library* is a good starting point to find work on health-related interventions and therapies. The results retrieved by a search are summarised under the names of the resource classes within the *Cochrane Library*.

After the *Cochrane Library*, this chapter suggests that one turns to the *PubMed* databases (including the *MEDLINE* database). Here one searches the primary topic and then uses the *PubMed* system's quality presaved search strategies to filter and retrieve any documents for:

- meta-analyses;
- systematic reviews;
- aetiology clinical queries;
- diagnosis clinical queries;
- therapy clinical queries;
- prognosis clinical queries.

Although the clinical queries groups are distinct theoretically, in practice for any given topic, depending on the research perspective, there may be overlap in the usefulness of the documents retrieved by the relevant *PubMed* filters.

The two major information resource groups that are mentioned above (in this section) and used to provide the examples in this chapter have been selected because of their general accessibility and their commitment to evidence-based filtering. Speak to your affiliated information consultant or librarian to determine the extent of evidence-based filters for any locally available licensed resources such as the *OvidSP* or the *ISI Web of Knowledge* versions of *MEDLINE*.

Table 2.5 Expansion and contraction logic

Document pool relationship	Expansion	Contraction	Exclusion*
Intra-pool	OR	AND	NOT
Complementary concept pools (inter-pool)	OR	–	–
Distinct non-complementary concept pools	–	AND	NOT

*Note (caution): exclusion of a concept using the connector NOT will exclude *all* documents which mention that concept (i.e. even those documents also focused on concepts that are indeed of interest).

3. Concepts and their relationships

The result of a literature search is references to a virtual pool of documents. The needs identification table (see Table 2.1) identifies relevant concepts within a topic. Notice that virtually each row in Table 2.1 potentially represents a distinct concept pool, some of which overlap in complementary ways. Each concept pool corresponds in a literature database with a potentially overlapping pool of documents.

It is important to prioritise concepts and, by extension, pools of retrieved documents. In particular, one must decide which single pool of documents represents the basic set or foundation of a particular search design. The so-called PICO clinical query subject analysis system is one means of doing this (Forrest *et al.* 2009). In this system, the condition or disease of the patient or population is normally the primary topic. Then one plans how to manipulate this primary set of documents. Thus, for the sample topic mentioned in this chapter, one would prioritise the concepts as follows:

- primary topic: single-tooth implants;
- secondary topic: longevity.

Immediately, within an evidence-based context, one should be alert to the need for 'longevity' to be considered through a 'hierarchy of evidence'. A useful discussion of levels of evidence is provided online by the Centre for Evidence-Based Medicine. Systematic reviews and meta-analyses (secondary sources) and reports of randomised controlled trials (primary sources) take precedence in approaches to the secondary concept.

3.1 Expansion and contraction management

There are basically two types of processes in literature searching:

- expansion strategies and processes;
- contraction strategies and processes.

Expansion and contraction processes are managed by use of two types of concept pool relationships:

- intraconcept pool relationships;
- interconcept pool relationships.

Table 2.6 Complementary search statements

ss #	Search statement typed as query	Terminology type
#1	Dental Implants, Single-Tooth[MeSH Terms]	*MeSH* controlled for use in the *MEDLINE* database
#2	single AND tooth AND (implant OR implants)	Text words free/natural for *PubMed In process* file
#3	#1 OR #2	*MeSH* OR Text words

Notes:
1. Some particular documents are found by both ss#1 and ss#2. One of these duplicated records is dropped by *PubMed* in ss#3.
2. In *PubMed* the *In process* file contains new records awaiting *MeSH* subject descriptors.

One uses the device of concept pools to logically group concepts prior to searching. In order to establish distinct concept pools, carefully consider the relationships between concepts as listed in the requirements table (Table 2.1). Table 2.5 and to some extent Table 2.6 summarise relationship patterns. Section 4 discusses search techniques and terminology used carefully to express these relationships in the process of a search inquiry. Concept pools may be either:

- complementary (expanding: same, similar or related concepts which have been pooled for convenience), or
- non-complementary (contracting: logically distinct concepts)

The scope of a literature search and usually the volume of results may be expanded through both the complementary intra-pool and the complementary inter-pool types of relationships. By contrast, in the non-complementary type of relationship, normally each added distinct concept pool successively narrows the search design and reduces results quantitatively. They should also qualitatively improve results, particularly when quality search filter options available from various launch points in information systems are used as a means of contraction. Relationships between concept pools are expressed in search statements (search queries) by Boolean connector words (see Section 4.1). It is helpful to make notes (including diagrams, sketches and tables) to assist progress through search design (e.g. in Section 3 above and Section 4).

4. Terminology for concepts and relationships

After organising the concepts into distinct and coherent 'concept pools', identify and refine appropriate terminology for the ideas within and between each concept pool. The aim is twofold: (i) to retrieve the most relevant records from our information source; and (ii) to avoid loss of relevant records due to unresolved terminology issues and illogical use of relationship indicator/connector terms. There are three types of terminology relevant to search design:

- Boolean connector words (OR, AND, NOT), which express relationships;
- controlled vocabulary (specific for database, such as *MeSH* for *MEDLINE*);
- free or natural vocabulary (as a complement or substitute for lack of controlled vocabulary, e.g. for very new records).

4.1 Boolean connector words

Boolean connectors are used as needed within and between search statements in a search design. Some information systems provide inquiry launch options for search design elements that have inbuilt Boolean logic, as discussed in Section 5. The logic of expansion or contraction in literature searching is known as Boolean logic. Explanations of (and tutorials on) Boolean logic are easily obtained (see Section 10.7). In summary:

OR = expansion by addition (of words/concepts/options)

AND = contraction by addition (of words/concepts/options)

NOT = contraction by subtraction (of words/concepts/options)

When used to express Boolean logic (relationships) the meaning of these connector words differs from that in 'everyday' language in quite specific ways; for example 'OR' within a search statement is used to retrieve any (i.e. *all*) documents in a literature source that mention any of the concepts listed. In contrast, the Boolean word 'AND' reduces retrieval. Use 'AND' to find records that consider a relationship between distinct non-complementary concepts and thus to eliminate those that do not. Finally, one must be aware that it is easy inappropriately to use 'NOT' in a search statement and to consequently and unintentionally lose relevant references from results. It is used only when one definitely wants to eliminate all references containing the discarded concept, including any that happen also to contain information about relevant and needed concepts. Boolean

'NOT' is however useful to manage (separate) results at the end of a search design; for example separation of the most recent references into a separate pool of documents is possible (see Section 7).

4.2 Controlled vocabulary

Search design for retrieval from the *Cochrane Library* and the *MEDLINE* database must take into account terms used by various relevant authors and by the *MeSH* controlled vocabulary (*MeSH Thesaurus*). *MeSH* descriptors (subject headings) have context built into them via their *MeSH Tree* category numbering system. On the other hand, natural vocabulary terms do not necessarily have context built into them; for example on their own, the terms 'crown' and 'oral' have various meanings, depending on the discipline within which they are being discussed (dentistry, medicine, pharmacy, etc.).

In the *Cochrane Library*, the *Keywords* field in records is linked to the *MeSH Search* function. In the *PubMed MEDLINE* database the *MeSH* headings field in database records is linked with the *Search MeSH* function (then one proceeds to *Search PubMed* via *Links*). The basic guideline for indexers (and therefore users) of *MeSH* is to seek out and choose from the thesaurus the most specific term/s that are available and suitable for topics represented in a document/article. This is an important principle to remember as one designs a literature search. The *MeSH* system exists to facilitate systematic searching and to overcome variations in the language used by different authors; for example some authors refer to 'implant-supported single crowns', others to 'single tooth implants', 'implant supported missing teeth', 'ISCs' and 'implanted SCs'. These variations are all covered by one preferred *MeSH* descriptor term, which is recorded in the *MeSH* headings field of each reference or document in the *MEDLINE* database to which it has been currently applied:

Dental Implants, Single-Tooth

This is currently the exact phrase (including inversion, spacing and punctuation) that we use in *PubMed*. Although this term may be found via the *Search MeSH* database function in *PubMed* (see Section 5), it also may be typed directly into the *PubMed* search query box in one of the forms below:

Dental Implants, Single-Tooth[MeSH Terms]

The following form is used via the *Focus to major topic* option and contracts results (see Table 2.7):

Dental Implants, Single-Tooth[Major MeSH Term]

When typed into the *PubMed* query box, the statement should appear without a space before the square bracketed phrase [MeSH Terms]. Then click on *Search*. Such

Table 2.7 Search elements and launch points in *PubMed*

Navigate via	Launch points	Functions
From *Search PubMed* **v** use drop down menu and choose *MeSH*	*MeSH* term: enter term and click on *Search*	Auto-explosion (default): finds documents about a selected general topic *plus* its specialties (see *MeSH Tree*) Use *Links* (right side of screen) to return to *PubMed* and complete the search
Advanced Search/Search Builder	ALL fields searching	(Default): searches in all the available fields (parts) of records in database
Advanced Search/Clinical Queries	*Clinical Queries* search box at top for systematic reviews	Uses saved searches to filter out documents that do not qualify according to criteria for systematic reviews
Advanced Search/Clinical Queries	*Clinical Queries* for clinical study categories	Change question type via drop down menu to search diagnosis, aetiology, therapy or prognosis and drop **v** to switch between *Broad* and *Narrow* strategies
Limits	Chose from options	Limits results to selected criteria: type of article (e.g. Meta-Analysis, Clinical Trial), Date ranges, Age groups, Gender, Species, Journal type (e.g. Dentistry list), Language, etc.
From *Search PubMed* **v** use drop down menu and choose *MeSH*	*MeSH* term: focus to major topic using *MeSH*	Limits results to documents with chosen *MeSH* term coded as major focus of document Use *Links* (right side of screen) to return to *PubMed* and complete the search
From *Search PubMed* **v** use drop down menu and choose *Search MeSH*	*MeSH* term: select *MeSH* subheading (qualifier) category	Limits results to documents with selected *MeSH* term/ subheading (qualifier) Use *Links* (right side of screen) to return to *PubMed* and complete the search
From *Search PubMed* **v** use drop down menu and choose *Search MeSH*	*MeSH* term: Select *Do not explode this term*	Limits results to documents at selected general topic in *MeSH Tree* (excludes articles about more specific topics in the same *MeSH Tree*) Use *Links* (right side of screen) to return to *PubMed* and complete the search
Advanced Search/Search Builder **v** drop down menu	Choose field (part of record) specified	Limits results to matches in a particular field (e.g. author, title, abstract, etc.)

Notes:
1. Once in *PubMed*, at the top left of the homepage above the main search query box, we may select other files to search such as *MeSH* (see via the drop down menu) instead of *PubMed*.
2. *PubMed* now simultaneously searches for systematic review and clinical study category.
3. Avoid unintentional use of a limit on subsequent search statements. A *Limit* should be deactivated after each relevant search statement to avoid contamination of following search statements. They do not deactivate automatically.
4. An alternative service *OvidSP* from Wolters Kluwer Health provides an Explode *MeSH* term option (i.e. *MeSH* term explosion is not the default setting in that service, unlike in *PubMed*).

queries are assigned a session search statement # by the *PubMed* system and results are displayed.

4.3 Free or natural or text word vocabulary

So-called 'free' or 'natural' terminology is also known as 'text word' vocabulary and is devised by the search designer. Text word vocabulary must be included at the appropriate point in search design to retrieve references that:

- lack controlled vocabulary, for example because they are very recent and not yet indexed (i.e. for use in the *PubMed In process* non-*MEDLINE* database);

- include controlled language descriptors that describe a more general topic for various reasons (e.g. article focus).

The principle 'less gives more' is relevant to search design, so one may use the following simple search statement:

single AND tooth AND (implant OR implants)

Type this string exactly as above (with spaces and punctuation) into the *PubMed* search query box and click on *Search*. It is assigned an online session search statement

by the system. A text word form of search statement aims to retrieve recent matching records in the *PubMed In process* (non-*MEDLINE*) database and any old records not tagged with the current most specific heading. Note that when searching in the *OvidSP* service provided by Wolters Kluwer Health (not *PubMed*), select directly or change to the database called *Pre-MEDLINE* to find most recently added records.

The word 'single' has other contextual meanings but here the situation is controllable because the word 'tooth' provides context in this search statement. Use both the singular and plural forms of the noun 'implant' and nest them within parentheses. This nesting device shows that the terms contained therein should be processed as an internal expansion of terms using 'OR'; that is, before being combined with the other two words in a process of contraction. It is not possible to truncate at implant* because (like 'dent*') it retrieves too many results in diverse disciplines. One expects that this statement will be effective without using the other word forms of 'implant' (verbs, adjectives and participles).

For contraction place the Boolean operator word 'AND' between the three elements. This is also because at the exploration stage of our work we have noticed that they do not necessarily appear together nor in that order in title, abstract or other text. *PubMed* does not offer an adjacency search facility. The abbreviations 'ISC' and 'SC' mentioned above are problematic as search elements (sometimes used in the singular and sometimes in the plural and have other meanings in other contexts). For example, 'SC' is an abbreviation used in *MEDLINE* for the *MeSH* qualifier term (subheading): 'secondary'.

To recapitulate, when one uses 'text word' or 'natural' language in a search statement it usually needs to be manipulated for expansion of retrieval. In general, the most commonly used forms of manipulation for text word expansion are: synonyms, alternative spellings, truncation (using truncation symbol according to provider instructions, e.g. the symbol *). In other words, these are basically search expansion devices in text word natural language search mode. In the cases where another discipline uses the same text words, we need to provide contraction through word/s that give our discipline's context. Commonly, search statements using 'natural language' (text words) are a compromise. Table 2.6 shows an example of one search statement (ss#1) constructed from a controlled *MeSH* term for use in the *MEDLINE* database file and one search statement (ss#2) constructed from text words for use in the *In process (non-MEDLINE)* database file. These are complementary search statements that would be expected to retrieve overlapping document pools. They may be combined into a third search statement (ss#3), which drops one copy of previously duplicated records (de-duplication).

Various combinations of controlled and free vocabulary may be very effective in search design in certain circumstances. This may be viewed in action if one accesses examples of pre-expanded and saved search strategies (filters) in *PubMed* (see Section 10.6). Information specialists and librarians at institutions using the *OvidSP* service may design and save expert filter searches for use by their customers.

There is a general overlap between the two categories of controlled and free vocabulary in that search designers work with both types of search language when appropriate and manipulate them in accordance with system rules (see the example in Table 2.6). This requires some basic knowledge of the database protocols, for example that information is broken down, labelled and coded into designated parts known as fields within the references recorded in an information resource.

5. Search design elements and launch points

Search elements may be whole search statements or parts of search statements. Launch points are various system-provided search options available at the user interface level of an information resource system that correspond with various common search elements. They take into account opaque features of a database, such as data structure and indexing guidelines. Table 2.7 summarises some common search design elements and their corresponding launch points as provided by the *PubMed* information system. There may be more than one navigation route to a particular launch point. If a system launch point exists for a particular concept then use this option (i.e. instead of typing a search term with a Boolean construction into the search dialog box on the screen). In effect, electronic search engines provide us with search options that apply Boolean operators. It is important to be familiar with their role and understand the logic they use 'behind the scenes'. One must ask: Does this option apply 'OR' or 'AND' Boolean logic between the concepts mentioned?

These launch features are likely to vary from search platform to platform (e.g. *PubMed* versus the licensed *OvidSP* system) and from software upgrade to upgrade within such systems over time. Commonly, an information system will present options to us that address the data formats, indexing and field tagging that are particular to a specific database. A user new to such an information resource (or a casual user) may be unaware of relevant data structure, information system protocols, rules and specifications and consequently be unable to access and retrieve relevant documents.

In summary, an information system provides various search launch points (options). There are similarities and differences between the appearance and function of options available from various providers. Beware of simultaneously using too many contractions within a single search design and thus losing relevant references. Contraction launch points may not apply to records with a 'prior to indexing' status, such as the most recently acquired references in the *PubMed's In process* (non-*MEDLINE*) database.

6. Refinement and choice of search designs

This stage of search design includes terminology testing and also trialling of a series of search designs. One is looking for 'best fit' situations in terms of results. We start with terms from the primary concept pool: single-tooth implants. The hierarchy of evidence framework suggests that a series of search designs should be executed. Some of the designs overlap and potentially may be combined. However, because one must be wary of illogical and unwieldy combinations, they are expressed as separate searches in this chapter.

The search series suggested below may be terminated at any point. This normally occurs in the clinical situation when one judges that one has retrieved enough high-quality references (best evidence). On the other hand, in the case of really comprehensive searching required to underpin a research proposal for a higher degree, a comprehensive literature review would normally require one to work through a larger series of search designs. Suggestions for stepping through these search design series are set out below and recorded as search histories in Tables 2.8–2.11. The general strategy suggested here is first to search for:

1. high-quality evidence-based secondary sources such as systematic reviews and meta-analyses; then
2. primary sources such as randomised controlled trials (via elements in search designs to employ evidence-based filters).

Table 2.8 Search history: Section 6.1

ss#	Search details
#1	MeSH descriptor Dental Implants, Single-Tooth explode all trees

Note: Use *Search History* function to view summary of search session.

Table 2.9 Search history: Section 6.2.1

ss#	Search details
#1	Dental Implants, Single-Tooth[MeSH Terms]
#2	single AND tooth AND (implant OR implants)
#3	#1 OR #2
#4	#3 AND Limits: Meta-Analysis
#5	#3 AND systematic[sb]
#6	#3 AND (Therapy/Narrow[filter])

Notes:
1. Remember to deactivate *Limits* after #4.
2. Via *Advanced Search* ss#5 – #ss6 are retrieved simultaneously.
3. If useful, results for meta-analyses may be removed from ss#5 by another search statement thus: #5 NOT #4.
4. Randomised controlled trials are retrieved by ss#6.
5. Most recent and oldest results may be isolated by the search statement: #2 NOT #1.

6.1 *Cochrane Library*

We begin in the *Cochrane Library* databases

1. Aim: to find *Cochrane Reviews, Other Reviews and Clinical trials* in the *Cochrane Library* resource by navigating via: *Advanced Search/MeSH Search* [type exact *MeSH* term for topic]/*Go To MeSH Trees/View Results/*. *Library* resource files are simultaneously searched and results are displayed in groups as follows:
   - *Cochrane Reviews*;
   - other reviews;
   - clinical trials;
   - technology assessments;
   - economic evaluations.
   Cochrane Library results are also accessible via its *Search History* facility (see Table 2.8).
2. If there is insufficient retrieval (results) from the search above, we may also scan the Cochrane Oral Health Group's list of reviews and protocols (reviews in progress) before we move on to the *PubMed* service.

6.2 *PubMed* databases, including *MEDLINE*

Each of the following search designs is shown in a search history format in Tables 2.9–2.11.

Table 2.10 Search history: Section 6.2.2 (1)

ss#	Search details
#1	Dental Implants, Single-Tooth[MeSH Terms]
#2	single AND tooth AND (implant OR implants)
#3	#1 OR #2
#4	Dental Restoration Failure[MeSH Terms]
#5	Survival Analysis[MeSH Terms]
#6	Treatment Outcome[MeSH Terms]
#7	Longitudinal Studies[MeSH Terms]
#8	#4 OR #5 OR #6 OR #7
#9	#3 AND #8

Note: Use of the phrase [MeSH Terms] eliminates *In Process file* (including most recent) records that do not have *MeSH* descriptors.

Table 2.11 Search history: Section 6.2.2 (2)

ss#	Search details
#1	Dental Implants, Single-Tooth[MeSH Terms]
#2	single AND tooth AND (implant OR implants)
#3	#1 OR #2
#4	#3 AND (Prognosis/Broad[filter])
#5	#3 AND (Aetiology/Broad[filter])
#6	#3 AND (Therapy/Broad[filter])
#7	#3 AND (Diagnosis/Broad[filter])
#8	#4 OR #5 OR #6 OR #7

Notes:
1. Clinical trials are retrieved by ss#6.
2. ss #8 assumes multiple time perspectives are acceptable.

6.2.1 *Evidence-based search sequence*

1. Aim: to find meta-analyses (via *Limits*, see Table 2.9). Before proceeding to the next design we remember to click *Remove* to deactivate the limit used in this design.
2. Aim: to find systematic reviews (via *Advanced Search/More Resources/Clinical Queries/Systematic Reviews*, see Table 2.9). Note that the results of this design include those of the preceding narrower search.
3. Aim: to find randomised controlled trials (via *Advanced Search/More Resources/Clinical Queries/Clinical Study Categories/Therapy/Narrow*). Remember to select *Narrow* from the drop down menu at *Therapy*. The default *Broad* may be used in a later design (see Table 2.9 and Table 2.11).
4. Aim: To find the most recent information (including records in the *In process (non-MEDLINE* database). Via option to *Display Settings* use drop down menu (top left of screen) to ensure references are sorted by *Recently Added* for ss#3 and then view (see Table 2.9).

6.2.2 *Searching extensions*

In addition to the above, we may also proceed as follows:

1. Aim: to identify any references missed by the above strategies by using other *MeSH* terms found (e.g. attached to useful references): *Dental Restoration Failure, Treatment Outcome, Dental Health Surveys, Survival Analysis, Longitudinal studies* (see Table 2.10).
2. Aim: to find (via *Advanced Search/More Resources/ Clinical Queries/Clinical Study Categories*) all relevant work in the following search filter categories (see Table 2.11):
   - aetiology/etiology clinical queries;
   - diagnosis clinical queries;
   - therapy/intervention clinical queries;
   - prognosis clinical queries.
3. Aim: to identify older results in *PubMed* go to last pages of displayed records for ss #3 and work backwards.

7. Search history and display of references (records)

To reuse a search statement in another search query without retyping it into the search box, ascertain its search statement number (ss#) by scrolling down to view the *Search History*. As noted in Section 6, examples of search histories are given in Tables 2.8–2.11. It is useful to note that there are some other handy techniques to manage results. For example, the Boolean operator word 'NOT' may be used if for some reason you wish to view the references picked up by the text word search strategy rather than the *MeSH* term search strategy. Type into the search dialogue box:

#n NOT #n (e.g. #2 NOT #1) [Search]

The Boolean operator word 'OR' may be used to combine several results to eliminate overlap (de-duplicate references). For example, the results of several *PubMed Clinical Study Categories* searches may be combined into a single pool of documents for visual scanning purposes.

If the results retrieved consist of only a few references from a high-quality search design, it may be better to scan visually to select those of interest than to contract the results by addition of another concept.

8. Evaluation of results

Critical evaluation of results is another skill required for the practice of evidence-based dentistry. There are several good resources for self-instruction in this area. The Centre for Evidenced-Based Medicine provides resources on critical appraisal via its *EBM Tools* tab at www.cebm.net. A new edition of an important series of articles on evaluation of the literature has been prepared by Guyton *et al.* (2008). This material is also updated and available electronically at the website www.jamaevidence.com/resources/520. The Cochrane Collaboration's *Handbook for systematic Reviews of Interventions* (2010) gives an insight into the preparation of systematic reviews published in the *Cochrane Library*. The CONSORT Group's *CONSORT Statement*, which aims to improve the reporting of two-parallel design randomised controlled trials, is also of interest to readers of randomised controlled trials.

9. Conclusion and caveats

Each new topic requires a new search design. There is no such thing as a 'one size fits all' search design. It all depends on context and purpose, topic and availability of references in the literature. There is a hierarchy of information resources and search designs and how far down the hierarchy a searcher ventures depends on results of a design higher up the search hierarchy. Accept that despite best efforts, one can never guarantee to have retrieved all relevant documents from a literature search. A major factor here is discrepancies between concepts and terminology (including spelling) used by ourselves, the authors and indexers. A good search design aims to reduce the effect of such discrepancies. Otherwise, unintentional loss of relevant retrieval is a potential consequence. Most topics may require the construction of several search designs. This is usually inevitable for changes from one information system or resource to another. We must aim to design search strategies that withstand peer review.

10. Further assistance (information/ help/tutorials)

Information system assistance tends to be oriented to new users and/or to experienced users. Return regularly to *Help* pages linked to the websites and develop the required skills; for example gradually absorb details of data formats, computer record field tagging and indexing rules. The ability to construct more efficient and effective search designs depend on such study. A subject information librarian is a source of expertise and advice on search design for particular topics.

10.1 Centre for Evidenced-Based Medicine

EBM Tools: Asking focused questions, *Finding the evidence* and *Critical appraisal* (http://www.cebm.net, accessed 24 August 2010).

10.2 Cochrane Collaboration

Training (http://www.cochrane.org/Training, accessed 24 August 2010).

10.3 *Cochrane Library*

LEARN [and] *HELP* [Tabs] [and] *SEARCH TIPS* [sidebar] (http://www.thecochranelibrary.com, accessed 24 August 2010).

10.4 *MeSH*

Fact Sheet: Medical Subject Headings (MeSH) (http://www.nlm.nih.gov/pubs/factsheet/mesh.html, accessed 24 August 2010).

Also use various links at the *MeSH* homepage (http://www.nlm.nih.gov/mesh/meshhome.html, accessed 24 August 2010).

MeSH tutorials via *PubMed* homepage include *PubMed/More Resources/MeSH Database* (http://www.ncbi.nlm.nih.gov/mesh, accessed 24 August 2010).

10.5 *PubMed*

PubMed/Using PubMed/PubMed Quick Start
   PubMed/Using PubMed/Tutorials

Tutorials are available via the *PubMed* homepage (http://www.ncbi.nlm.nih.gov/pubmed, accessed 24 August 2010).

10.6 *PubMed/Clinical Queries*

To view pre-expanded and saved expert filter search design strategies follow the links from the *PubMed* homepage: *PubMed Tools/Clinical Queries.*

Search Strategy used to create the Systematic Reviews Subset on PubMed (http://www.ncbi.nlm.nih.gov/bsd/pubmed_subsets/sysreviews_strategy.html, accessed 24 August 2010)

Clinical Queries using Research Methodology Filters– see link at *PubMed/PubMed Tools/Clinical Queries/ Clinical Study Categories/filter* citations (accessed 24 August 2010).

10.7 Boolean and Venn diagram logic (expression of relationships)

Go to your library's website to see if a Boolean logic tutorial is available. Use a general search engine on the inter-net to find an introduction to Boolean logic (and Venn diagrams) for literature searching. Boolean logic is used in other contexts than literature searching, for example in mathematics. An example for literature searching is http://internettutorials.net/boolean.asp (accessed 24 August 2010).

10.8 General

There are also various introductions to literature searching in the health sciences (e.g. Jankowski 2008).

References

Centre for Evidenced-Based Medicine. EBM tools (http://www.cebm.net, accessed 18 August 2010).

Cochrane Collaboration. Homepage (http://www.cochrane.org, accessed 24 August 2010).

Cochrane Database of Systematic Reviews In: *Cochrane Library.* Homepage (http://www.thecochranelibrary.com or http://www.cochrane.org, accessed 18 August 2010).

Cochrane Handbook for Systematic Reviews of Interventions (http://www.cochrane-handbook.org, accessed 24 August 2010).

Cochrane Library. Homepage (http://www.thecochranelibrary.com or http://www.cochrane.org, accessed 18 August 2010).

Cochrane Oral Health Group. Homepage (http://www.ohg.cochrane.org, accessed 18 August 2010).

CONSORT Group. CONSORT statement (http://www.consort-statement.org/consort-statement, accessed 18 August 2010).

Forrest, J.L., Miller, S.A., Overman, P.R. *et al.* (2009) *Evidence-based Decision Making: A Translational Guide for Dental Professionals.* Wolters Kluwer, Philadelphia.

Guyton, G., Drummond, R., Meade, M.O. *et al.* (2008) *Users' Guides to the Medical Literature: Essentials for Evidence-based Clinical Practice*, 2nd edn. McGraw-Hill, New York. Also available at http://www.jamaevidence.com/resource/520 (accessed 16 August 2010).

Health on the Net Foundation. HONcode (http://www.hon.ch/HONcode/Pro/intro.html, accessed 25 August 2010).

ISI Web of Knowledge (http://www.isiwebofknowledge.com, accessed 8 December 2010).

Jankowski, T.A. (2008) *The Medical Library Association Essential Guide to Becoming an Expert Searcher: Proven Techniques, Strategies, and Tips for Finding Health Information.* Neal-Schuman, New York.

Jung, R.E., Pjetursson, B.E., Glauser, R. *et al.* (2008) A systematic review of the 5-year survival and complication rates of implant-supported single crowns. *Clinical Oral Implants Research*, 19 (2), 119–130.

MEDLINE (see under *PubMed*).

MeSH Browser (http://www.nlm.nih.gov/mesh/MBrowser.html, accessed 18 August 2010).

NLM Gateway (http://gateway.nlm.nih.gov/gw/Cmd, accessed 18 August 2010).

Pjetursson, B.E., Bragger, U., Lang, N.P. *et al.* (2007) Comparison of survival and complication rates of tooth-supported fixed dental prostheses (FDPs) and implant-supported FDPs and single crowns (SCs). *Clinical Oral Implants Research*, 18 (Suppl. 3), 97–113.

Ovid. Homepage by Wolters Kluwer Health includes information on the *OvidSP* search platform (http://www.ovid.com, accessed 24 August 2010).

PubMed (http://www.pubmed.gov or http://www.ncbi.nlm.nih.gov/sites/entrez?db=pubmed, accessed 24 August 2010).

Torabinejad, M., Anderson, P., Bader, J. *et al.* (2007) Outcomes of root canal treatment and restoration, implant-supported crowns, fixed partial dentures, and extraction without replacement: a systematic review. *Journal of Prosthetic Dentistry*, 98 (4), 285–311.

Section 2

Treatment Planning

3

Consent and Clinician–Patient Relationships

Diana Kingston and Iven Klineberg

Patient consent in oral and general health care is multi-faceted and may be discussed from various, often overlapping, perspectives. These include academic and theoretical discourse, legal and regulatory frameworks, bioethics and clinical ethics, guidelines for professional conduct, professional education, institutional and administrative practices, decision-making processes, information management, communication processes, relationships, psychology and various sociocultural issues.

1. Bioethics and consent

Bioethics concerns the treatment of ethical questions that arise in health care and other related disciplines. Bioethics has a long history. Its origins can be dated from the Hippocratic Oath. There is a large body of literature and it comprises many strands. Strands relevant to our present discussion include medical ethics (including its clinical and philosophical branches) and professional ethics (Grodin 1995). Professional ethics is a branch of ethics that focuses on professional responsibility and conduct, and aims to be practical, realistic and responsive to the problems of practitioners (such as health clinicians). Various professional and regulatory bodies, including dental associations and jurisdictional registration boards, promulgate codes of ethics and professional conduct and other guidelines. Examples from the Canadian Dental Association (1997), American Dental Association (2010), Dental Board of Australia (2010) and the General Dental Council (Great Britain) (2005) are in the reference list. There are various regional approaches to these issues outlined in the literature, for example the Canadian setting (Fisher 2009) and the Europe approach (Gastmans et al. 2007). Kerridge et al. (2009, p.94) set out a model for ethical decision-making which proposed that relevant ethical principles for consideration were autonomy, beneficence, non-maleficence, justice, confidentiality/privacy and veracity. Many authors, including Rule and Veatch (2004) have discussed ethical questions in dentistry.

An important milestone for this topic was the adoption in 2005 and publication in 2006 by UNESCO of its *Universal Declaration on Bioethics and Human Rights* (UNESCO 2006). Various Articles in the Universal Declaration are relevant to dental practice and research. A recent UNESCO publication provides material on the background, principles and application of the *Universal Declaration* (Have et al. 2009).

Article 6 of the *Universal Declaration* is devoted to *Consent*. Surrounding Articles are also relevant to patient consent in the health professions, including dentistry (e.g. see Articles 3–5 and 7–11). These latter Articles deal with: Human dignity and human rights; Benefit and harm; Autonomy and individual responsibility; Persons without the capacity to consent; Respect for human vulnerability and personal integrity; Privacy and confidentiality; Equality, justice and equity; and Non-discrimination and non-stigmatisation.

Sections 2–3 of Article 6 relate to consent in a research environment, while Section 1 of Article 6 states:

> 'Any preventive, diagnostic and therapeutic medical intervention is only to be carried out with the prior, free and informed consent of the person concerned, based on adequate information. The consent should, where appropriate, be express and may be withdrawn by the person concerned at any time and for any reason without disadvantage or prejudice.'

2. Clinical decision-making

It has been suggested that the complex interaction between health-care professionals and patients at the time of decision-making is at the core of consent (Kerridge et al. 2009). The clinician–patient relationship ultimately becomes a key focus in the consent process. Elements related to the patient include competence, understanding of information and voluntary decision-making. Jonsen et al. (2006) suggested a structured approach to ethical decision-making in a medical clinical

Oral Rehabilitation: A Case-Based Approach, First Edition. Edited by Iven Klineberg, Diana Kingston.

setting. This approach listed four groups of questions to be considered by a clinician, which are also relevant to dentistry:

- indications for intervention, including indicated and non-indicated interventions;
- preferences of patients, including informed consent, decisional capacity, beliefs, truthful communication and competent refusal of treatment;
- quality of life, including enhancing quality of life;
- contextual features, including role of other parties, confidentiality, economics, influence of religion, role of ethics committees and the law.

3. Consent and the law

The concept of valid or informed patient consent provides congruence between ethics and the legal framework within which a clinician is operating and is a concept accessible to lay people (Goodman 2003, p.68). Health care is delivered within a legal and regulatory environment that significantly regulates and determines standards of care and the rights and obligations of both providers and recipients of health care (Forrester & Griffiths 2010). Health law controls not only what is expected of institutions and professionals but also what they must refrain from doing in practice. An understanding of health law in a particular setting is fundamental to the provision of safe and competent patient care and is a resource for professional decision-making. Since health law varies with jurisdiction, it is important that dentists and other health professionals have an understanding of the relevant legal systems within which they are working. This includes sources of law, categories of law, other major features as well as court hierarchy.

In common law countries such as Australia, Canada, England and New Zealand, sources of law are parliamentary law, delegated legislation and common law based on judges' decisions in court cases. In Australia, for example, categories of law include industrial, contract, criminal (includes assault), tort (includes negligence, negligent misrepresentation and trespass to person), constitutional law, statutory arrangements between the federal and state governments and also commitment to international treaties. Various legal issues in Australia are affected by the different law-making powers of state and federal governments. This intergovernmental framework can be the subject of change, for various reasons. For example, from 1 July 2010 a national registration and accreditation scheme was introduced in Australia to cover 10 health professions, including dentistry. Prior to that, the individual state and territory regulation and registration boards played a central role in those functions.

The constitutional and legal systems in the United States of America (and in other countries) are different from those of the countries mentioned above in various significant ways. A considerable body of literature on health law in the United States of America is relevant to dentists in jurisdictions there (e.g. see Sanbar *et al.* 2007). In the United States of America there are variations in consent laws between states. Clinicians must be responsible regarding their own jurisdiction's consent laws (Lewis & Tamparo 2007). Various authors, including Pollack (2002), have discussed law and risk management in dental practice in the United States of America.

In England, there are similar categories of law to the Australian categories that have been referred to above. However, in addition there are various influences on English law from European law. Mitchell and Mitchell (2009) summarised for dentists in England and elsewhere in the United Kingdom information regarding legal processes, complaint procedures, contracts, consent, negligence, professional indemnity, defence organisations, General Dental Council and registration, wise precautions and how to avoid litigation. Maclean (2009) has written on autonomy, informed consent and the law. Earlier, Lambden (2002) considered the relationship between dental law and ethics and D'Cruz *et al.* (2006) discussed legal aspects of dental practice.

4. Clinical confidentiality and privacy

The concepts of confidentiality of patient information and the privacy of patients are basic elements of professional health-care provision (Forrester & Griffiths 2010). The rule of clinical confidentiality dates back at least to the Hippocratic Oath. There are practical benefits from clinical confidentiality for diagnosis and treatment. Patients and clients are more likely to exchange relevant and sensitive information if they feel assured that it will remain confidential. Within a particular legal and jurisdictional context, confidentiality of patient information is maintained through statutory provisions and, where applicable, common law and equitable principles. There are also international standards related to the management of patient records. A search for International Organization for Standardization (ISO) standards on health informatics retrieves several pages of results (http://www.iso.org).

Article 9 of the *Universal Declaration* states:

'The privacy of the persons concerned and the confidentiality of their personal information should be respected. To the greatest extent possible, such information should not be used or disclosed for purposes other than those for which it was collected or consented to, consistent with international law, in particular international human rights law.'

There are two types of patient records: those of an institutional (administrative) nature and individual patient treatment records. Patients may give specific consent to access by other parties to their records or the information therein.

5. Consent, autonomy and competence

Maclean (2009, p.80) discussed consent as permission and consent as agreement and noted that professionals control resources, such as information on treatment choices and access to other professionals, which are necessary for the patient to exercise their autonomy. This leads to a consideration of autonomy within the professional–patient relationship (see Section 7).

Article 5 of the *Universal Declaration* states:

'The autonomy of persons to make decisions, while taking responsibility for those decisions and respecting the autonomy of others, is to be respected. For persons who are not capable of exercising autonomy, special measures are to be taken to protect their rights and interests.'

White (1994) considered capacities that define competence to give a free and informed consent and stated that informed consent is neither morally nor legally valid without patient competence to consent. Bielby (2008, p.16) identified two types of decisional competence and noted that humans possess such competence by degree. In addition, clinicians must be aware of legal aspects of competence relevant within their jurisdiction, including types of competence, tests of competence and parties that may legally act as substitute decision-makers for those with low or impaired decision-making capacity.

Informed consent was introduced to make the responsibility of information sharing a more patient-centred process, as it regularises patient communication about treatment. It also empowers patients to be engaged in the process, facilitates communication between clinician and patient and encourages patients to ask questions on any matter relating to their treatment. In this way patients become engaged in the process of decision-making to determine the optimum treatment choice for them.

Consent can be given in writing, verbally or be implied. In the jurisdiction to which they are referring, Mitchell and Mitchell (2009) commented briefly on these three forms of consent and also referred to consent for children and for adults who are not competent to give consent. As summarised, treatment without any consent may result in assault on the patient. Further, treatment after general consent only, and without explanation of what is involved, may result in a finding of negligence against the clinician. Written consent to a specific form of treatment is preferable, particularly if it discloses what the clinician expects to be able to deliver. Consent may be withdrawn at any time.

6. Negligence and standards of care

The concept of a normal standard of professional care is often considered when questions of negligence arise. In the United Kingdom, professional negligence is defined as a failure to exercise reasonable care in one's professional capacity (Mitchell & Mitchell 2009). Normally, it must be established that a particular clinician had a duty of care to a particular patient (had a particular patient–clinician relationship) and that this duty was breached causing injury or damage. These authors identified three

additional types of negligence: criminal (e.g. assault as a result of treatment without consent), contributory (on the part of the patient) and vicarious (e.g. when an institution is held responsible in relation to the actions of a particular clinician).

7. Dentist–patient relationship

It is crucial that the dentist–patient relationship be patient centred. A great deal of care must be taken by the clinician as part of the process of explanation of treatment options and in gaining the confidence of the patient. Although this is a relationship between two parties, the dentist and the patient, it exists within a legal and institutional context. Maclean (2009) considered the balance required by the clinician to respect both the patient's autonomy and the patient's welfare. He mentions three duties: to benefit the patient's health; respect the patient's agency/autonomy; and not to favour one patient over another. Mutual trust is crucial to the patient–professional relationship. The clinician must try to understand the patient as a person, avoid manipulation and deception and be sensitive to the patient's vulnerabilities. Respect for the patient's autonomy requires a clinician to be open, honest and empathetic. As Maclean (2009, p.109) pointed out, to facilitate the relationship, patients should be open and honest, willing to listen to professional advice and to explain their decisions.

Various guidelines on giving information to patients are available, for example those by the NHRMC (2004). Kerridge *et al.* (2009, p.283) list 10 requirements for information transfer in clinical practice and five modifying factors to be taken into account during that process. In summary, the dentist should explain to the patient the diagnosis, prognosis, uncertainties regarding diagnosis and prognosis, treatment options, burdens and benefits of investigations and treatments, whether the intervention is conventional or experimental, who will perform the intervention, consequences of choice, significant expected outcomes (short- and long-term), and the time and cost involved. Information given may be modified by the seriousness of the patient's condition, nature of the intervention, degree of possible harm, likelihood of risk and patient factors such as need, attitudes and understanding.

Oral care rehabilitation needs to embrace an oral health related quality of life approach. There should be recognition that treatment can be transformational in terms of a patient's psychosocial profile and personal well-being.

References

American Dental Association. *Principles of Ethics and Code of Professional Conduct*, updated 2010 (http://www.ada.org, accessed 6 July 2010).

Bielby, P. (2008) *Competence and Vulnerability in Biomedical Research*. Springer, Dordrecht.

Canadian Dental Association (1997) *Code of Ethics* (http://www.cda-adc.ca, accessed 7 July 2010).

D'Cruz, L. (2006) *Legal Aspects of General Dental Practice.* Churchill Livingstone, Edinburgh.

Dental Board of Australia. *Code of Conduct for Registered Health Practitioners* (http://www.dentalcouncil.net.au, accessed 7 July 2010).

Fisher, J. (2009) *Biomedical Ethics: a Canadian Focus.* Oxford University Press, Oxford.

Forrester, K. & Griffiths, D. (2010) *Essentials of Law for Health Professionals*, 3rd edn. Mosby Elsevier, Sydney.

Gastmans, C., Diericks, K., Nys, H. *et al.* (eds) (2007) *New Pathways for European Bioethics.* Intersentia, Antwerp.

General Dental Council (Great Britain) (2005) *Principles of Patient Consent: Standards Guidance.* General Dental Council, London (http://www.gdc-uk.org, accessed 7 July 2010).

Goodman, K. (2003) *Ethics and Evidence-based Medicine: Fallibility and Responsibility in Clinical Science.* Cambridge University Press, Cambridge.

Grodin, M.A. (ed.) (1995) *Meta Medical Ethics: The Philosophical Foundations of Bioethics.* Kluwer Academic, Dordrecht.

Have, H.A.M.J.ten & Jean, M.S. (eds) (2009) *The UNESCO Universal Declaration on Bioethics and Human Rights: Background, Principles and Application.* UNESCO, Paris.

International Organization for Standardization (http://www.iso.org, accessed 7 July 2010).

Jonsen, A.R., Siegler, M. & Winslade, W. (2006) *Clinical Ethics: A Practical Approach to Ethical Decisions in Clinical Medicine.* McGraw-Hill, New York.

Kerridge, I., Lowe, M. & Stewart, C. (2009) *Ethics and Law for the Health Professions*, 3rd edn. The Federation Press, Annandale, NSW.

Lambden, P. (ed.) (2002) *Dental Law and Ethics.* Radcliffe Medical Press, Oxford.

Lewis, M.A. & Tamparo, C.D. (2007) *Medical Law and Ethics*, 6th edn. F.A. Davis, Philadelphia.

Maclean, A. (2009) *Autonomy, Informed Consent and Medical Law: A Relational Challenge.* Cambridge University Press, Cambridge.

Mitchell, D.A. & Mitchell, L. (2009) *Oxford Handbook of Clinical Dentistry*, 5th edn, pp. 703–722. Oxford University Press, Oxford.

NHMRC (2004) *General Guidelines for Medical Practitioners on Providing Information to Patients.* National Health and Medical Research Council (Australia), Canberra.

Pollack, B.R. (2002) *Law and Risk Management in Dental Practice.* Quintessence, Chicago.

Rule, J.T. & Veatch, R.M. (2004) *Ethical Questions in Dentistry.* Quintessence, Chicago.

Sanbar, S.S. and American College of Legal Medicine Textbook Committee (eds) (2007) *Legal Medicine*, 7th edn. Mosby/Elsevier, Philadelphia.

UNESCO (2006) *Universal Declaration on Bioethics and Human Rights.* United Nations Educational, Scientific and Cultural Organization, Paris.

White, B.C. (1994) *Competence to Consent.* Georgetown University Press, Washington DC.

4

An Approach to Treatment Decision-Making

Iven Klineberg

1. Treatment philosophy

Clinical assessment, planning and management need to recognise and emphasise the biology of the jaw muscle system (Baum 1991, 2003) as a requirement for best practice. The biological framework of the stomatognathic (jaw–muscle) system, within which all treatment is centred, has a remarkable adaptive capacity that also needs to be acknowledged (Sessle 2005).

In recognition of the above, the continual change in soft tissues, bone as well as tooth orientation and position is an accepted reality of long-term management requirements. As a result, a focus on simple, conservative and minimally invasive procedures is strongly recommended in acknowledgement of each patient's oral health needs, recognising the desirability to maintain, where possible, natural teeth and tissues.

Complex treatment may be indicated, but needs to be carefully considered within the context of two important paradigms – form and function:

- *Form and aesthetic enhancement.* Aesthetics includes facial form, facial profile, lip form and smile, which are integrated with tooth position, shape, orientation and colour. These features have profound significance on patient psychosocial well-being, social confidence and social interaction, and are directly related to the informed consent that drives the decision to proceed with a particular treatment plan.
- *Function.* Function of mastication and swallowing bear directly on diet and nutrition and as a result have implications for long-term oral health of both soft tissues as well as hard tissues of teeth and bone. In addition and of special significance is the impact that mastication and swallowing have on general health.

The impact of mastication on cognition has been comprehensively reviewed by Weijenberg *et al.* (2010) and Ono *et al.* (2010); these were the first definitive reviews on the topic. Data from animal and human studies confirm a causal relationship between mastication and executive cognition with particular concerns for the elderly. However, evidence is also reported from animal and human data for young subjects and clearly indicates that optimising mastication enhances cognitive functions. Studies confirm that mastication develops enhanced concentration and memory with more rapid information processing, and spatial and numeric recall, which enhance learning. The possible mechanisms underlying these direct neuroplastic changes include many areas of the brain involved with cognition as well as sensorimotor functions. Executive function representation is linked to the prefrontal cortex and the striatum (Salat *et al.* 2004), while memory and recall are linked to the hippocampus (Viard *et al.* 2009); when the hippocampus is impaired, memory recall is affected. In addition, the ascending activating system appears to drive general arousal, which may also be reduced with impaired mastication.

These remarkable correlates with mastication and their implications for nutrition as well as cognition and executive cerebral function, place the very significant responsibility of oral rehabilitation in the hands of the clinician with appropriate training to optimise mastication and swallowing. These data add to the evidence base that emphasises the importance of oral rehabilitation for general health across young and older adult populations.

1.1 Best practice

Best practice requires a patient-centred approach to patient care where each patient's concerns, expectations and social circumstances are important components of informed consent, case planning, treatment agreement and optimum treatment delivery. Decision-making in clinical practice delivering oral health care is complex and is based on:

1. the clinician's level of knowledge and ability, supplemented by a search of the relevant evidence base for the decisions required;

Oral Rehabilitation: A Case-Based Approach, First Edition. Edited by Iven Klineberg, Diana Kingston.
© 2012 Blackwell Publishing Ltd. Published 2012 by Blackwell Publishing Ltd.

2. applying these generalised data for patient-specific needs;
3. with this information, addressing each patient's wishes and expectations.

1.2 Occlusal scheme

Occlusal scheme requirements include:

- determination of the optimum occlusal vertical dimension;
- provision of stable tooth contacts across the dental arch;
- development of appropriate lateral and protrusive tooth guidance to support fluent functions of mastication, swallowing (see above) and speech;
- design of an anterior tooth arrangement to optimise lip support, smile and facial form, to meet each patient's aesthetic and psychosocial expectations.

1.3 Patient assessment

At the commencement of treatment, patient assessment provides an opportunity to evaluate patient expectations and to acknowledge matters that may impact on outcomes.

Of necessity, a comprehensive assessment needs to include:

- general medical history, use of specific medications, their dose and their implications for oral health and function;
- understanding of each patient's psychological framework in which assessment, planning and treatment is centred, using a psychometric assessment such as the SCL-90-R questionnaire (Derogatis & Melisaratos 1983), which seeks answers to 90 behavioural questions as components of nine behavioural domains.

These details provide information about personality and patient characteristics, of which the clinician would otherwise be totally unaware and which may be of particular importance for case management. The information may bear directly on patient acceptance of treatment and its outcomes in the short and long term.

1.4 Outcome assessment

Outcome assessment at the conclusion of treatment is valuable and ensures that there is an opportunity for each patient to provide feedback on the specific management provided and their treatment experience, as distinct from the clinician's opinion.

The outcome assessment is directly influenced by:

- the patient's psychosocial status at the commencement of treatment;
- the ability of the clinician to provide the explanatory information to allow informed consent;
- the patient's experiences during treatment.

These patient-derived benefits are independent of the technical quality of treatment but are dependent on the quality of the patient–clinician interaction.

Positive outcomes are based on:

- the engagement of each patient's interest in their oral health status and the rehabilitation requirements planned;
- the awareness of their personal well-being and their enhanced psychosocial confidence and self-esteem, which also includes aesthetic benefits from treatment.

The overall positive outcome defines what is now recognised as improved oral health related quality of life.

1.5 Adaptation

Adaptation to treatment is a complex behavioural response and is founded on the patient's consent to treatment, their understanding and acceptance of what is planned, and their belief in the clinician as an ethical professional in whom they trust to provide optimum service for them.

This psychological component is of particular importance, and is supported by a neurophysiological response of central neuroplasticity. Neurological adaptation occurs to small and large modifications to the intraoral environment, which may include tooth adjustment and restoration, tooth loss, the provision of fixed dental prostheses (FDPs) and removable dental prostheses (RDPs), and the rehabilitation of the edentulous state. The implications for optimising mastication to support and enhance cognitive function with its complex neurophysiological interactions is another dimension to general health care.

Both the psychological and the neurophysiological components are important elements that underline each patient's acceptance of, and adaptation to, treatment (Sessle *et al.* 2009, Weijenberg *et al.* 2010).

2. Treatment planning – a comprehensive strategy for optimising outcomes

Treatment planning requires a standardised approach for data collection and the use of a template ensures that all relevant aspects are considered for each patient.

2.1 Patient assessment

Patient assessment includes details of the medical, social and dental history and it is recommended that this order of information gathering is followed to emphasise the importance of medical and social backgrounds and their implications for oral rehabilitation.

Importantly, the influence of medical conditions on oral health needs to be determined and the influence of oral health and jaw function on general health needs to be recognised. An emphasis on a biological approach in treatment design, delivery and outcomes, recognises this medical–dental interrelationship as a crucial element of integrated health care.

Also important is the commitment to the management of oral infections and diseases as an integral part of preliminary treatment, following an overall assessment of patient requirements. This includes, in particular, plaque control and oral hygiene instruction and monitoring as well as management of dental caries and periodontal disease. Careful periodontal assessment includes:

- soft tissues – mucosal thickness, height, presence of keratinised mucosa and its height and papilla fill of interproximal spaces;
- alveolar bone height and width and bone crest levels;
- radiographic assessment.

Patient assessment requires assessment of the whole mouth and jaw-muscle system, as well as assessment of teeth and supporting soft and hard tissues. This includes:

- soft tissues (muco-periosteum, tongue, fauces, cheeks, lips);
- hard tissues (base bone and alveolar bone);
- teeth (dental caries, status of restorations, missing teeth, occlusal plane levels and tooth surface loss);
- periodontium and temporomandibular joints (TMJs) (mobility, sounds).

The following summary is useful:

1. Assess medical background and implications, especially of medications on oral health (note the specific doses).
2. Assess aesthetics and consider facial form and symmetry, smile line and high lip line, dental centre lines, occlusal vertical dimension (OVD) and anterior tooth relationships, occlusal plane level and its orientation (anteroposteriorly and laterally), particularly in relation to smile line and aesthetics.

   Anatomical landmarks give a structural context to case planning and management decision-making in oral rehabilitation and relate planning to patient-specific features that are of particular importance with increasing treatment complexity (Mack 1996). Consideration of anatomical landmarks ensures a structural approach to management of each patient's specific aesthetic (dental, facial, psychosocial) and functional (occlusal, neuromuscular and TMJ) needs.

   Clinical application includes the accurate transfer of clinical features to an articulator to progress laboratory stages of planning and treatment that requires face bow and maxillomandibular transfer records. A face bow transfer is a simple record that correlates the relationship of the patient's temporomandibular condyles, maxillary occlusal plane and a third facial point of reference to appropriately orientate the maxillary diagnostic and working casts within the centre of the articulator.

The value of the face bow has been questioned by Carlsson (2006, 2008). However, for complex treatment planning and delivery, the three-dimensional (3D) transfer of the maxillary cast to an adjustable articulator in the appropriate anatomical orientation is a realistic procedural step. Furthermore, until accurate 3D computer modelling replaces articulators in treatment planning, such devices will be required together with a patient-specific face bow record.

The maxillomandibular transfer records the clinical relationship of the mandibular and maxillary dental arches to a reproducible position of the temporomandibular condyles bilaterally. This record orientates the mandibular diagnostic and working casts to the maxillary arch with transfer to an articulator. Articulators continue to be a requirement of prosthodontic rehabilitations (both RDPs and FDPs) and allow a realistic approximation of the relationships of the patient's dental arches and TMJs for laboratory diagnostic, planning and treatment.

The occlusal plane anteroposteriorly relates to the ala-tragal line bilaterally and the interpupillary line frontally; it is integrated with the patient's facial profile proportions to develop an anatomically pleasing relationship where the lower and middle thirds of the face are approximately equal. The importance of proportionality of facial form is more obviously recognised where there is disproportion that arises from reduced lower face height in association with gross tooth wear, occlusal collapse with tooth loss, as well as skeletal anomalies of jaw and arch size discrepancy.

3. Recognise age-specific features and realistic possibilities.
4. Be cognisant that each patient's preferences may be significantly influenced by unfiltered internet information, discussion with friends and with other clinicians, and media promotion about desirable and achievable aesthetics. Instead, focus on an optimum blend of form with function and a mature and rational consideration of needs and options. Patient views need to be tempered by the evidence base for optimising outcomes, a cost–benefit analysis for the case and realistic expectations of clinician and patient.
5. Recognise and assess changes in occlusal form (primarily attritional wear and erosion) within the context of the dynamic structural relationships of the stomognathic/dentofacial system, which constantly changes throughout life, with adaptation of lower face height to maintain speaking space. This was first comprehensively documented by the long-term studies of Tallgren (1957) and reviewed by Crothers (1992).

   It is acknowledged that in a biological system, compensatory tooth eruption occurs in response to tooth wear to maintain an effective OVD. Murphy (1959) reported compensatory mechanisms that prevent loss of OVD of the order of 60%. With an increase in treatment for OVD, jaw muscle adaptation occurs with muscle lengthening and the addition of sarcomeres in series to maintain an effective 'freeway' or 'speaking' space. This biological response to an increase in OVD, which is often overlooked as a component of biological adaptation, was described from animal studies more than 35 years ago by Goldspink (1976).

6. Recognise that the concept of the shortened dental arch (SDA) is a valid treatment option and that clinical outcomes of SDAs have confirmed no long-term side effects (Witter *et al.* 1999, 2007, Kanno & Carlsson 2006). However, patient-specific requests for posterior tooth replacement are a clear determinant of when an SDA treatment plan is not a viable option

2.2 Treatment options

Treatment options are an important consideration of informed patient consent and allow judicious presentation and discussion of the evidence base of the expected clinical outcomes. A presentation and discussion of the case-specific treatment options follows information gathering.

A determination of the evidence base may require time to collect published clinical data and to consider the information relevant for each option. Such an approach ensures that the clinician is well prepared to advise their patients and to comment on inevitable questions and possible concerns relating to patients' need for advice, guidance, confirmation of uncertainties, and depending on their interest and use of the internet, to address confusion and misinformation.

In this context, a commitment to advising each patient on which treatment is most likely to ensure an optimal outcome is desirable. This may be achieved by providing the most rational but not necessarily the 'ideal' treatment for each patient's particular oral health needs.

As a component of informed consent, and in relation to possible treatment options to optimise outcomes, a detailed risk–benefit analysis is needed to define treatment effectiveness in the long term. To consolidate the data required for a rational approach to case planning, risk–benefit should be linked with advice on the costs of the various options.

In order to provide this detailed information, preliminary imaging, including an orthopantomogram (OPG), periapical radiographs and study casts correctly articulated on an anatomical articulator, provide a focus for discussion. In addition, this information and the opportunity for patients to examine casts of their own mouth and their specific tooth arrangement, is of inestimable benefit in their understanding and is a forerunner of patient consent.

In cases where additional information is needed to specifically address aesthetic concerns, a diagnostic wax-up of the articulated study casts is an added benefit and may serve as a template for a clinical 'mock-up' of anterior tooth form, and for defining subsequent provisional restorations.

A decision-making protocol for decision analysis for implant treatment has been comprehensively presented by Flemmig and Beikler (2009). In this approach, the evidence base of relevant options is considered within the framework of the impact on the remaining dentition, masticatory function and patient satisfaction. Decision trees are proposed to logically determine survival and success estimates to allow a risk assessment of outcomes through prognostic modelling.

Complex treatment requires written information on treatment options, a risk–benefit analysis and costing and, once there is acceptance of an agreed treatment option, detailed clinical data are collected.

2.3 Provisional restorations

Provisional restorations, particularly when based on diagnostic preparations of tooth form and position, serve to confirm the clinician's evidence-based proposals.

Where an increase in OVD is needed, it is often desirable and appropriate to build on the existing dental situation with a variety of approaches. These may include:

- composite resin addition to remaining teeth or existing restorations;
- modification of existing complete or partial dental prostheses with acrylic resin;
- provision of occlusal splints with full-arch coverage for monitoring patient-specific responses;
- the use of an anterior appliance of composite resin.

The latter may be an addition to anterior teeth to encourage posterior tooth eruption, which provides an increase in anterior space for restorative crown lengthening (Dahl & Krogstad 1982, 1985). Each approach is valuable in specific treatment planning as a guide for informed decision-making to more realistically define outcomes.

2.4 Summary

It is important to recognise that oral health is an integral component of general health, and that clinical and patient-mediated success requires that simple or complex oral rehabilitation treatment blends as a seamless component of the biology of the jaw-muscle system.

Prosthodontics has a significant influence on general health as well as oral health. General health benefits from improved function allowing optimised diet and nutrition, with improvement in general health and cognition. Improved nutrition and general health also encourage improved psychosocial well-being and self-confidence, which are empowering patient benefits and are encapsulated in improved oral health related quality of life. The interaction and integration of general well-being and enhanced quality of life with optimising oral health through function and aesthetics is of inestimable importance to individuals, where the integrated benefit far outweighs the individual benefits of treatment components.

In the context of best evidence for decision-making, normative values are at the core of a successful patient–clinician relationship as they accept a range of values that are embodied in the variability of the general population: a theoretical or textbook ideal of tooth arrangements is for textbooks and is not a realistic concept of individual form and function as a reflection of community variability.

Finally, simple approaches are likely to be effective and are readily accepted; furthermore, they provide an opportunity to reassess and retreat as time requires.

3. Treatment sequencing

The treatment planning guide shown in Figure 4.1 defines a sequence of steps that allows:

- logical data collection;
- its analysis to define the patient-specific problem list;
- decision-making to consider treatment options and an optimum treatment plan for each patient's specific needs;
- informed patient-centred understanding based on discussion;
- patient consent on the decision (see Chapter 3).

This initial procedural sequence is desirable for both complex rehabilitations and simple treatments. It provides a professional approach and a basis for ethical decisions and a realistic justification to meet patient-specific needs. A sequence such as this ensures that

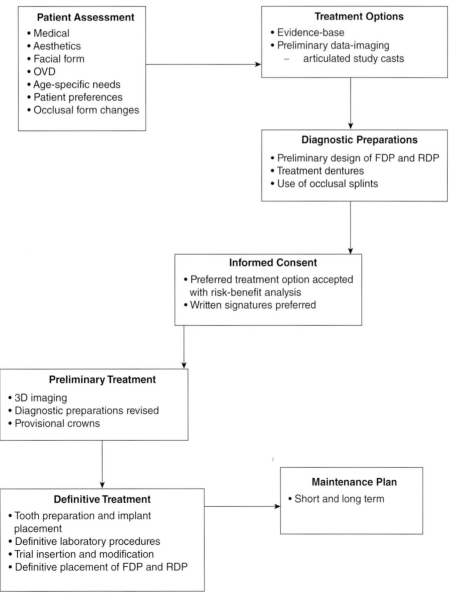

Figure 4.1 Treatment plan flow chart. FDP, fixed dental prostheses; OVD, occlusal vertical dimension; RDP, removable dental prostheses.

informed patient consent is achieved logically to justify definitive treatment. These preparatory procedures need to be detailed in each patient's clinical case notes as well as the clinical and laboratory stages; the use of photographic details to record preparatory and procedural stages are a valuable adjunct to record-keeping.

3.1 Outline (16 phases)

3.1.1 Data collection

The first information that needs to be asked for, understood and then recorded in the patient's case notes is the reason for their presentation for consultation. Although it may appear elementary, addressing the patient's specific concerns and wishes is crucial to meeting each patient's expectations and providing optimum oral health care. Understanding this requirement logically progresses to documentation of specific patient-based information.

Phase 1. History: medical, social and dental

Medical history includes past and present conditions, medications and implications for oral health such as effects on saliva quality, for example buffering capacity and quantity (Forde *et al.* 2006; Koka *et al.* 2006), with implications for tooth surface loss (Bartlett & Smith 1996; Scully 2003, 2009, Moazzez *et al.* 2004; Bartlett *et al.* 2008).

Dental history needs to determine the presence of disease and the initial aim of management is to arrest oral disease and prevent its reoccurrence. To achieve this, consider the patient's oral health awareness and their oral hygiene status as an indicator of their understanding of the need for, and their compliance with, an appropriate home-care routine. The presence of plaque at the time of consultation is often confronting as it indicates that the first step to oral health – the maintenance of an oral hygiene routine – is not understood or implemented. An assessment of the teeth includes those present, their orientation mesiodistally and labiolingually/labiopalatally, their orientation to the occlusal plane, the presence of dental caries, restorations and their status, and tooth surface loss (attrition, erosion and abrasion).

Social history includes:

- nutrition – carbohydrate intake and the balance of protein, fruit and vegetables;
- smoking, alcohol intake, general fluid intake – water, tea, coffee;
- health awareness is linked with general hygiene, diet, physical fitness – exercise/sport;
- social confidence and social interaction.

Phase 2. Extraoral examination

The facial profile is assessed with the patient upright to determine postural vertical dimension (lower face height) with face relaxed and with smile. Note high smile line as this has aesthetic implications. Assess occlusal vertical dimension and 'speaking space' (free-way space [FWS]).

Phase 3. Intraoral examination

- Frontal – intercuspal position, jaw opening.
- Lateral – right/left.
- Occlusal plane frontal and lateral – maxilla/mandible.

Phase 4. Imaging

- OPG, full mouth periapical radiographs.
- Implant treatment needs cone-beam computed tomography (CT) and 3D manipulation in an appropriate software program (e.g. NobelGuide, Med 3D, Simplant).

Phase 5. Periodontal assessment and charting

Gingival pocket depth is an indicator of periodontal health/disease and the presence of bleeding on probing confirms inflammation. A variety of simple or more advanced interventions are available and need to be determined and implemented for each case (Bengazi *et al.* 1996, Cardaropoli *et al.* 2006).

Referral to a periodontist is desirable as a routine and is essential where there is established disease for interdisciplinary collaboration, which is important in optimising outcomes of rehabilitation and the long-term prognosis (Hardt *et al.* 2002).

3.1.2 Data analysis and decision-making

Phase 6. Problem list

A problem list should be specified, as assessed from the detailed analysis of patient-specific data.

Phase 7. Articulated study casts and diagnostic wax-up

Articulated study casts and diagnostic wax-up of an optimised occlusal scheme are required to define the rehabilitation. This information is crucial as it is an essential and detailed view of the proposed change and a guide for informed patient discussion. Additional information is needed about specific fixed and/or removable restorations and implants where appropriate, both of which are needed to support the discussion on treatment options.

Phase 8. Treatment options

Treatment options need to focus on viable alternative treatments relevant to each case, which provide a blend of functional and aesthetic rehabilitation to meet each patient's expectations. The use of photographic records is often advantageous to assist in understanding the aesthetic modifications required but needs to be tempered with appropriate age-matched features of form (degree of incisal wear, flattening of cusps, etc.) and colour (blend of colour change with varying incisal, gingival and interproximal staining) to capture the presentation of intact teeth and reflect age- and gender-matched features.

Phase 9. Treatment plan risk assessment and informed consent

Templates such as the Objective Aesthetic Criteria in Dentate Patients (Magne & Belser 2002) and the Aesthetic Risk Assessment for edentulous sites, *ITI Treatment Guide* (Table 4.1) (Martin *et al.* 2007), are an

Table 4.1 *ITI TREATMENT GUIDE* (from Martin *et al.* 2007, with permission from Quintessence Publishing)

Aesthetic risk factors	Low	Medium	High
Medical status	Healthy patient and intact immune system		Reduced immune system
Smoking habit	Non-smoker	Light smoker (<10 cigarettes/day)	Heavy smoker (>10 cigarettes/day)
Patient's aesthetic expectations	Low	Medium	High
Lip line	Low	Medium	High
Gingival biotype	Low-scalloped, thick	Medium scalloped, medium thick	High scalloped, thin
Shape of tooth crowns	Rectangular		Triangular
Infection at implant site	None	Chronic	Acute
Bone level at adjacent teeth	≤5mm to contact point	5.5–6.5 to contact point	≥7mm to contact point
Restorative status of neighbouring teeth	Virgin		Restored
Width of edentulous span	1 tooth (≥7mm)[1] 1 tooth (≥5.5mm)[2]	1 tooth (<7mm)[1] 1 tooth (<5.5mm)[2]	2 teeth or more
Soft-tissue anatomy	Intact soft tissue		Soft-tissue defects
Bone anatomy of alveolar crest	Alveolar crest without bone deficiency	Horizontal bone deficiency	Vertical bone deficiency

[1]Standard Plus implants, regular neck.
[2]Standard Plus implants, narrow neck.

excellent means of ensuring that all details are considered to guide decision-making and for patient discussion. The focus on aesthetics is usually an important driver of patient decision-making; however, the clinician needs to emphasise the crucial outcomes of function (i.e. mastication, swallowing and speech) as the guidelines for optimising oral rehabilitation. The importance of enhanced function as the determinant of nutrition and general health along with confident speech, especially where public speaking is a work expectation, cannot be underestimated.

In addition, a treatment sequence such as that summarised in Figure 4.2 (Magne *et al.* 1996) will help the clinician to specify treatment plan details and the patient to understand the complexity of the rehabilitation and the overall timeline for each stage.

Phase 10. Management of oral disease and dysfunction
This includes management of dental caries, periodontal disease, angular cheilitis, denture sore mouth and other mucosal lesions (see Scully 2009), orofacial pain and temporomandibular disorder (Greene 2010).

3.1.3 Definitive procedures
Phase 11. Definitive diagnostic procedures
Definitive diagnostic procedures are:

- 3D imaging for bone assessment where implants are to be used;

- diagnostic preparations, revised and refined following earlier patient discussions;
- provisional crown preparation; this may be preceded by the application of composite resin to duplicate anterior crown form from the diagnostic preparations as a clinical trial, which provides a realistic patient opportunity to assess aesthetics of tooth position and form, as well as lip contour and speech.

Phase 12. Tooth preparations
For details of tooth preparations and implant placements, see Chapter 6.

Phase 13. Laboratory stages
For details of laboratory stages, see Figure 4.2.

Phase 14. Trial insertion
Trial insertion of FDPs and/or RDPs involves the following stages:

1. complete a detailed assessment of marginal contour fit and gingival appearance;
2. check axial contour on the labial to provide realistic tooth form to blend with overall facial form and contour of remaining natural teeth where present;
3. check space of buccal corridor and the aesthetic impact and interproximal contour – check contact point location and gingival papilla contour;

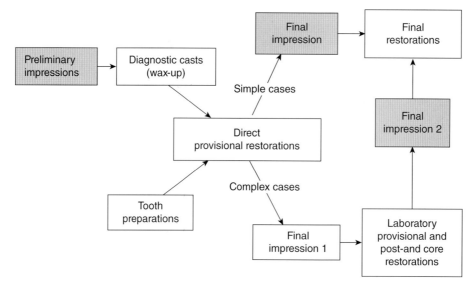

Figure 4.2 Laboratory stages (from Magne *et al.* 1996, with permission from Quintessence Publishing).

4. check occlusal contact distribution and occlusal plane orientation with facial landmarks;
5. finally, check facial form and frontal view of crown form, centre line, individual tooth form, lip support, profile and lateral views.

Phase 15. Final insertion
Check frontal and lateral contours, occlusal view and contact distribution as before.

3.1.4 Maintenance plan
Phase 16. Recall plan and discussion
Recall plan and discussion of short- and long-term needs as a likely scenario based on the evidence, as a reinforcement of what was already discussed in relation to informed consent, is an important follow-up strategy and a reinforcement of clinician–patient responsibility. It is also a confirmation for the patient of the ethical and professional responsibility of the clinician.

References
Bartlett, D.W. & Smith, B.G. (1996) The dental relevance of gastro-oesophageal reflux: Part 2. *Dental Update*, 23 (6), 250–253.

Bartlett, D., Ganss, C. & Lussi, A. (2008) Basic erosive wear examination (BEWE): a new scoring system for scientific and clinical needs. *Clinical Oral Investigations*, 12 (Suppl. 1), S65–S68.

Baum, B.J. (1991) Has modern biology entered the mouth? The clinical impact of biological research. *Journal of Dental Education*, 55 (5), 299–303.

Baum, B.J. (2003) Can biometrical science be made relevant in dental education? A North American perspective. *European Journal of Dental Education*, 7 (2), 49–55.

Bengazi, F., Wennström, J.L. & Lekholm, U. (1996) Recession of the soft tissue margin at oral implants. A 2-year longitudinal prospective study. *Clinical Oral Implants Research*, 7 (4), 303–310.

Cardaropoli, G., Lekholm, U. & Wennström, J.L. (2006) Tissue alterations at implant-supported single-tooth replacements: a 1-year prospective clinical study. *Clinical Oral Implants Research*, 17 (2), 165–171.

Carlsson, G.E. (2006) Facts and fallacies: an evidence base for complete dentures. *Dental Update*; 33 (3), 134–142.

Carlsson, G.E. (2008) Critical review of some dogmas in prosthodontics. *Journal of Prosthodontic Research*, 53 (1), 3–10.

Crothers, A.J. (1992) Tooth wear and facial morphology. *Journal of Dentistry*, 20 (6), 333–341.

Dahl, B.L. & Krogstad, O. (1982) Effect of a partial bite raising splint on the occlusal face height. An x-ray cephalometric study in human adults. *Acta Odontologica Scandinavica*, 40 (1), 17–24.

Dahl, B.L. & Krogstad, O. (1985) Long-term observations of an increased occlusal face height obtained by a combined orthodontic/prosthetic approach. *Journal of Oral Rehabilitation*, 12 (2), 173–176.

Derogatis, L.R. & Melisaratos, N. (1983) The Brief Symptom inventory: an introductory report. *Psychological Medicine*, 13 (3), 595–605.

Flemmig, T.F. & Beikler, T. (2009) Decision making in implant dentistry: an evidence-based and decision-analysis approach. *Periodontology 2000*, 50, 154–165.

Forde, M.D., Koka, S., Eckert, E. *et al.* (2006) Systemic assessments utilizing saliva: part 1 general considerations and current assessments. *International Journal of Prosthodontics*, 19 (1), 43–52.

Goldspink, G. (1976) The adaptation of muscle to a new functional length. In: *Mastication: Proceedings of a Symposium on the Clinical and Physiological Aspects of Mastication held at the Medical School, University of Bristol on 14–16 April 1975* (eds D.J. Anderson & B. Mathews), pp. 90–99. John Wright, Bristol.

Greene, C.S. (2010) Diagnosis and treatment of temporomandibular disorders: emergence of a new care guidelines statement. *Oral Surgery, Oral Medicine, Oral Pathology, Oral Radiology and Endodontology*, 110 (2), 137–139.

Hardt, C.R, Gröndahl, K., Lekholm, U. *et al.* (2002) Outcome of implant therapy in relation to experienced loss of periodontal bone support: a retrospective 5-year study. *Clinical Oral Implants Research*, 13 (5), 488–494.

Kanno, T. & Carlsson, G.E. (2006) A review of the shortened dental arch concept focusing on the work by the Käyser/Nijmegen group. *Journal of Oral Rehabilitation*, 33 (11), 850–862.

Koka, S., Forde, M.D. & Khosla, S. (2006) Systemic assessments utilizing saliva: part 2 osteoporosis and use of saliva to measure bone turnover. *International Journal of Prosthodontics*, 19 (1), 53–60.

Mack, M.R. (1996) Perspective of facial esthetics in dental treatment planning. *Journal of Prosthetic Dentistry*, 75 (2), 169–176.

Magne, P. & Belser, U. (2002) *Bonded Porcelain Restorations in the Anterior Dentition: A Biomimetic Approach*. Quintessence, Chicago.

Magne, P., Magne, M. & Belser, U. (1996) The diagnostic template: a key element to the comprehensive esthetic treatment concept. *International Journal of Periodontics & Restorative Dentistry*, 16 (6), 560–569.

Martin, W.C., Morton, D. & Buser, D. (2007) Pre-operative analysis and prosthetic treatment planning in esthetic implant dentistry. In: *ITI Treatment Guide*, Vol. 1, (eds D. Buser, U. Belser & D. Wismeijer), p.20. Quintessence, Berlin.

Moazzez, R., Bartlett, D. & Anggiansah, A. (2004) Dental erosion, gastro-oesophageal reflux disease and saliva: how are they related? *Journal of Dentistry*, 32 (6), 489–494.

Murphy, T. (1959) Compensatory mechanisms in facial height to functional tooth attrition. *Australian Dental Journal*, 4, 312–323.

Ono, Y., Yamamoto, T., Kubo, K.Y. *et al.* (2010) Occlusion and brain function: mastication as a prevention of cognitive dysfunction. *Journal of Oral Rehabilitation*, 37 (8), 624–640.

Salat, D.H., Buckner, R.L., Snyder, A.Z. *et al.* (2004) Thinning of the cerebral cortex in aging. *Cerebral Cortex*, 14 (7), 721–730.

Scully, C. (2003) Drug effects on salivary glands: dry mouth. *Oral Diseases*, 9 (4), 165–176.

Scully, C. (2009) *Oral and Maxillofacial Medicine*, 2nd edn, pp.79–86. Churchill Livingstone, Edinburgh.

Sessle, B.J. (2005) Biological adaptation and normative values. *International Journal of Prosthodontics*, 18 (4), 280–282.

Sessle, B.J., Klineberg, I. & Svensson, P. (2009) A neurophysiologic perspective on rehabilitation with oral implants and their potential side effects. In: *Osseointegration and Dental Implants* (ed. A. Jokstad), pp. 333–344. Wiley-Blackwell, Ames, Iowa.

Tallgren, A. (1957) Changes in adult face height due to ageing, wear and loss of teeth and prosthetic treatment. *Acta Odontologica Scandinavica Supplementum*, 15 (24), 63–75.

Viard, A, Lebreton, K., Chetelat, G. *et al.* (2009) Patterns of hippocampal–neocortical interactions in the retrieval of episodic autobiographical memories across entire life-span of aged adults. *Hippocampus*, 20 (1), 153–165.

Weijenberg, R.A. Scherder, E.J. & Lobbezoo, F. (2010) Mastication for the mind – the relationship between mastication and cognition in ageing and dementia. *Neuroscience and Biobehavioral Reviews*, 6, 1–15.

Witter, D.J., van Palenstein Helderman, W.H., Creugers, N.H. *et al.* (1999) The shortened dental arch concept and its implications for oral health care. *Community Dentistry & Oral Epidemiology*, 27 (4), 249–258.

Witter, D.J., Kreulen, C.M., Mulder, J. *et al.* (2007) Signs and symptoms related to temporomandibular disorders – follow-up of subjects with shortened and completed dental arches. *Journal of Dentistry*, 35 (6), 521–527.

5

Orofacial Pain and Temporomandibular Disorders

Chris Peck

1. Introduction

Orofacial pain and temporomandibular disorders (TMDs) are prevalent conditions that need to be considered when planning and undertaking oral rehabilitation. Orofacial pain occurs in a quarter of the population and can significantly impact an individual's family, social and work activities (Macfarlane *et al.* 2002). Pain in the oral and facial regions frequently originates from the dentition and associated structures and is mostly well managed in dental practice. Other important sources of orofacial pain include the local nervous and musculoskeletal systems, and pain referred from nearby and distant sites. While TMDs involve the jaw muscles and TMJs and are a common source of orofacial pain, they also include non-painful disorders that impair jaw function.

Pain is an unpleasant sensory and emotional experience associated with actual or potential tissue damage or described in terms of such damage (International Association for the Study of Pain 1994). Pain does not necessarily need pathology or a noxious (i.e. tissue-damaging or potentially tissue-damaging) stimulus, as individuals can experience pain without tissue damage or nociception (transmission of nerve signals resulting from noxious/damaging stimulation). It is a higher brain process, an experience *per se*, and does not necessarily need peripheral nervous system activity. Furthermore, the pain experience is unique to an individual and two people with similar pathology can each describe their pain very differently. This multidimensional nature of pain comprises sensory-discriminative (pain's location, intensity, duration, quality), motivational-affective (unpleasant emotional experience that motivates avoidance, escape behaviour, catastrophising/excessive focus on pain), and cognitive-evaluative (beliefs based on previous experiences) dimensions.

2. Orofacial pain and temporomandibular disorder classification

Although a number of clinical groups have proposed classification systems for orofacial pain, no single system has

been considered the benchmark. For example, the International Headache Society has as one of its 13 headache categories, headache or facial pain, attributed to a disorder of cranium, neck, eyes, ears, nose, sinuses, teeth, mouth, or other facial or cranial structures (International Headache Society 2004). The American Academy of Orofacial Pain have eight diagnostic categories: intracranial pain disorders, primary headache disorders, secondary headache disorders, neuropathic pain disorders, intraoral pain disorders, TMDs, cervical pain disorders, associated structures and axis II mental disorders (Leeuw 2008). The classification systems can be confusing as many of the groups do not have clearly defined diagnostic criteria, are largely related to topographic distribution of symptoms which frequently overlap between groups and likely have different underlying pathophysiological mechanisms. Woda and colleagues have proposed a system based on clustering signs and symptoms in the hope that these clusters have similar pathophysiological mechanisms (Woda *et al.* 2005). In this classification system, there are acute and chronic orofacial pains with a somatic aetiology (e.g. pulpitis, periodontitis, myositis) and chronic orofacial pains without simple somatic aetiologies. This latter category is then subdivided into:

- neuralgia (post-injury neuralgia, trigeminal neuralgia);
- primary headache disorders (tension-type, migraine and cluster headaches);
- persistent idiopathic orofacial pain (burning mouth syndrome, TMDs, atypical facial pain).

For TMDs there are also multiple systems, although the research diagnostic criteria for TMDs (RDC/TMD) has become the standard (Dworkin & LeResche 1992). This system uses a dual axis with diagnoses made on physical and psychosocial axes. This system's advantage is that it fits with the biopsychosocial concept of pain, and indeed the psychosocial axis of this classification system is likely applicable for any orofacial pain. The physical (axis I) diagnostic groups (Box 5.1) are not mutually exclusive

---

Oral Rehabilitation: A Case-Based Approach, First Edition. Edited by Iven Klineberg, Diana Kingston.
© 2012 Blackwell Publishing Ltd. Published 2012 by Blackwell Publishing Ltd.

Box 5.1 Types of temporomandibular disorders
Common temporomandibular disorders

Myofascial pain presents with a history of pain in the jaw muscle region and pain on palpation of the muscles. Mouth opening may be restricted but can be increased with clinician assistance.

Disc displacements present with either joint sounds, with jaw movement indicating the disc repositioning from an anteriorly displaced position, or a history of joint sounds that is replaced with severely reduced mouth opening, indicating a disc that remains anteriorly displaced. With the latter, opening improves over time, although it tends not return to the original maximum gape.

Arthralgia presents with a history of pain in the TMJ region and pain on palpation of the joint.

Osteoarthritis presents with joint crepitus (gratey, gravelly sounds on movement) and degenerative changes confirmed by imaging of the joint.

Less common temporomandibular disorders

Developmental disorders (e.g. hyperplasia, hypoplasia), which are typically painless but may impact jaw function.

Muscle splinting/trismus (protective reflex rigidity) usually presents as a limitation of jaw motion, usually with an obvious, associated, pain-related cause (e.g.

painful joint/pericoronitis). The 'splinting' muscles are often painful and the 'splinting' decreases when the cause is removed. The restricted jaw motion cannot be increased when assisted by the clinician.

Muscle spasm (involuntary, painful, muscle contraction) presents as severe muscle pain and restricted jaw motion due to acute involuntary muscle contraction (shortening). There may be observable fasciculation of muscle parts, or even of the entire muscle.

Myositis (painful, general inflammation, usually of the entire muscle) presents with a history of muscle trauma or infection, prominent pain of the entire muscle, restricted jaw motion that can be increased with clinician assistance, and possibly swelling.

Muscle contracture (involuntary shortening without motor activity) presents with a chronic history of restricted jaw motion resulting from rearrangement of intramuscular collagen over time, plus soft tissue tightness, joint ankylosis and weak antagonist muscles.

Subluxation/dislocation presents with the condyle anterior to the articular eminence at maximum opening and either a transient (but self-reducing) inability to close jaw (subluxation), or a more enduring inability to close the jaw (dislocation), which frequently cannot be self-reduced.

---

and patients can have one or more diagnoses. The psychosocial (axis II) group includes the graded chronic pain scale, which assesses pain-related disability, psychological measures and jaw function impairment (see International RDC-TMD Consortium website). TMDs also include other relatively rare conditions (Box 5.1).

2.1 Common orofacial pains

Common orofacial pains include the following:

- *Intraoral pain disorders* of dental pulp, periodontium, mucogingival tissues. These are largely managed in dental practice.
- *Headaches* may be primary (e.g. migraine, tension type, cluster) or secondary to other pathology (e.g. giant cell arteritis).
- *Neuropathic pain* is pain initiated or caused by a primary lesion or dysfunction in the nervous system (International Association for the Study of Pain 1994). The more common orofacial neuropathic pains include post-traumatic (from dental treatment such as tooth extraction or pulpectomy, orthognathic surgery resulting in nerve injury) and trigeminal neuralgia (episodic brief electric shock-like pain, abrupt in onset and termination, limited to the distribution of one or more divisions of the trigeminal nerve). Other neuropathic pains include glossopharyngeal neuralgia (severe transient

stabbing pain experienced in the ear, base of the tongue, tonsillar fossa or beneath the angle of the jaw) and post-herpetic neuralgia resulting from acute herpes zoster infection with viral inflammation of the dorsal root and ganglion, which destroys myelinated fibres.

- *Pain from associated structures*, including sinuses (e.g. sinusitis), salivary glands (e.g. sialolithiasis, sialadenitis), and referred and radiating pain from ears, nose, throat and eyes.
- *Systemic disease*, including ischaemic heart disease, fibromyalgia and painful systemic arthritic disease.
- *TMDs*, as outlined above, are the major cause of non-odontogenic orofacial pain. Risk factors for TMDs include trauma, clenching, third molar removal, somatisation (predisposition to report numerous non-specific symptoms) and female gender (Huang *et al.* 2002). Also, there are predictors for the development of a chronic TMD, including a history of widespread pain and anxiety (Aggarwal *et al.* 2010), muscle pain and high pain intensity (Epker *et al.* 1999).

3. Orofacial pain and temporomandibular disorder assessment
3.1 Pain assessment

Pain is a complex, multidimensional and unique experience that can only be assessed indirectly. The patient's

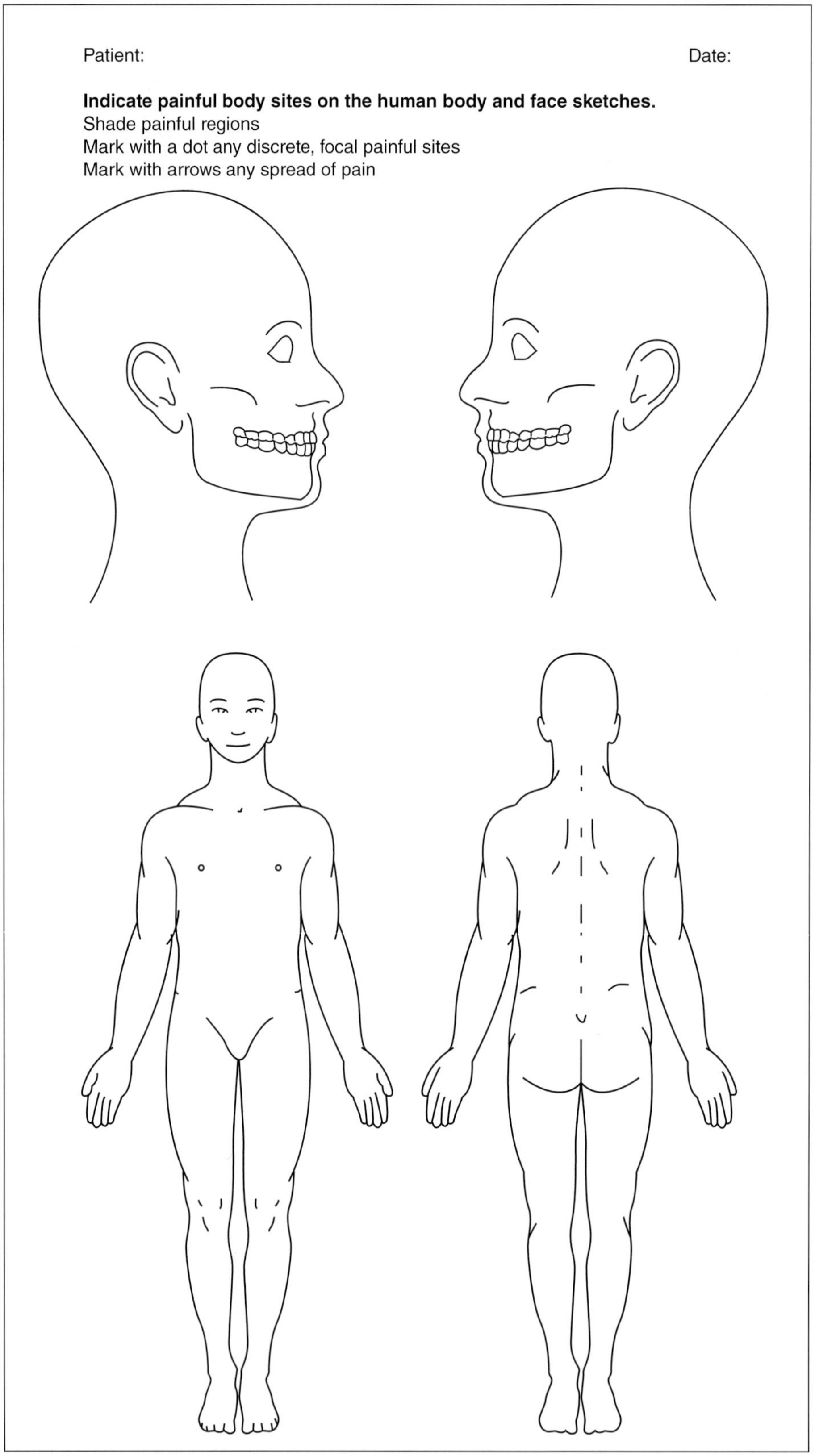

Patient: Date:

Indicate painful body sites on the human body and face sketches.
Shade painful regions
Mark with a dot any discrete, focal painful sites
Mark with arrows any spread of pain

Figure 5.1 Pain location map.

history is the most important component of pain assessment. This can be unsettling to some clinicians who have consequently sought more objective measures for pain. However, the relationship between objective measures (e.g. pathology, physical strength, range of motion) are at best weakly correlated with pain reports (Turk & Melzack 1992, 2001) and also pathology may be present frequently in asymptomatic individuals.

3.2 Key elements of a pain-related history

The goals of the pain-related history are to obtain information to help with diagnosis, assess the patient's psychological, legal, vocational and disability status, recognise barriers to assessment and management, and help determine further tests and clinical examinations (Figure 5.1 & Table 5.1).

The history is obtained with a patient interview, which allows the clinician to develop a rapport with the patient, supplemented with the use of standardised questionnaires, which ensures specific history questions are asked (see below). It is important to build a trusting relationship with the patient, perform the interview in a private setting and use open-ended questions and not be overly directive during the interview.

The interview includes both verbal and behavioural communication; listening to the patient's exact words and their sequence and observing body language are important. The history should broach biological and psychosocial components (Box 5.2). The evaluation varies with specific circumstances; for example an acute pain history may focus largely on the sensory components, whereas with the chronic pain history the psychosocial components will likely have increasing importance.

3.3 Clinical examination

The clinical examination will be guided by the findings in the patient history and may include extraoral examination of the musculoskeletal structures (see below), cranial nerve testing and intraoral examination of hard and soft tissues. Examination findings will frequently confirm the provisional diagnosis derived from the patient's history.

3.4 Other tests

Other tests may be indicated following the history and examination, including laboratory (e.g. blood tests for systemic arthropathies), imaging and diagnostic neural blockade. Importantly, imaging is the only diagnostic test recommended in addition to the history and examination of a patient with TMD (Greene 2010).

Imaging is used to confirm or exclude specific diagnoses (e.g. trigeminal neuralgia secondary to a central lesion, sinusitis, periapical pathology), confirm the extent of known disease and evaluate the progression of disease (e.g. TMJ osteoarthritic changes) or treatment. The sites imaged in orofacial pain and TMDs include hard and soft tissues of intraoral structures (e.g. dentition and jaws, salivary glands and ducts) and the TMJs, the sinuses and

other craniofacial structures. There are no guidelines for imaging chronic orofacial pain apart from TMJ imaging (Brooks *et al.* 1997), and recently reliable image analysis criteria have been presented for diagnosing osseous and non-osseous TMJ components using computerised tomography and magnetic resonance imaging, respectively (Ahmad *et al.* 2009). Panoramic radiographs are frequently used as a screening tool and, while they provide a good overall view of the jaws, condyles and maxillary sinuses,

Table 5.1 McGill pain descriptors (adapted from Melzack 1975)

Select those words from the following group that best describes your pain. Note that at most one word from each group should be chosen			
1	2	3	4
Flicking Quivering Pulsing Throbbing Beating Pounding	Jumping Flashing Shooting	Pricking Boring Drilling Stabbing Lancinating	Sharp Cutting Lacerating
5	6	7	8
Pinching Pressing Gnawing Cramping Crushing	Tugging Pulling Wrenching	Hot Burning Scalding Searing	Tingling Itchy Smarting Stinging
9	10	11	12
Dull Sore Hurting Aching Heavy	Tender Taut Rasping Splitting	Tiring Exhausting	Sickening Suffocating
13	14	15	16
Fearful Frightful Terrifying	Punishing Gruelling Cruel Vicious Killing	Wretched Blinding	Annoying Troublesome Miserable Intense Unbearable
17	18	19	20
Spreading Radiating Penetrating Piercing	Tight Numb Drawing Squeezing Tearing	Cool Cold Freezing	Nagging Nauseating Agonising Dreadful Torturing

Groups 1–10: Sensory descriptors: a patient's sensation of pain.
Groups 11–15: Affective descriptors: a patient's reaction to pain.
Group 16: Evaluative descriptors: pain intensity.
Groups 17–20: General descriptors.
In each group, the words are arranged in order of increasing pain.

Box 5.2 Key components of a pain history

Presenting complaint: Determines why the patient is seeking care and ensures that the complaint is applicable to the clinician's area of expertise.

Length of illness: Discriminates acute from chronic conditions.

Progression since onset: Reviews complaint over time.

Pain site: Provides the sensory distribution of pain. Multiple pain sites may indicate a patient with more than one pain condition, or a more generalised problem. Assess for extracranial pain. A pain map diagram may be used (see Figure 5.1).

Spread of pain – location and extent: Determines if there is pain radiation or referral to near or distant sites. This may help discriminate peripheral and central pain mechanisms.

Quality: Pain descriptors can help differentiate pain conditions. Where patients find it difficult to describe the pain quality, it may be beneficial to provide a list of pain descriptors (Melzack 1975) from which the patient selects those words that best describe their pain (see Table 5.1).

Severity: Pain severity can be assessed with a number of instruments, including scales where patients rank their pain between no pain and worst possible pain on a 100 mm line (visual analogue scale) or between 0 and 10 (numerical rating scale). Composite scores that average individual scores (such as worst pain, least pain, current pain, average pain) may be more reliable over time. Pain severity is often used as a measure for treatment outcome, although in chronic pain other psychosocial measures also need to be assessed (see below).

Frequency: Pain frequency may be indicative of specific painful conditions and relate to the degree of suffering and aggravating factors.

Duration: This, together with pain quality and frequency, can help diagnose specific chronic conditions (Lance 1993).

Temporal pattern: Does the pain demonstrate a daily, seasonal or other cyclical pattern?

Time of onset: Is pain onset variable or is it at the same time of day/week/season?

Mode of onset: Is the pain spontaneous, related to an injury or are there premonitory symptoms? This may provide diagnostic validity for certain pain states (e.g. migraine is sometimes preceded by focal neurological symptoms (Lance 1993).

Precipitating and aggravating factors: What variables (e.g. jaw function, stressful events) trigger or aggravate the pain complaint?

Relieving factors: No relieving factors may suggest a serious disorder.

Previous treatments: Obtain previous treatments and their success or failure. This may help exclude/include conditions in a differential diagnosis; however, it must be noted that ineffective treatments may be the result of inappropriate use.

Associated features: Is this complaint discrete and localised or widespread? Perform a system review to rule out serious conditions such as space-occupying lesions and to assess the health of the patient.

Past health: Are there previous conditions that may be associated with the present complaint? Previous trauma, chronic recurring conditions (e.g. sinusitis) may provide diagnostic clues.

Family history: Investigate for a familial tendency for systemic illnesses that may relate to the presenting complaint.

Occupation: Is this contributing to the complaint either physically or mentally (e.g. lack of job satisfaction, stressors)?

Functional activities: Are there reports of generalised functional impairment and impairment localised to the jaw system?

Pain behaviours: Assess facial expressions (grimacing), motor activity (slow movement), verbal reports (reports of hopelessness), paralingual vocalisations (moan, sigh), behaviours to reduce pain (medication use, health-care use, using protective devices, e.g. neck collar), body postures (shifting posture frequently, rubbing affected area), functional limitations (stopping to rest, moving in a guarded manner).

Psychological aspects: Assess suffering (e.g. interpersonal disruption, economic distress, occupational problems). Is the patient demonstrating anxious or depressed behaviour?

the view is oblique and only gross structural changes are observable.

3.5 Assessment of temporomandibular disorders

The RDC/TMD assessment outlined above has been reviewed and a revised set of criteria is being developed that will have increased clinical utility (Schiffman *et al.* 2010). Importantly, such specific assessments do not replace a comprehensive pain assessment, but are complementary and should be utilised when the clinician is confident that the patient's complaint is a TMD.

The RDC/TMD assessment uses a standardised questionnaire and examination for which clinicians have been trained, calibrated and assessed (see International RDC-TMD Consortium website). The questionnaire has a major focus on the psychosocial domain by assessing pain-related disability, jaw function impairment and the common psychological disorders associated with chronic pain: depression and somatisation. The examination focuses on the range of movement, joint sounds and palpation tenderness of the jaw muscles and joints.

3.6 Occlusion and temporomandibular disorders

The role of the dental occlusion in the development of TMDs is hotly debated, although many of the arguments are based on uncontrolled clinical anecdotes rather than the current scientific literature.

Dental occlusion is defined as the dynamic biological relationship of the components of the masticatory system that determine tooth relationships (Klineberg & Jagger 2004) and there is enormous individual variation. Stable occlusal relationships are the norm in humans. There is significant overlap of occlusal features between individuals with and without jaw disorders and the dental occlusal scheme is not a predictor of disease (Pullinger & Seligman 2000, Seligman & Pullinger 2000). While in these studies some occlusal variables were associated with TMDs (e.g. overjet >5.25 mm, unilateral posterior cross-bite, centric relation to intercuspal position [ICP] slides >1.75 mm), the associations were weak. Importantly, an association does not imply a cause–effect relationship where particular occlusal schemes cause TMDs. There are instances that suggest the opposite, that is, that TMJ changes cause a change to the occlusion; for example, the TMJ degenerative changes in advanced osteoarthritis can lead to a clinically observable anterior open-bite. Also, the introduction of experimental masseter muscle pain affects the ability to close into a retruded contact position, resulting in an occlusal change with a shift of tooth contacts more anteriorly (Stohler 2006).

The introduction of occlusal interferences has not resulted in the development of a TMD (Clark et al. 1999), and avoidance behaviour and reduction of tooth contact is the expected response with any tooth discomfort. Humans have very high interocclusal discriminatory ability, which is partly due to low-threshold periodontal mechanosensitivity, resulting in the ability to detect thicknesses as small as 8 μm between the teeth (Kogawa et al. 2010). This discrimination is reduced in TMD subjects, which is likely a consequence rather than the cause of the TMD (Kogawa et al. 2010). It is also hard to understand how the dental occlusion could be responsible for the extracranial pain that is commonly seen with TMDs, or for fibromyalgia, as 75% of these individuals also have a TMD (Plesh et al. 1996). Current evidence-based assessment systems for TMDs do not assess the dental occlusion; they focus on measuring the range of jaw movement and palpating for muscle and joint pain and articular sounds (Dworkin & LeResche 1992). The scientific evidence simply does not support that dental occlusion plays an aetiological role in TMDs (Luther 2007).

Further, if dental occlusion played a large role in the onset of TMDs, it would be expected that occlusion-based treatments would resolve these problems. A systematic review of 18 randomised controlled trials showed equivocal results for occlusal appliance use for TMDs. The study concluded that there were, at best, modest outcomes compared with other conservative management strategies and that occlusal adjustments are not indicated in management (Forssell & Kalso 2004). Extensive occlusal adjustment cannot be justified preventively, or in the presence of a TMD, since occlusion may change in the presence of pain or disease activity. As outlined above, any occlusal changes are likely the result of pain and impaired jaw function. Those with severe, unremitting pain may demand occlusal therapy to alleviate symptoms, especially in the presence of a malocclusion. An American Association of Dental Research policy statement (Greene 2010) recommends that TMD treatment be initially based on conservative, reversible and evidence-based modalities. This does not include treatment of the occlusion, including irreversible occlusal adjustments. Treatment must focus on pain and other comorbidities and be patient centred and not symptom specific. With improvement, local management of the dental occlusion then may be considered for functional or aesthetic reasons.

In summary, the risk that occlusal features will lead to the development of TMDs is low to very low (Pullinger & Seligman, 2000). Patients' beliefs about the role of the dental occlusion in the cause of TMDs need to be challenged, and in particular this includes any suggestion of a simple cause–effect model between occlusion and the TMD.

4. Orofacial pain and temporomandibular disorder management

The goals for management are to:

- reduce or eliminate pain;
- restore comfortable jaw function;
- reduce health-care utilisation;
- improve quality of life.

Typical strategies include pharmacotherapy, physical medicine, behavioural management and prevention.

4.1 Management steps

4.1.1 Explanation and reassurance

Explain pain and its impact in lay terms. It is important to reassure patients by acknowledging their pain and informing them that management is available. Clinical psychologists may be used to help with this. It is important to motivate patients to 'own' their problem and to explain that passive or maladaptive coping strategies such as hoping, withdrawal, resting and the use of medication are associated with increased pain, depression and disability. These should be replaced by adaptive strategies such as exercise, dealing directly with stressful events and positive statements that the pain can be dealt with (Peres & Lucchetti 2010).

4.1.2 Pain reduction

Medication is frequently required. Analgesics used for mild to moderate pain include paracetamol, aspirin or non-steroidal anti-inflammatory drugs (e.g. ibuprofen). Chronic use needs to be considered carefully as do contraindications. Topical analgesics, including non-steroidal anti-inflammatory drugs, as an alternative for localised muscle or articular pain have demonstrated effectiveness for acute pain (Massey et al. 2010) and do not have the same adverse events as the orally administered drug. Topical capsaicin (the active component of chilli peppers) is also used for localised neuropathic or musculoskeletal pain (Padilla et al. 2000). The required three- to four-times daily applications cause an initial burning sensation and precautions must be taken to avoid the eyes and mucosal surfaces. If used intraorally, a polyvinyl cover extending over the application site is essential to limit spread of capsaicin.

Combination analgesics (e.g. paracetamol–codeine) and the opioids may be used for more severe pain but consideration must be given to the risk of dependence, drowsiness, nausea and vomiting.

Co-analgesics are drugs that have been developed primarily to treat other conditions but demonstrate analgesic properties. The main classes are antidepressants and anticonvulsants. Amitriptyline, a tricyclic antidepressant, has been extensively studied (Saarto & Wiffen 2005) for chronic pain management. It is used at sub-antidepressant doses and its analgesic effect is faster than its antidepressant effect. A number of adverse events, including dry mouth, drowsiness and blurred vision, need to be monitored and caution must be taken, especially in those with diseases such as cardiovascular conditions, hyperthyroidism and glaucoma. Anticonvulsants include carbamazepine, which is the gold standard for treatment of trigeminal neuralgia, and gabapentin, which is indicated for neuropathic pain. Muscle relaxants, including diazepam, can be used short term for acute orofacial pain with accompanying muscle splinting but care needs to be taken with the risk of dependency.

4.1.3 Regain function

A major goal is to reduce pain-related disability; for orofacial pain, this not only includes a focus on family, social and work activities but also on jaw function. Impaired jaw function is frequently associated with orofacial pain or a major complaint with TMDs. To overcome this, simple jaw movements extending the range of motion and a graded return to jaw function by, for example, gradually increasing the hardness and consistency of foods often improves jaw function.

Physiotherapy can help with regaining function and management may include patient education, jaw exercises, manual therapy, pain reducing modalities, cervical posture and strengthening exercises (Medlicott & Harris 2006).

Pain is associated with a number of psychological states, including anxiety (frequently seen with acute pain), depression (frequently seen with chronic pain) and somatisation (Dworkin 2001). These can lead to a number of behaviours, including sleep problems, isolation, avoidance and extensive health-care use, and furthermore lead to poorer treatment response (Turner & Dworkin 2004). Thus, it is imperative that patients undergo a psychosocial assessment and their management targets dysfunction in this area. Strategies may include relaxation therapy to produce physiological affects opposite to those of anxiety, pacing to regain function, desensitisation to feared activities and cognitive behavioural therapy. For TMD patients with high levels of psychosocial dysfunction, a brief programme of cognitive behavioural therapy has demonstrated effectiveness in the short term (Dworkin et al. 2002).

4.1.4 Review

Patient review provides an opportunity to assess the patient's progress, encourage gains, reinforce appropriate management and discourage maladaptive behaviours. It provides the patient with a single source for management and helps reduce inappropriate health-care use. Review should include assessment tools to monitor progress. Interim reviews (e.g. telephone, e-mail) provide patients with reassurance that they have an empathetic, personal and humane health-care provider.

4.1.5 Future prevention

It is important that any gains achieved are not lost. Particularly with chronic orofacial pain, there is a need for patients to be encouraged to maintain management strategies, including exercises and other behaviours, and reduce maladaptive habits. It is important for patients to be educated on how to minimise jaw functions that may exacerbate orofacial pain. For example, dental appointments frequently need to be modified (Box 5.3).

4.2 Pain and temporomandibular disorder management in the context of oral rehabilitation

Pain and impaired jaw function can significantly impact oral rehabilitation and need to be considered and managed in the initial phase of treatment planning and then monitored throughout the subsequent oral rehabilitation of the patient. Oral rehabilitation treatment plans may need to be modified, depending on pain and jaw function status and its impact on the patient. Wherever possible, oral rehabilitation should be delayed until the patient feels in control of their pain and has acceptable range of jaw movement for dental treatment. Strategies to reduce the risk of exacerbating orofacial pain or TMDs from dental treatment need to be considered (Box 5.3). The use of

Box 5.3 Dental procedures for patients with temporomandibular disorders

Patients with symptomatic TMDs may not tolerate wide mouth opening required for dental procedures. They may also experience increased symptoms following a dental procedure. The following suggestions may reduce the stress placed on the temporomandibular structures should a dental procedure be necessary. The appropriateness of their use will have to be determined for each individual.

Prior to the procedure

1. Apply moist heat to the sides of the face for 10–15 minutes before the procedure.
2. Reduce chewing and wide-opening for several days prior to the procedure.
3. Consider prescribing a non-steroidal anti-inflammatory drug prior to the procedure (e.g. ibuprofen 400 mg) if no contraindications exist.
4. Consider prescribing a muscle relaxant prior to the procedure (e.g. diazepam 2–5 mg) if no contraindications exist. Be aware that muscle relaxants are sedative and will affect the patient's state of alertness.
5. Schedule the procedure in the morning, when the patient's reserve is generally greater.
6. Shorter appointments spread over a longer period are generally preferable to longer appointments.

During the procedure

1. To support the jaw, use a *child-size* rubber surgical mouth prop on the side opposite the operative field. This should be inserted to the opening that is comfortable for the patient and *not* used to increase the mouth opening. The prop should be removed momentarily every 10–15 minutes to allow the jaw to move around and thus prevent stiffness.
2. Rest periods for the jaw during the procedure will help reduce strain.
3. Apply moist heat to the jaw muscles and joints to reduce strain.
4. *Gentle* massage of the masseter and temporalis muscles may be helpful.
5. Rely on the patient's report of jaw pain to assess whether strain is occurring.

After the procedure

1. Recommend a soft diet and limitation of wide opening.
2. Prescribe moist heat applications for 10–20 minutes two to three times daily.
3. Consider prescribing a muscle relaxant (e.g. diazepam 2–5 mg at night).
4. Consider prescribing an non-steroidal anti-inflammatory drug (e.g. ibuprofen 400 mg qid) or a mild analgesic (e.g. paracetamol 500–1000 mg qid).
5. Report any persisting symptoms (e.g. pain, limited jaw movement, new joint noise, difficulty chewing).

provisional restorations and appliances is important to help assess whether oral rehabilitation aggravates pain or impairs jaw function, and this provisional treatment phase may be longer than in patients without pain.

Bruxism needs to be considered in oral rehabilitation as it is common, being reported by over 30% of adults, and increases the risk of orofacial pain and impaired jaw function (Ciancaglini *et al.* 2001) and can damage the dentition and restorations. While a definitive diagnosis is through sleep studies, this is impractical for most patients and self-report and evidence of excessive tooth wear are the main criteria. There is a distinction between awake and sleep bruxism; awake bruxism tends to be limited to voluntary or semi-voluntary clenching, while sleep bruxism is likely a central nervous system disorder associated with microarousals and can include both tooth clenching and grinding. Management focuses on reducing possible contributory factors, including emotional stress, cigarette smoking and alcohol use, and protecting the dentition. While behavioural therapy focusing on stress reduction and reduction of environmental factors (e.g. smoking, alcohol) is frequently indicated, patient compliance tends to be poor. Occlusal appliances are frequently used to protect the teeth and, with extensive oral rehabilitation, should be considered in patients who have a history of bruxism.

Dental occlusal appliances have also been advocated as a management strategy for TMDs; they protect the dentition and may modify jaw behaviour and help reduce orofacial pain (Capp 1999). Of note is that individuals suffering widespread muscle pain do not improve as well as those with localised jaw muscle pain (Raphael & Marbach 2001). They are comparable with physical medicine, behavioural medicine and acupuncture in the short term; however, in the long term behavioural therapy is better (Fricton 2006). Consequently, it is recommended that appliances be used as an adjunct for pain management rather than definitive treatment and as a habit management aid and protection of the dentition in sleep bruxism (Dao & Lavigne 1998). There are many appliance designs, although when compared to appliances covering a limited number of teeth, full coverage acrylic appliances will minimise tooth movement and localised occlusal forces and can be both stable and retentive.

References

Aggarwal, V.R., Macfarlane, G.J., Farragher, T.M. *et al.* (2010) Risk factors for onset of chronic oro-facial pain – results of the North Cheshire oro-facial pain prospective population study. *Pain*, 149 (2), 354–359.

Ahmad, M., Hollender, L., Anderson, Q. *et al.* (2009) Research diagnostic criteria for temporomandibular disorders (RDC/TMD): development of image analysis criteria and examiner reliability for image analysis. *Oral Surgery, Oral Medicine, Oral Pathology, Oral Radiology and Endodontology*, 107 (6), 844–860.

Brooks, S.L., Brand, J.W., Gibbs, S.J. *et al.* (1997) Imaging of the temporomandibular joint: a position paper of the American Academy of Oral and Maxillofacial Radiology. *Oral Surgery, Oral Medicine, Oral Pathology, Oral Radiology and Endodontology*, 83 (5), 609–618.

Capp, N.J. (1999) Occlusion and splint therapy. *British Dental Journal*, 186 (5), 217–222.

Ciancaglini, R., Gherlone, E.F. & Radaelli, G. (2001) The relationship of bruxism with craniofacial pain and symptoms from the masticatory system in the adult population. *Journal of Oral Rehabilitation*, 28 (9), 842–848.

Clark, G.T., Tsukiyama, Y, Baba, K. *et al.* (1999) Sixty-eight years of experimental occlusal interference studies: What have we learned? *Journal of Prosthetic Dentistry*, 82 (6), 704–713.

Dao, T.T. & Lavigne, G.J. (1998) Oral splints: the crutches for temporomandibular disorders and bruxism? *Critical Reviews in Oral Biology & Medicine*, 9 (3), 345–361.

Dworkin, S.F. (2001) The dentist as biobehavioral clinician. *Journal of Dental Education*, 65 (12), 1417–1429.

Dworkin, S.F. & LeResche, L. (1992) Research diagnostic criteria for temporomandibular disorders: review, criteria, examinations and specifications, critique. *Journal of Craniomandibular Disorders*, 6 (4), 301–355.

Dworkin, S.F., Turner, J.A., Mancl, L. *et al.* (2002) A randomized clinical trial of a tailored comprehensive care treatment program for temporomandibular disorders. *Journal of Orofacial Pain*, 16 (4), 259–276.

Epker, J., Gatchel, R.J. & Ellis, E. 3rd (1999) A model for predicting chronic TMD: practical application in clinical settings. *Journal of the American Dental Association*, 130 (10), 1470–1475.

Forssell, H. & Kalso, E. (2004) Application of principles of evidence-based medicine to occlusal treatment for temporomandibular disorders: are there lessons to be learned? *Journal of Orofacial Pain*, 18 (1), 9–22.

Fricton, J. (2006) Current evidence providing clarity in management of temporomandibular disorders: summary of a systematic review of randomized clinical trials for intra-oral appliances and occlusal therapies. *The Journal of Evidence-Based Dental Practice*, 6 (1), 48–52.

Greene, C.S. (2010) Managing the care of patients with temporomandibular disorders: a new guideline for care. *Journal of the American Dental Association*, 141 (9), 1086–1088.

Huang, G.J., LeResche, L. & Critchlow, C.W. (2002) Risk factors for diagnostic subgroups of painful temporomandibular disorders (TMD). *Journal of Dental Research*, 81 (4), 284–288.

International Association for the Study of Pain. Task Force on the Taxonomy (1994) *Classification of Chronic Pain: Descriptions of Chronic Pain Syndromes and Definitions of Pain Terms*, 2nd edn. IASP Press, Seattle.

International Headache Society. Headache Classification Subcommittee (2004) *The International Classification of Headache Disorders*, 2nd edn. *Cephalalgia* 24 (Suppl. 1) 8–160.

International RDC-TMD Consortium website (http://www.rdc-tmdinternational.org, accessed 15 December 2010).

Klineberg, I. & Jagger, R. (2004) *Occlusion and Clinical Practice: An Evidence Based Approach*. Wright, Edinburgh.

Kogawa, E.M., Calderon, P.D., Lauris, J.R. *et al.* (2010) Evaluation of minimum interdental threshold ability in dentate female temporomandibular disorder patients. *Journal of Oral Rehabilitation*, 37 (5), 322–328.

Lance, J.W. (1993) *Mechanism and Management of Headache*, 5th edn. Butterworth-Heinemann, Oxford.

Leeuw, R. de (2008) *Orofacial Pain: Guidelines for Assessment, Diagnosis, and Management*, 4th edn. Quintessence, Chicago.

Luther, F. (2007) TMD and occlusion Part II. Damned if we don't? Functional occlusal problems: TMD epidemiology in a wider context. *British Dental Journal*, 202 (1), E3.

Macfarlane, T.V., Blinkhorn, A.S., Davies, R.M. *et al.* (2002) Oro-facial pain in the community: prevalence and associated impact. *Community Dentistry & Oral Epidemiology*, 30 (1), 52–60.

Massey, T., Derry, S., Moore, R.A. *et al.* (2010) Topical NSAIDs for acute pain in adults. *Cochrane Database Systematic Reviews* (6), CD007402.

Medlicott, M.S. & Harris, S.R. (2006) A systematic review of the effectiveness of exercise, manual therapy, electrotherapy, relaxation training, and biofeedback in the management of temporomandibular disorder. *Physical Therapy*, 86 (7), 955–973.

Melzack, R. (1975) The McGill Pain Questionnarie: Major properties and scoring methods. *Pain*, 1 (3), 277–299.

Padilla, M., Clark, G.T. & Merrill, R.L. (2000) Topical medications for orofacial neuropathic pain: a review. *Journal of the American Dental Association*, 131 (2), 184–195.

Peres, M.F. & Lucchetti, G. (2010) Coping strategies in chronic pain. *Current Pain & Headache Reports*, 14 (5), 331–338.

Plesh, O., Wolfe, F. & Lane, N. (1996) The relationship between fibromyalgia and temporomandibular disorders: prevalence and symptom severity. *Journal of Rheumatology*, 23 (11), 1948–1952.

Pullinger, A.G. & Seligman, D.A. (2000) Quantification and validation of predictive values of occlusal variables in temporomandibular disorders using a multifactorial analysis. *Journal of Prosthetic Dentistry*, 83 (1), 66–75.

Raphael, K.G. & Marbach, J.J. (2001) Widespread pain and the effectiveness of oral splints in myofascial face pain. *Journal of the American Dental Association*, 132 (3), 305–316.

Saarto, T. & Wiffen, P.J. (2005) Antidepressants for neuropathic pain. [update in *Cochrane Database of Systematic Reviews*, 2007, (4):CD005454] *Cochrane Database of Systematic Reviews* (3), CD005454.

Schiffman, E.L., Ohrbach, R., Truelove, E.L. *et al.* (2010) The Research Diagnostic Criteria for Temporomandibular disorders. V: methods used to establish and validate Axis I diagnostic algorithms. *Journal of Orofacial Pain*, 24 (1), 63–78.

Seligman, D.A. & Pullinger, A.G. (2000) Analysis of occlusal variables, dental attrition, and age for distinguishing healthy controls from female patients with intracapsular temporomandibular disorders. *Journal of Prosthetic Dentistry*, 83 (1), 76–82.

Stohler, C.S. (2006) Management of dental occlusion. In: *Temporomandibular Disorders: an Evidence-Based Approach to Diagnosis and Treament* (eds D.M. Laskin, C.S. Greene & W.L. Hylander), pp. 403–411. Quintessence, Chicago.

Turk, D.C. & Melzack, R. (eds) (1992) *Handbook of Pain Assessment*. Guilford Press, New York.

Turk, D.C. & Melzack, R. (eds) (2001) *Handbook of Pain Assessment*, 2nd edn. Guilford Press, New York.

Turner, J.A. & Dworkin, S.F. (2004) Screening for psychosocial risk factors in patients with chronic orofacial pain: recent advances. *Journal of the American Dental Association*, 135 (8), 1119–1125.

Woda, A., Tubert-Jeannin, S., Bouhassira, D. *et al.* (2005) Towards a new taxonomy of idiopathic orofacial pain. *Pain*, 116 (3), 396–406.

Section 3

Management

6

Diagnostic Planning and Tooth Preparation Technique: A Biological Approach

Robin Hawthorn

1. Introduction

Concepts of diagnostic planning have changed to embrace the use of implants for replacement of missing teeth. No longer is traditional bridgework the first choice, as abutments may be structurally compromised and offer poor prognosis for FDPs. The latter still provide a treatment option, but limitations of traditional bridgework have become apparent with clinical experience and long-term clinical outcome data. Before the concept of fixed-free design, success in bridgework was dependent on core strength of the abutment teeth and their solidarity (lack of mobility) supported by the periodontium and adequate bone.

The following examples illustrate this aspect of diagnostic planning:

1. A three-unit FDP has been successful (Figure 6.1a, b) for 12 years, until as a result of its fixed design, one of the abutments fractured at the gingival margin. This failure was attributed to progressive change in the remaining dentition with eventual overloading through the lever effect on one of the abutments. The progressive differential loss of periodontal support allowed a cantilever load to be applied to the more rigid abutment. The failure may have been avoided if the design had encompassed the fixed-free concept, so that mobility that may develop in one abutment unit would not have the same cantilever load effect on the stronger abutment.

2. Figure 6.1c, d illustrates an FDP involving teeth 17–23 that has been in place for 24 years as a nine-unit prosthesis supported by three abutments 17, 13, 23. It has been successful because the abutments are well-supported periodontally, there is no mobility and the occlusal load has been sustained wholly by the prosthesis. The figures illustrate a slight change in gingival level over the 24 years but because of excellent core strength, retentive form and the preservation of abutment rigidity, the prosthesis has remained successful.

3. A third FDP design in Figure 6.2 illustrates splinted abutments in both anterior segments supporting a four-unit pontic section that has been in place for 29 years. The preparations were robust and appropriately aligned and home care was excellent; in addition, potential changes in occlusal loading were monitored by the clinician. The concern was that one of the splinted abutments would de-bond, without notice initially, leading to failure of that abutment. This FPD design would not be contemplated today because of the potential risk of changes in abutment rigidity over time with the potential for de-bonding. Success in this case resulted from careful maintenance, preservation of good posterior occlusal support and careful adjustment of the occlusion to minimise parafunctional overloading. The initial preparation of vital teeth was undertaken with a conservative approach with an emphasis on retentive form.

4. Figure 6.3 illustrates failure, which is frequently encountered when mobile abutments are rigidly splinted. Figure 6.3a shows the preparations after periodontal treatment with retentive form established through parallel preparations. Figure 6.3b shows the final bridge in position supporting a removable partial denture and Figure 6.3c, d indicate that tooth 33 has de-bonded. This outcome raises the question: which of these four teeth was the most rigidly supported? Tooth 33 was the strongest succumbing to cantilever loading of the six-unit rigid FDP.

A change in design principle was described by Jacobi *et al.* (1985), emphasising the importance of incorporating a fixed-free design to account for differing tooth mobility and changing occlusal loading through tooth wear.

The introduction and acceptance of all-ceramic FDPs may reintroduce problems of differing tooth mobilities and increasing failure.

Treatment options have changed with the availability of implants and experience, and professional responsibility directs the clinician to wisely assess the

Oral Rehabilitation: A Case-Based Approach, First Edition. Edited by Iven Klineberg, Diana Kingston.
© 2012 Blackwell Publishing Ltd. Published 2012 by Blackwell Publishing Ltd.

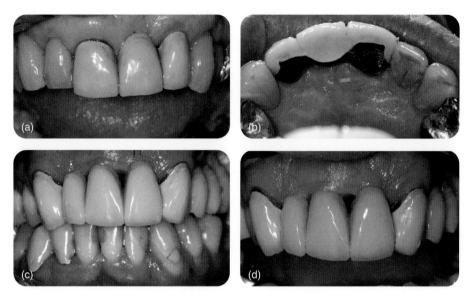

Figure 6.1 (a, b) A three-unit fixed dental prosthesis (FDP) has been successful for 12 years until, as a result of its fixed design, one of the abutments fractured at the gingival margin. (c, d) An FDP involving teeth 17–23.

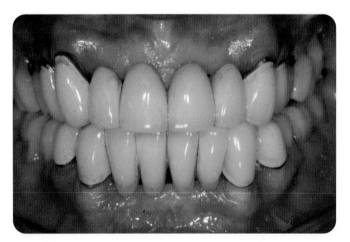

Figure 6.2 Splinted abutments in both anterior segments supporting a four-unit pontic section that has been in place for 29 years.

need for preparation of abutments with loss of tooth structure with the availability and broad application of dental implants.

5. The following case (Figure 6.4a–d), which was referred for specialist advice, is an example of poor treatment planning, particularly with the availability and success of implant procedures. In this case, a young female patient with traumatic loss of a central incisor was provided with a treatment plan that may be regarded as verging on malpractice. The option of a single tooth implant was ignored and the alternative FDP design involved unnecessary abutments rigidly splinted and based on poor crown preparation. The outcome for this young female was a clinical disaster.

6. Figures 6.5–6.8 illustrate steps in a zirconia-based implant-supported fixed bridge, extending from 21 to 23 (Figure 6.5a), progressing through stages of impres-

sion, proformer construction, scanning, try-in and refining of the initial porcelain, final prosthesis and placement with gingival contouring. The important features are: (i) the locking of the impression copings for rigidity of the implant relationship (Figure 6.5b); and (ii) fabrication of the FDP mock-up to become the zirconia pro-forma that follows the intraoral try-in (Figure 6.5c, d & 6.6a). The bridge mock-up is fabricated in laboratory composite, which may be readily modified intraorally to optimise soft tissue approximation and aesthetic contour.

The intraoral mock-up illustrates its shaping and final duplication on the master cast to determine labial reduction for future porcelain addition (Figure 6.6a–d). The final transition from the mock-up to the zirconia pro-forma for scanning is shown in Figure 6.7a, b). Adjustment (Figure 6.1c,d) ensures that adequate space is provided for porcelain layering to achieve the desired aesthetic result. Figure 6.7c, d) illustrates the computer-aided design (CAD)–computer-aided manufacturing (CAM) phase of image capture and digitisation.

The first age of porcelain fabrication and trial fitting is shown in Figure 6.8a, which illustrates tailoring of the porcelain and in particular gingival contour to define the final gingival outline. The final fabrication and placement with minor gingival recontouring at initial issue is shown in Figure 6.8b–d. During the post-placement period, the gingival tissue response is monitored over several weeks and minor additions of porcelain to provide support for soft tissues and to guide tissue form may be required.

2. Tooth preparation technique

The following outlines an approach to crown preparation that has been developed utilising principles often seen in the art world, where the influence of the left brain (the

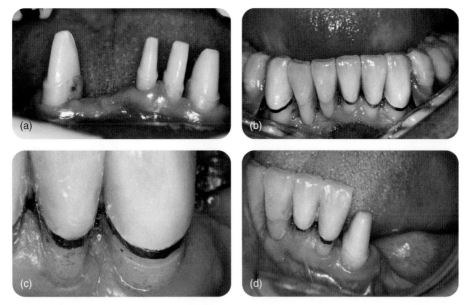

Figure 6.3 Failure is frequently encountered when mobile abutments are rigidly splinted. (a) Preparations after periodontal treatment. (b) Final bridge in position supporting a removable partial denture. (c, d) Tooth 33 has de-bonded.

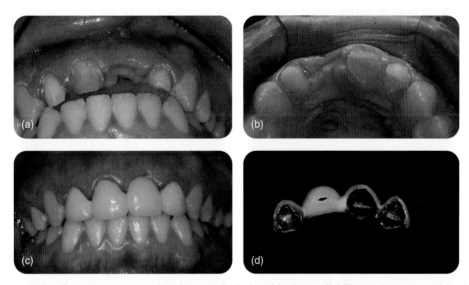

Figure 6.4 (a–d) An example of poor treatment planning, particularly with the availability and success of implant procedures.

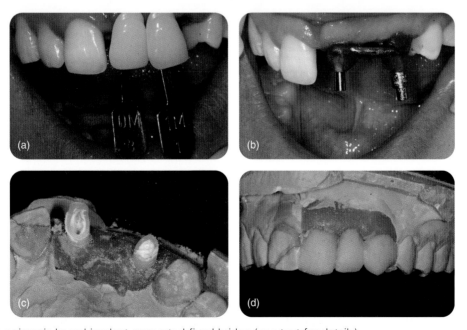

Figure 6.5 Steps in a zirconia-based implant supported fixed bridge (see text for details).

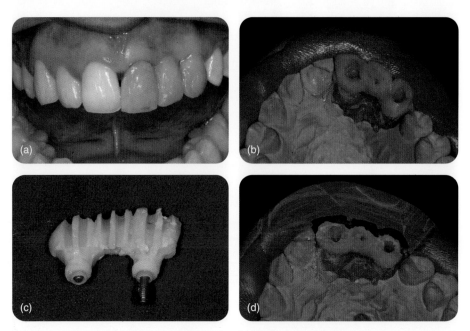

Figure 6.6 (a–d) Steps in a zirconia-based implant-supported fixed bridge: intraoral mock-up (see text for details).

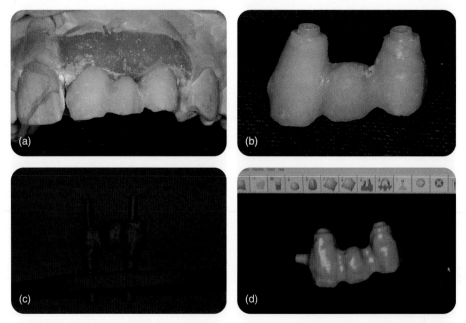

Figure 6.7 Steps in a zirconia-based imported-supported fixed bridge. (a, b) Final transition from the mock-up to the zirconia pro-forma for scanning. (c, d) The CAD–CAM phase of image capture and digitisation.

verbal, logical and analytical hemisphere) is trained to be less dominant than the right hemisphere three-dimensional conceptual and imaginative areas.

Sperry (1974), who investigated the lateral specialisation of cerebral function, found that 'verbal' and 'non-verbal' communication were located in the left and right hemispheres, respectively.

Edwards (1999) graphically demonstrated the benefits of this approach in teaching art. 'Inside 97' students were taught to draw the side of a vase rather than the side of the face and this eliminated preconceptions and emphasised the need to work spatially.

The speciality programme in prosthodontics has used simulation, a key element of which is an operating microscope used to demonstrate sequential steps in crown preparation. Figures 6.9–6.13 illustrate the stages of tooth preparation for the labial, lingual, interproximal and incisal regions. Teaching these procedures in a 'segmental' manner provides a focus of attention on specific aspects of preparation, rather than relying on a preconceived concept of crown preparation. This sequential approach improves the standard of tooth preparations and emphasises the development of desirable retentive and resistance form. Graduate students often have a

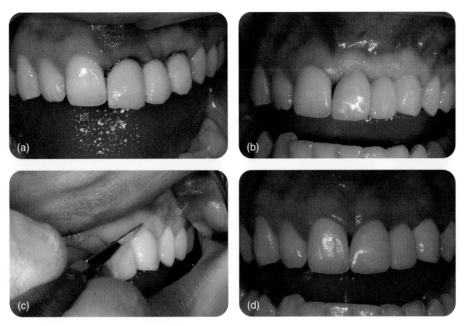

Figure 6.8 Steps in a zirconia-based implant-supported fixed bridge. (a) The first stage of porcelain fabrication and trial fitting. (b–d) The final fabrication and placement with minor gingival recontouring at initial issue.

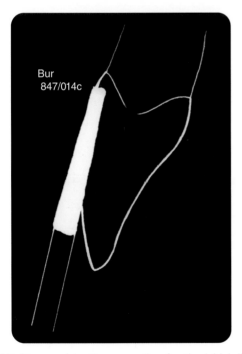

Figure 6.9 Stages of tooth preparation for the labial, lingual, interproximal and incisal regions. The labial reduction.

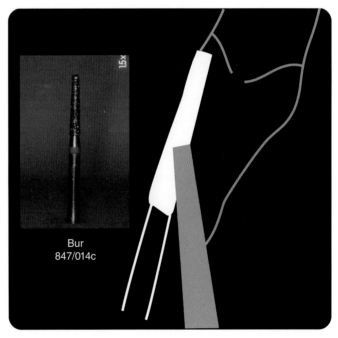

Figure 6.10 Stages of tooth preparation for the labial, lingual, interproximal and incisal regions. The incisal reduction.

poor concept of crown form and this approach addresses this by encouraging them to relate crown preparation to local landmarks that generally have been planned while preparing a diagnostic wax-up. Therefore, crown form is not simply a preconceived preparation but is tailored to tooth position and shaped to provide the specific retention and resistance form required for particular teeth.

Figure 6.14 illustrates an all-ceramic crown preparation (either zirconia or alumina) and shows how this preparation differs from a traditional ceramo-metal preparation. The primary differences are the greater reduction required for the ceramic layering on the lingual aspect and the preparation angles, which should be rounded to avoid stress concentration.

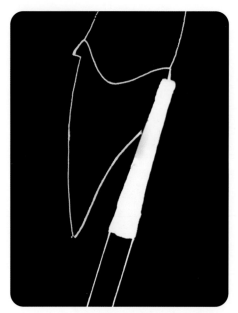

Figure 6.11 Stages of tooth preparation for the labial, lingual, interproximal and incisal regions. The lingual reduction.

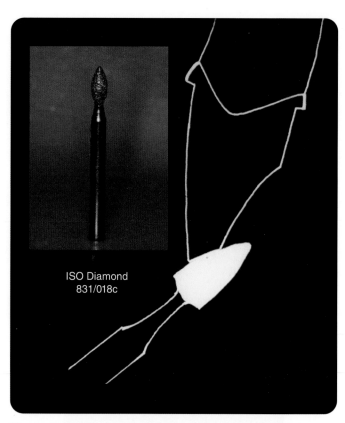

ISO Diamond
831/018c

Figure 6.13 Stages of tooth preparation for the labial, lingual, interproximal and incisal regions. The final gross reduction phase is the preparation of the incisal or occlusal area for adequate porcelain (and gold) thickness.

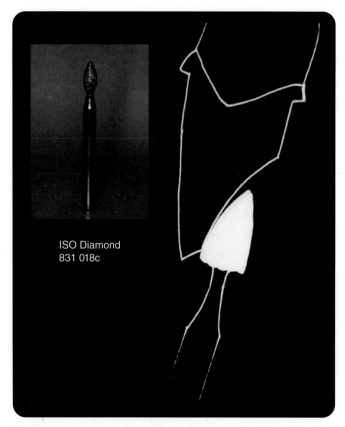

ISO Diamond
831 018c

Figure 6.12 Stages of tooth preparation for the labial, lingual, interproximal and incisal regions. The second part of the lingual reduction is carried out above the cingulum.

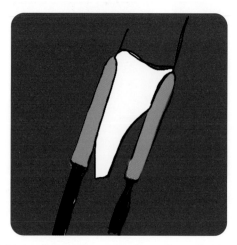

Figure 6.14 In all-ceramic restorations, the reduction is slightly greater lingually and all line angles are slightly rounded.

The labial reduction (Figure 6.9) is the most critical step. This reduction determines the aesthetic quality of the final crown, as sufficient space is required for porcelain layering. The reduction should be made in two steps:

1. The first step is parallel to the tooth axis, which is a depth cut that requires an understanding of how much reduction is required as tooth position may modify this. The axial reduction, in particular the reduction in the area of the gingival margin, should be less than the width of the tip of the bur to avoid over-reduction and weakening of the tooth core.
2. The second step is the incisal reduction – this region is parallel to the labial face of the tooth and to reduce the prominence of the preparation in the incisal region, the amount of reduction necessary will depend on tooth position relative to the adjacent teeth (Figure 6.10). Preparing the labial reduction in this way creates adequate space for porcelain layering and, more importantly, helps to establish the retentive form of the preparation and maintain the core strength.

The next reduction is lingual reduction (Figure 6.11), which should be carried out initially by preparing minimal reduction below the cingulum area and parallel to the axis of the tooth. This is where retentive form is established, as this reduction is parallel to the first part of the labial reduction. The depth of reduction is dependent on the type of crown, with the all-ceramic crown requiring greater reduction. The second part of the lingual reduction is then carried out above the cingulum (Figure 6.12) to adequately clear the opposing occlusion, the amount of reduction varying to suit the type of crown being prepared.

The interproximal reduction follows and requires a thinner diamond bur so that the parallel nature of the preparation is maintained. If the traditional gross reduction bur is used for this step, the preparation will lose significant retentive form as it is impossible to prepare the interproximal reduction with a larger bur without over-reducing the preparation. As a precaution and until adequate skill is developed, protection of the interproximal areas of the adjacent teeth is recommended.

The final gross reduction phase is the preparation of the incisal or occlusal area for adequate porcelain (and gold) thickness. Figure 6.13 illustrates this step. The incisal reduction is only made when reduction is actually required; for example, an occlusal vertical dimension change negates the need for incisal reduction and its associated loss of retention.

In all-ceramic restorations, the reduction is slightly greater lingually and all line angles are slightly rounded (Figure 6.14). The lingual reduction must be greater to accommodate the thickness required for the ceramic material. The bur type is changed to a chamfer bur shape only after the gingival retraction is achieved and margin finalisation is commenced.

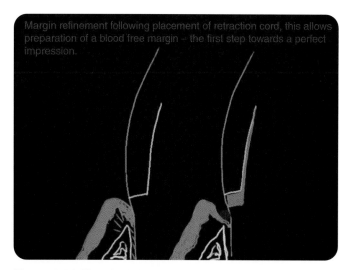

Figure 6.15 The gingival margin is moved away from the preparation area.

At this stage the gross reduction is complete.

The next phase is margin finalisation, which may be regarded as a first step in the impression process (Figure 6.15). Retraction cord is placed to protect gingival tissues from the preparation bur. This prevents soft tissue abrasion as bleeding from gingival tissue trauma adds to the difficulty of the impression procedure.

A two-cord technique may be used, with the first cord being placed at this stage (a fine 'size 0' cord to displace the soft tissue margin apically and to move the gingival margin away from the preparation area). The crown margin is then finalised with fine grit diamond burs and hand instruments.

With completion of the preparation margin, a second strand of retraction cord is placed and should be left in position for 5 minutes to ensure that gingival retraction is effective.

The second strand is carefully removed and the preparation inspected and any minor improvements in preparation form carried out. There should be no hurry to take the impression, as the retraction should allow adequate time for minor preparation modifications. If there is a bleeding point, haemostasis can be achieved with a product that has a local haemostatic effect, such as Expasyl.

A light body impression material (an addition silicone) is carefully syringed around the preparation, initially at the gingival crevice and then extended to cover the whole preparation, attempting to avoid incorporation of air bubbles. Once the preparation is covered, an air syringe is used to blow and spread the material to check that this preparation surface has been completely wet by light body material. More light body material may then be syringed around the preparation and finally the heavy body material in combination with putty silicone placed in a standard tray, is seated over the light body material.

If a standard disposable plastic tray is used, care should be taken to release any pressure on the tray after it is fully seated, as any distortion of the plastic tray will create inaccuracy when the impression is removed.

The accompanying DVD graphically illustrates a recommended sequence of specific steps in this segmental technique of crown preparation. It also illustrates other helpful hints that have been developed as a logical teaching protocol to make this technique-sensitive procedure a little easier to undertake.

References

Edwards, B. (1999) *The New Drawing on the Right Side of the Brain.* pp. 50–65. Putnam, New York.

Jacobi, R., Shillingburg, H.T. Jr & Duncanson, M.G. Jr (1985) Effect of abutment mobility, site, and angle of impact on retention of fixed partial dentures. *Journal of Prosthetic Dentistry*, 54 (2), 178–183.

Sperry, R.W. (1974) Lateral specialization in the surgically separated hemispheres. In: *The Neurosciences: Third Study Program* (eds F.O. Schmitt & F.G. Worden), pp. 5–19. MIT Press, Cambridge, MA.

7

Provisionalisation in Fixed Prosthodontics

Max Guazzato, Robert Santosa and Johnson P.Y. Chou

1. Introduction

The role of the provisional restorations, or interim treatment, is crucial in the success of fixed prosthodontic treatment (Burns *et al.* 2003). Virtually all teeth receiving indirect restorations require provisional restorations. However, the role played by the interim procedures varies according to the clinical situation. Provisional restorations are used primarily for:

1. Short-term provisional FDPs to restore single tooth/ implants or a group of missing teeth. The provisional restorations fit within the dental arch, which provides reference for their occlusion, contour and aesthetic needs (Magne *et al.* 1996). These provisional restorations protect pulpal tissues and stabilise the tooth until the permanent FDP is completed.
2. Provisional FDPs may be a reference for the entire prosthesis (Magne *et al.* 1996). Where several teeth are missing, the provisional treatment is to protect pulpal tissue and for diagnostic purposes (e.g. to re-establish a correct maxillary–mandibular relationship). The term 'interim treatment' has been used to indicate complexity and different treatment objectives. With interim treatment, provisional restorations are used longer until treatment objectives are achieved. The rationale, the construction and the materials used for long-term provisional restorations are often different from those of short-term restorations (Preston 1976, Burns *et al.* 2003).

The literature describing construction of provisional restorations is extensive but is primarily case reports describing a particular technique. Few articles address differences between short- and long-term provisional restorations (Galindo *et al.* 1998). Burns *et al.* (2003) reviewed provisional restorations comprehensively and their article is the basis for describing differences in the rationale,

technique and materials used for short- and long-term provisionals.

Any tooth prepared for an indirect FDP needs to be protected and stabilised with a provisional restoration. In single tooth or partially edentulous spaces, a provisional restoration may also be fitted before the definitive FDP.

The provisional restoration protects the pulpal tissues and restores acceptable aesthetics and function while the definitive FDP is fabricated.

2. Short-term provisional fixed dental prostheses

2.1 Rationale for use

Where tooth preparation involves exposure of dentine, alteration of form must be protected and stabilised with provisional restorations that resemble the planned definitive treatment (Federick 1975). The objective of short-term provisional FDPs is to protect, sedate pulpal tissue, protect teeth from dental caries, restore aesthetics and function, prevent tooth migration and stabilise the dentition by immediately replacing prepared tooth structure and missing teeth (Federick 1975, Burns *et al.* 2003) (Figure 7.1a–e).

In implant dentistry, a short-term provisional FDP may be used at the time of implant placement or after appropriate healing, before delivery of the definitive restoration. The term 'immediate restoration' is used when the prosthesis is fixed to implants within 48 hours and without achieving full occlusal contact with the opposing dentition (Figure 7.2a–i), whereas 'immediate loading' is when the prosthesis is fixed to the implants and is in occlusion within 48 hours (Morton *et al.* 2004) (Figure 7.3a–g). Immediate provisionalisation provides improved comfort and function during implant healing compared with a conventional denture (Wohrle 1998). This procedure is likely to reduce postoperative denture adjustments without tissue conditioning or relining. Implant-supported

Oral Rehabilitation: A Case-Based Approach, First Edition. Edited by Iven Klineberg, Diana Kingston.
© 2012 Blackwell Publishing Ltd. Published 2012 by Blackwell Publishing Ltd.

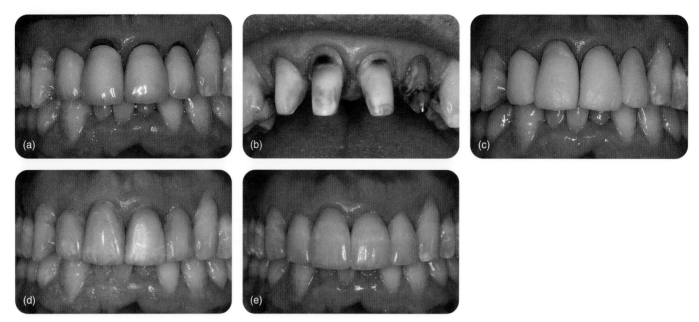

Figure 7.1 (a) The patient requested the replacement of existing ceramo-metal crowns (CMCs) because of poor aesthetics (exposure of the metal margins). (b) The CMCs have been removed and repreparation of the teeth has been completed. (c) Temporary single crowns were made with Protemp (3M ESPE) using a lab-putty key. The monochromatic shade and the reproduction of the shade of the previous crowns do not provide clinician and patient with any diagnostic information. (d) The Protemp (3M ESPE) temporary crowns are cut back and layered with light-cured direct composite resin material to match shape and shade of the adjacent teeth. The temporary crowns have been characterised with orange and white staining. (e) The orange and white staining and the simulation of the root surface exposure are minimised in the definitive all-ceramic crowns to achieve a younger and cleaner look without compromising the match with the adjacent dentition.

provisional FDPs also prevent migration of adjacent teeth and stabilise the occlusion.

2.2 Materials used for fabrication

Short-term provisional FDPs are used for as long as required to fabricate and issue the permanent prostheses. Materials and techniques used to fabricate provisional restorations should meet functional, biological and aesthetic needs as listed in Box 7.1. Furthermore, considering that provisionals are used for short periods, the techniques and materials used to fabricate these restorations should be easily applied and relatively inexpensive. Although there is no ideal material, resin and composite materials have been used successfully. Their advantage is the ease with which they may be altered with additions and subtractions (Skurow & Nevins 1998). The most common provisional crown materials are (Burns *et al.* 2003):

- methyl methacrylate (Jet acrylic – Lang Dental);
- ethyl methacrylate (Trim – Harry J. Bosworth);
- bis-acrylic composite – auto-polymerised (Protemp – 3M ESPE);
- bis-acrylic composite – dual-polymerised (Luxatemp Solar – Zenith/DMG);
- urethane dimethacrylate composite – light-polymerised (Triad – Dentsply).

Most composite materials, for example Protemp (3M-ESPE), are supplied with an auto-mix delivery system similar to impression materials that allows quick and easy use. In addition, unlike methacrylate resins, they do not produce residual free monomers after polymerisation, which explains why there is reduced tissue toxicity compared with methacrylate resins. However, Diaz-Arnold *et al.* (1999) confirmed a general decrease in mechanical properties over time for two out of three composite materials tested. Furthermore, the monochromatic shade of his material strongly limits its application in aesthetic areas without the use of layering materials that improve the appearance of the provisional restoration (Figure 7.1c). The literature indicates that despite the ease of fabrication of provisional restorations with auto-polymerised composite materials, methyl methacrylate resins are often the preferred material. Despite their tissue toxicity, methacrylate resins have better mechanical properties and colour stability. Although there are some differences among the resin and composite materials, the literature clearly indicates that all materials have deficiencies in terms of marginal accuracy, plaque adherence causing inflammation of the gingival tissue, and lack of colour stability. These concerns are exaggerated when a direct technique is used (Tjan *et al.* 1997, Luthardt *et al.* 2000).

A major concern of FPDs is gingival tissue response. Donaldson (1974) reported that provisional restorations

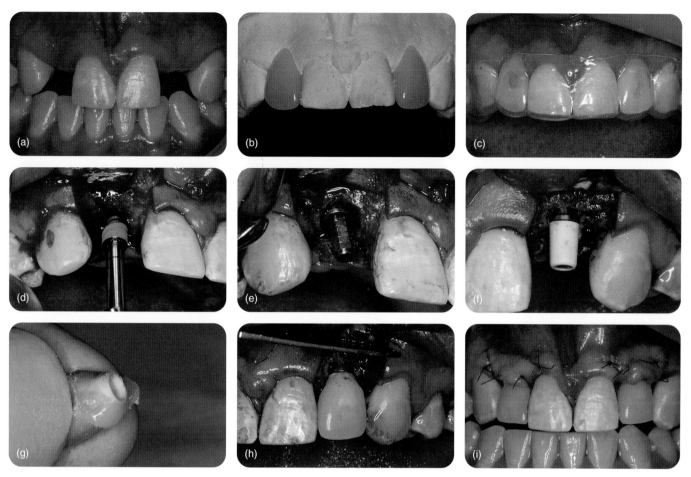

Figure 7.2 (a) The patient presented with congenitally missing maxillary lateral incisors and had orthodontic treatment to create sufficient space to restore the missing teeth with dental implants. (b) Two plastic shell provisional crowns have been adapted to the study cast. (c) A vacuum-pressed template was made to support the provisional crowns in the correct position. (d) Two Nobel Biocare implants were inserted. (e) Two immediate temporary abutments (Nobel Biocare) have been mounted on the implants. (f) The corresponding plastic cap was adapted to the immediate temporary abutment. (g) The shell provisional crown was filled with acrylic resin to 'pick up' the plastic cap adapted to the immediate temporary abutment. (h) The provisional crown has been finished and its adaptation is checked before suturing the flap. (i) The flaps were sutured and the occlusion checked to ensure that at least 1 mm clearance was present in intercuspal position as well as protrusive and laterotrusive movements.

led to recession at approximately 80% of the free gingival margin and that an anatomically contoured provisional restoration caused less recession than a non-anatomically contoured one. In contrast, MacEntee *et al.* (1978) reported no detectable change in gingival tissue associated with provisional restorations treatment over a 3-week period. This matter was resolved by Shavell (1988) who stated that 'the brand of provisional material and method of fabrication are not as important as the devotion, skill, and attention to detail of the dentist'.

2.3 Techniques used for fabrication

In general, provisional restorations may be made with a preformed material or alternatively customised using direct or indirect techniques.

Burns *et al.* (2003) reported that three techniques encompass most of the literature on direct provisional restorations:

- Use of a premanufactured provisional shell: preformed provisional crowns or matrices usually consist of tooth-shaped shells of plastic, cellulose acetate or metal. These may be relined with acrylic resin to provide a custom fit before cementation. Preformed provisional crowns are limited to the restoration of a single tooth or implant (Figure 7.2b).
- Use of an impression material or pressure- or vacuum-formed translucent matrix.
- Use of a custom prefabricated acrylic resin shell. The direct technique is indicated for single units and up to four-unit provisional FDPs.

The most common indirect technique consists of fabricating a matrix from a diagnostic wax-up of the planned tooth contours. Auto-polymerising acrylic resin or composite material may be packed into a matrix and fitted over the prepared tooth cast (Christensen 1996, Burns *et al.* 2003).

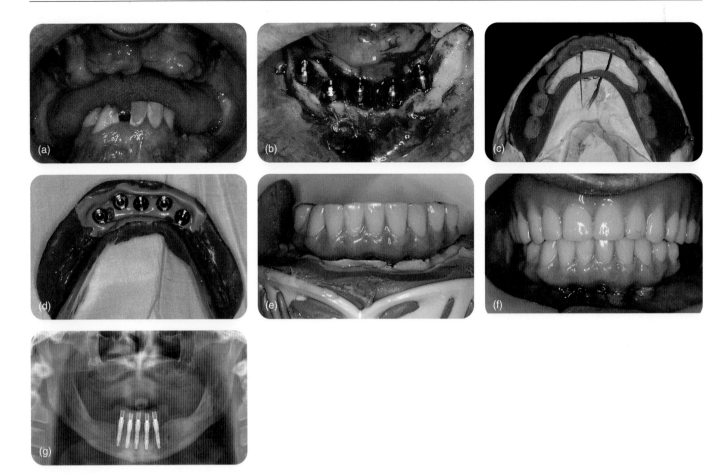

Figure 7.3 (a) The patient wore a removable complete maxillary denture, which was not functional because it was dislodged by the over-erupted mandibular anterior teeth. The patient requested restoration of the mandibular teeth with a fixed prosthesis. (b) The remaining teeth have been extracted and most of the sockets removed with an osteotomy to compensate for the over-eruption. Five implants were inserted in the interforaminal region and multi-unit abutments were placed on the implants. (c) An immediate mandibular denture fabricated before the surgical procedure has been modified on the lingual aspect to create space for temporary abutments. (d) The modified denture was used to take an abutment level impression with temporary abutments and polyether material. (e) Polyvinyl siloxane (PVS) material was used to make a model to hold the denture during its conversion from removable to provisional fixed prosthesis. (f) The acrylic provisional fixed prosthesis was screw-retained to the implants within hours after implant insertion. The implants in this case were immediately loaded. (g) A panoramic radiograph taken to verify the adaptation of all components.

The indirect method offers advantages compared with the direct technique and is the preferred method for multiple provisional restorations; Galindo *et al.* (1998) reported that indirect provisional restorations with methacrylate resins improved marginal accuracy, porosity and mechanical properties compared with direct methods. With an indirect technique, pulpal tissues are not exposed to monomer and the exothermal reaction during polymerisation.

Cement or screw-retained provisionals may be constructed over a healing implant (Santosa 2007). The decision whether to cement or screw-retain provisional or final implant restorations depends on the clinical situation and clinicians' preference.

Most implant companies have prefabricated abutments for cement-retained restorations that are available in various heights to allow space for the metal and porcelain in crown construction. They also have a slight taper and indexing component providing resistance form for the overlying restorations. The abutments are torqued on to the implants, left *in situ* and a complementing pick-up coping component may be used for the impression and transfer of abutment position to the master cast.

A plastic protection cap, usually cylindrical in shape, may be cemented to the prefabricated abutment until the delivery of the final prosthesis and is often used in non-aesthetic regions.

Aesthetic provisional FDPs can be constructed for such abutments between impression and prosthesis delivery (Priest 2006). The provisional FDPs may be made from a prefabricated custom shell (prefabricated preformed acrylic crowns, vacuum-formed template from the diagnostic wax-up, hollowed denture teeth; or a hollowed decoronated clinical crown). These are relined

Box 7.1 Requirements for provisional restorations (modified from Federick 1975 & Burns et al. 2003)

Good marginal adaptation

Good internal accuracy in order to guarantee adequate retention and resistance to dislodgment during normal masticatory function

Aesthetically acceptable shade selection

Colour stable; translucent tooth-like appearance

Non-porous, easy to clean

Non-irritating to pulp and other tissues

Relatively short setting time, easy to mix and load in the matrix, fabricate, reline and easy to remove and repair

Strong, durable, hard, able to be polished and dimensionally stable

Plaque- and stain-resistant surface

Easy to remove and re-cement by the dentist

using self- or light-cured resins intraorally to capture the abutment component and are then completed extraorally to fit the implant restorative margins (Figure 7.2a–i).

To facilitate treatment, the crown form can be waxed, or selected, sized and trimmed in advance to fit the edentulous site on the study cast (Figure 7.2b). Care should be taken during cementation where the implant crown margin is placed subgingivally, especially in the anterior region (Figure 7.2h). Access to a deeply placed implant shoulder is difficult and excess residual cement is difficult to clean and may cause peri-implant inflammation (Pauletto et al. 1999). Alternatively, a temporary meso-abutment would allow a machined connection at the implant shoulder and customised cement margin that may be modified to allow a slightly subgingival margin for ease of cement removal. This abutment can be modified intra- or extraorally and prepared using a diamond bur with accessible cement level placed just below the free gingival margin.

Screw-retained provisional restorations eliminate the possibility of temporary cement being present in the peri-implant tissues (Figure 7.4.a–g). This can be achieved using temporary cylinders directly on the implant, and the provisional crown is formed in the laboratory on the master cast or at chairside using auto-polymerising or light-cured resin or composite resin following the diagnostic wax-up. The temporary cylinder will need to be adjusted to the occlusion. The advantage of provisional restorations at the commencement of the restorative procedure is in shaping the peri-implant tissue (Chee & Donovan 1998, Priest 2006) (Figure 7.4b–g). This process establishes an aesthetic soft tissue contour for laboratory fabrication (Biggs 1996, Higginbottom et al. 2004, Sadan et al. 2004). Well-shaped peri-implant tissues involving interdental papillae facilitate seating of the final prosthe-

sis. In addition, the provisional restorations may be modified over several appointments to achieve the desired emergence profile.

In completely edentulous situations, the existing removable provisional acrylic denture may be modified into a screw-retained provisional hybrid FDP. The technique involves the placement of temporary cylinders on to implants and modification of the existing mandibular denture. The cylinders are luted to the denture with auto-polymerising resin and the denture is then converted into an immediately loaded, screw-retained provisional hybrid FDP, ensuring minimal cantilever and well-distributed occlusal contacts (Figure 7.3a–g).

3. Long-term provisional fixed dental prostheses as interim restorative treatment
3.1 Rationale for use

As discussed in the rationale for the use of short-term provisional restorations, the objectives of provisional fixed partial dentures are to protect pulpal tissue and to provide comfort, aesthetics and function by stabilising the dentition until the definitive prosthesis is completed. Patients who require complex prosthodontics or a combination of treatments, require provisional restorations to serve as a diagnostic and therapeutic guide in addition to a protective, functional and stabilising role. In these cases the term 'interim restorative treatment' is preferred.

Interim restorations can be used for diagnostic purposes where functional, occlusal and aesthetic parameters are developed to determine optimum treatment (Burns et al. 2003). Provisional restorations provide a template for defining tooth contour, aesthetics, proximal contacts and occlusion, and for evaluating an alteration in the occlusal vertical dimension (Galindo et al. 1998).

Interim treatment may assist with periodontal therapy by:

- stabilising mobile teeth during the evaluation of questionable abutments;
- providing a favourable environment to re-establish periodontal health;
- providing visibility and access to surgical sites when removed;
- providing a scaffold on which gingival tissues heal with defined soft tissue contour (Donovan & Cho 2001, Orsini et al. 2006).

3.2 Techniques and materials used for fabrication

The techniques and materials used for long-term provisional restorations are similar to those used for short-term restorations. As discussed for short-term restorations, it is important to use materials that allow alteration by addition or subtraction. In this way, tooth contour is easily modified to improve aesthetics, phonetics and occlusion. Composite and acrylic resins are used for long-term FDPs. Generally, composite and acrylic

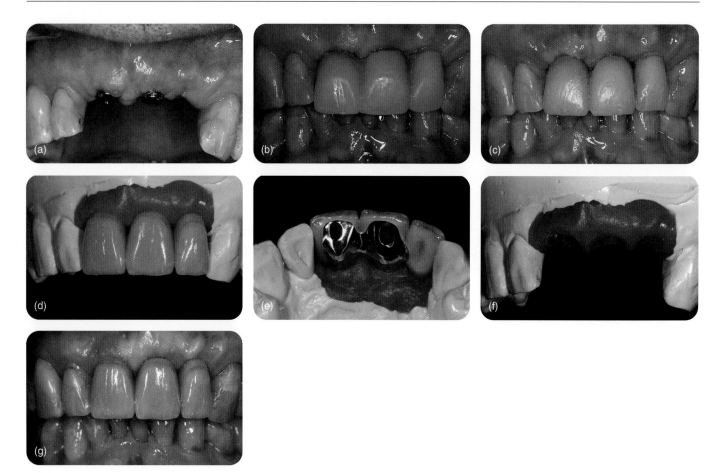

Figure 7.4 (a) Two implants have been inserted to restore the missing teeth 11, 21 and 22. (b) A provisional screw-retained partial denture has been made with temporary abutments, standard denture teeth and acrylic material. The aesthetics and contour of the provisional prosthesis as delivered by the laboratory was not satisfactory and needs to be modified. (c) The provisional screw-retained partial denture has been modified and was used to shape the soft tissue and test speech, occlusion and aesthetics prior to taking the final impression. (d) Labial view of the definitive metal–ceramic prosthesis on the master model. (e) Palatal view of the definitive metal–ceramic prosthesis on the master model showing the access holes for the screws retaining the prosthesis. (f) View of the soft tissue on the master model showing the formation of papillae achieved with the provisional prosthesis. (g) Intraoral view of the definitive prosthesis showing the natural appearance of the contour of soft tissue.

resins are brittle (Galindo *et al.* 1998) and mechanical properties may compromise the longevity of provisional restorations and the outcome of interim restorative treatment. Provisional prostheses may be strengthened using an indirect technique and/or by adding a framework to the composite or acrylic materials.

Long-term provisionals are fabricated on the basis of a diagnostic wax-up made on a copy of the patient's study casts. The wax-up is then used to fabricate a vacuum or a silicon template that is used to directly fit the existing teeth to assess aesthetics and function. Following tooth preparation, an impression is taken to fabricate the indirect provisional restorations in a laboratory (Galindo *et al.* 1998) and to allow processing of the acrylic resin under pressure and higher temperature. This process will optimise mechanical properties and minimise the risk of fracture (Galindo *et al.* 1998). However, it has been recommended that when the duration of the interim

restorative treatment is longer than 6 months, gold-band and acrylic resin restorations are more appropriate (Christensen 1997). Fibre-reinforced composite resins have also been proposed to improve mechanical properties and longevity of FDPs (Hamza *et al.* 2004, Chan *et al.* 2006).

Interim restorative treatment may be an RDP or complete denture, or be implant based, and used postextraction and throughout implant treatment. Construction is simple, relatively inexpensive and is readily adjusted by the surgeon or restorative clinician. Where staged treatment is required with serial extractions, teeth may be added to an existing RDP.

However, such an interim prosthesis may reduce the effectiveness of additional bone and gingival augmentation required to optimise the implant site. Care is needed to prevent the gingival portion of the interim dental prosthesis from contacting the healing soft tissues or an exposed healing abutment. Soft tissue borne prostheses used during healing may load the healing implant site and predispose to implant exposure, marginal bone loss and/or failure of implant integration. Interim RDPs need to be adjusted to minimise contact with the healing site. There are alternatives to tissue-supported interim restorative treatment. A removable, vacuum-formed appliance may be used as an interim treatment and this is also appropriate where there is limited interocclusal space or a deep anterior overbite (Sheridan *et al.* 1993, Moskowitz *et al.* 1997).

This prosthesis is constructed using an acrylic tooth bonded to a clear vacuum-formed material prefaced on a cast of the diagnostic wax-up. The prosthesis provides protection of the underlying soft tissues and implant site during healing. Limitations include the inability to mould surrounding soft tissues and, where there is lack of patient understanding or compliance, there may be rapid occlusal wear through the vacuum-formed material. In addition, some patients may not like to wear, or are unable to tolerate, a provisional RDP and in such cases a provisional FDP is required.

Fixed tooth-supported interim restorative treatment in the upper anterior region includes the use of orthodontic brackets and archwire on teeth adjacent to the implant site with an attached pontic. An alternative is a resin-bonded provisional pontic, which is tooth supported and retained by acid etching the contact surface of the abutment teeth. Small retentive grooves within enamel on the adjacent teeth may be used to increase pontic retention. The pontic can be an acrylic or porcelain tooth or a decoronated, extracted and obturated tooth. The resin-bonded acrylic resin or natural tooth may be reinforced with composite resin and/or ultra high molecular weight polyethylene ribbon (Ribbond, Ribbond, Seattle WA) (Smidt 2002, Priest 2006). These prostheses may continue to be reused as provisionals following implant healing. The archwire/resin retainer is removed and reattached between the surgical and prosthetic stages and can also be used to guide the surgeon during grafting and as a template for the final restoration. Resin-bonded, cast metal framework interim restorative treatment such as a resin-bonded bridge is suitable for long-term provisionalisation in the anterior region, especially in young patients (Priest 2006). This type of provisional is difficult to reuse during implant treatment as the bond strength between the metal retainer and the enamel is unpredictable during removal and reattachment. Furthermore, laboratory costs are relatively high and secondary caries may develop beneath the retentive element.

In extended partially edentulous areas where there are no or limited natural abutments to support interim restorative treatment, one or more transitional implants may be used (Babbush 2001). Transitional implants may be loaded immediately to support interim restorative treatment.

Care should be taken in planning the position of these implants and with their maintenance post-loading. They should not interfere with future implant sites, or be placed in poor-quality bone. When the depth of available bone is less than 14 mm or the amount of cortical bone is insufficient for primary stabilisation, immediate provisional implants may be contraindicated (Babbush 2001). Once the implants integrate, the supporting interim restorative treatment may be converted to an implant-supported interim prosthesis and the transitional implants removed.

4. Conclusion

Provisional FDPs or interim treatments play an important role in the success of prosthodontic treatment. Provisional restorations are valuable to:

- protect pulpal tissue of natural tooth abutments;
- restore an acceptable appearance and function during fabrication of the permanent prosthesis and guide development of optimal aesthetics;
- determine the correct maxillomandibular relationship and stabilise soft tissues.

Various materials and techniques may be used and the one selected needs to fulfil the requirements of treatment and ensure appropriate longevity of the restorations.

References

Babbush, C.A. (2001) Provisional implants: surgical and prosthetic aspects. *Implant Dentistry*, 10 (2), 113–120.

Biggs, W.F. (1996) Placement of a custom implant provisional restoration at the second-stage surgery for improved gingival management: a clinical report. *Journal of Prosthetic Dentistry*, 75 (3), 231–233.

Burns, D.R., Beck, D.A. & Nelson, S.K. (2003) A review of selected dental literature on contemporary provisional fixed prosthodontic treatment: report of the Committee on Research in Fixed Prosthodontics of the Academy of Fixed Prosthodontics. *Journal of Prosthetic Dentistry*, 90 (5), 474–497.

Chan, D.C., Giannini, M. & De Goes, M.F. (2006) Provisional anterior tooth replacement using nonimpregnated fiber and fiber-reinforced composite resin materials: a clinical report. *Journal of Prosthetic Dentistry*, 95 (5), 344–348.

Chee, W.W. & Donovan, T. (1998) Use of provisional restorations to enhance soft-tissue contours for implant restorations. *Compendium of Continuing Education in Dentistry*, 19 (5), 481–461; 488–489.

Christensen, G.J. (1996) Provisional restorations for fixed prosthodontics. *Journal of the American Dental Association*, 127 (2), 249–252.

Christensen, G.J. (1997) Tooth preparation and pulp degeneration. *Journal of the American Dental Association*, 128 (3), 353–354.

Diaz-Arnold, A.M., Dunne, J.T. & Jones, A.H. (1999) Microhardness of provisional fixed prosthodontic materials. *Journal of Prosthetic Dentistry*, 82 (5), 525–528.

Donaldson, D. (1974) The etiology of gingival recession associated with temporary crowns. *Journal of Periodontology*, 45, 468–471.

Donovan, T.E. & Cho, G.C. (2001) Predictable aesthetics with metal–ceramic and all-ceramic crowns: the critical importance of soft-tissue management. *Periodontology 2000*, 27 (2), 121–130.

Federick, D.R. (1975) The provisional fixed partial denture. *Journal of Prosthetic Dentistry*, 34 (5), 520–526.

Galindo, D., Soltys, J.L. & Graser, G.N. (1998) Long-term reinforced fixed provisional restorations. *Journal of Prosthetic Dentistry*, 79 (6), 698–701.

Hamza, T.A., Rosenstiel, S.F., Elhosary, M.M. *et al.* (2004) The effect of fiber reinforcement on the fracture toughness and flexural strength of provisional restorative resins. *Journal of Prosthetic Dentistry*, 91 (3), 258–264.

Higginbottom, F., Belser, U., Jones, J.D. *et al.* (2004) Prosthetic management of implants in the esthetic zone. *International Journal of Oral & Maxillofacial Implants*, 19 (Suppl.), 62–72.

Luthardt, R.G., Stossel, M., Hinz, M. *et al.* (2000) Clinical performance and periodontal outcome of temporary crowns and fixed partial dentures: a randomised clinical trial. *Journal of Prosthetic Dentistry*, 83 (1), 32–39.

MacEntee, M.I., Bartlett, S.O. & Loadholt, C.B. (1978) A histologic evaluation of tissue response to three currently used temporary acrylic resin crowns. *Journal of Prosthetic Dentistry*, 39 (1), 42–46.

Magne, P., Magne, M. & Belser, U. (1996) The diagnostic template: a key element to the comprehensive esthetic treatment concept. *International Journal of Periodontics & Restorative Dentistry*, 16 (6), 560–569.

Morton, D., Jaffin, R. & Weber, H.P. (2004) Immediate restoration and loading of dental implants: clinical considerations and protocols. *International Journal of Oral & Maxillofacial Implants*, 19 (Suppl.), 103–108.

Moskowitz, E.M., Sheridan, J.J., Celenza, F. *et al.* (1997) Essix appliances. Provisional anterior prosthesis for pre and post implant patients. *New York State Dental Journal*, 63 (4), 32–35.

Orsini, G., Murmura, G., Artese, L. *et al.* (2006) Tissue healing under provisional restorations with ovate pontics: a pilot human histological study. *Journal of Prosthetic Dentistry*, 96 (4), 252–257.

Pauletto, N., Lahiffe, B.J. & Walton, J.N. (1999) Complications associated with excess cement around crowns on osseointegrated implants: a clinical report. *International Journal of Oral & Maxillofacial Implants*, 14 (6), 865–868.

Preston, J.D. (1976) A systematic approach to the control of esthetic form. *Journal of Prosthetic Dentistry*, 35 (4), 393–402.

Priest, G. (2006) Esthetic potential of single-implant provisional restorations: selection criteria of available alternatives. *Journal of Esthetic and Restorative Dentistry*, 18 (6), 326–338.

Sadan, A., Blatz, M.B., Salinas, T.J. *et al.* (2004) Single-implant restorations: a contemporary approach for achieving a predictable outcome. *Journal of Oral & Maxillofacial Surgery*, 62 (Suppl. 2), 73–81.

Santosa, R. (2007) Provisional restoration options in implant dentistry. *Australian Dental Journal*, 52 (3), 234–242.

Shavell, H.M. (1988) Mastering the art of tissue management during provisionalization and biologic final impression. *International Journal of Periodontics & Restorative Dentistry*, 8 (3), 24–43.

Sheridan, J.J., Ledoux, W. & McMinn, R. (1993) Essix retainers: fabrication and supervision for permanent retention. *Journal of Clinical Orthodontics*, 27 (1), 37–45.

Skurow, H.M. & Nevins, M. (1988) The rationale of the preperiodontal provisional biologic trial restoration. *International Journal of Periodontics & Restorative Dentistry*, 8 (1), 8–29.

Smidt, A. (2002) Esthetic provisional replacement of a single anterior tooth during the implant healing phase: a clinical report. *Journal of Prosthetic Dentistry*, 87 (6), 598–602.

Tjan, A. H., Castelnuovo, J. & Shiotsu, G. (1997) Marginal fidelity of crowns fabricated from six proprietary provisional materials. *Journal of Prosthetic Dentistry*, 77 (5), 482–485.

Wohrle, P.S. (1998) Single-tooth replacement in the aesthetic zone with immediate provisionalization: fourteen consecutive case reports. *Practical Periodontics & Aesthetic Dentistry*, 10 (9), 1107–1114.

8

Maintenance and Long-Term Outcomes

Terry Walton

1. Considerations in the planning stage

Consideration of maintenance requirements should occur in the initial treatment-planning phase. As described in previous chapters, the prognosis and strategic nature of the remaining teeth need to be established. An expected 10-year prognosis for individual teeth is reasonable to provide an adequate benefit for the economic and personal (time, convenience, comfort) costs involved in treatment.

The retained teeth will inevitably have varied susceptibility to failure over the long term. The incorporation of implant-supported prostheses has improved the outcome of tooth-supported prostheses, as teeth with guarded prognoses need no longer be retained and healthy teeth need no longer be incorporated into extensive and long-span prostheses (Walton 2009a). The form and support of the individual teeth, their position in the arch, and the functional and parafunctional forces that will be applied, will have a bearing on the outcome.

Root-filled teeth have been reported to have a poorer prognosis than vital teeth (Tan et al. 2004). In a meta-analysis of the outcome of root-filled teeth, four conditions in descending order were found to significantly improve survival:

1. a crown restoration;
2. proximal contacts;
3. non-involvement as abutments in either FDPs or RDPs;
4. tooth type (Ng et al. 2010).

However, with the incorporation of implants, it has been shown that non-vital teeth in FDPs have the same outcome as vital teeth up to 10 years (Walton 2009b). It is the structural integrity of the teeth rather than the vitality status that impacts on their outcome.

There is increasing evidence that patients who are not responsive to supportive periodontal therapy will develop a higher incidence of peri-implant disease (Fardal & Linden 2008, De Boever et al. 2009). It is imperative that prostheses designs in these patients allow for effective hygiene and management of the supportive tissues. This may involve a compromise with aesthetic expectations.

Of significant importance is the recognition that the completed treatment functions in a dynamic environment. Differential wear of various natural and artificial materials, migration of teeth, and ongoing skeletal changes contribute to the direction and magnitude of applied biomechanical forces, both within a given patient and between patients. These forces must be dissipated without loss of structural integrity through the biological and artificial structures. Large forces, particularly associated with some parafunctional habits, command greater consideration. Prosthesis designs that incorporate effective resistance form (grooves, ferrules) and stress relief (non-rigid connection) can modulate these forces, reduce the incidence of disease (caries) and mechanical complications (loss of retention, veneer chipping and framework fracture) (Walton 2003) and facilitate retreatment (addition of teeth to a partial RDP).

Consideration of both the direction and extent of biomechanical forces will also have an influence on the form and design of prostheses. Cusp height and fossa depth should be flattened and incisal edges widened in a heavy bruxer to minimise increased tooth mobility, chipping and fracture of veneering materials, and tooth fracture. Tooth-supported prostheses that have compromised periodontal support and thus less resistance to lateral loading should have a similar cusp/fossa form. Splinting of adjacent implant-supported crowns may help resist rotational forces and minimise screw loosening, especially in molar regions and when maxillary anterior cantilever designs are employed.

Reliance on occlusal splints to dissipate parafunctional forces and preserve the integrity of prostheses is problematic. There are no studies of long-term compliance with prescribed splint use in 'non-pain' patients, but anecdotal evidence suggests it is low. In addition, interclinician reliability on judgements of bruxism severity is low (Marbach et al. 2003). Occlusal splints should not be used as a substitute for inadequate consideration of resistance

Oral Rehabilitation: A Case-Based Approach, First Edition. Edited by Iven Klineberg, Diana Kingston.
© 2012 Blackwell Publishing Ltd. Published 2012 by Blackwell Publishing Ltd.

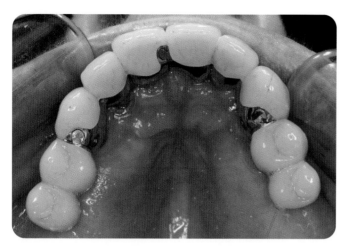

Figure 8.1 A maxillary periodontal prosthesis incorporating several design features to increase resistance form and facilitate future retreatment. These include: non-rigid connection between the central incisors to minimise tooth reduction to gain a common path of insertion thereby maintaining maximum resistance form of the periodontally compromised teeth; and removable premolar segments (cross-screws) to facilitate conversion of these cantilevered segments into a partial removable dental prosthesis (RDP) should the splinted anterior segment show ongoing increased mobility, or should sinus augmentation procedures be undertaken for future implant placement.

form of both the natural and artificial structures in prosthesis design. Nor should lack of compliance with splint use be used as a means of transferring the responsibility for prosthesis failure to the patient.

It is prudent to assume that complications and failure will occur and to try and predict the most likely retreatment scenarios. Prosthesis design might be modified to facilitate both maintenance and future retreatment (Figure 8.1). Screw access allows easy removal and replacement/repair of implant-supported prostheses. This would save considerable time and cost in patients who may also have a higher incidence of peri-implantitis; in patients who may be more susceptible to trauma (youth, sportsmen, bruxers); or in those who may experience continued facial growth. In tooth-supported prostheses, breaking up long-span, multi-abutment constructions with non-rigid connection facilitates less extensive replacement of an isolated failed segment.

2. The recall programme

The relative responsibility for ongoing assessment is a dilemma for the prosthodontist and the referring dentist. Recall visits could be considered mundane and less financially rewarding compared with operative procedures. However, it is the prosthodontist who will be required to take responsibility when complications occur. Diagnosis and treatment planning are the *raison d'être* for the prosthodontic specialty. In addition, only the treating clinician can be aware of the complexities of the

treatment provided. Acceptance of ongoing maintenance responsibility may avert more serious complications and consequences.

Some patients will require frequent professional oral hygiene treatments in addition to a review of prosthodontic treatment. This can be provided by either the referring dentist or dental hygienist. One advantage of the prosthodontist performing a prophylaxis is that it provides a second and potentially more effective examination, especially of subgingival and interproximal regions, when soft and hard deposits have been removed.

The recall programme should be tailored to individual patients. The timing of recall visits will be determined by several factors:

- The patient's susceptibility to disease. Preventive measures will require review and adjustment as changes in physical and mental condition occur with time.
- The complexity of the treatment. The more complex the treatment, the greater the frequency of reassessment.
- The biological, physiological and mechanical stability of the oral and associated extraoral tissues over time. As stability of the rehabilitation is demonstrated, the frequency of recall visits may be reduced.
- The patient's willingness and effectiveness in carrying out hygiene procedures. The need for hygiene reinforcement will vary with each patient's varying life complexities and responsibilities.

There is current debate concerning the relevance of traditional clinical parameters (probing depths and bleeding on probing) associated with implant-supported prostheses. Changes in these parameters, rather than specific measurements, are better indicators of pathology.

Differential wear of materials will result in altered occlusal contact patterns. Adjustments to both the natural and restored teeth may be indicated to maintain distribution of forces as widely as possible as these changes occur. Some changes may be acceptable and not require intervention.

Development of group function has been shown to occur with time (Beyron 1969). Although the preferred restored contact pattern may have incorporated canine disclusion for convenience and to facilitate physiological adaptation, a 'slow' development of group function following differential wear need not be modified – and indeed may be desirable, if it involves a wider distribution of forces. The proviso, however, is that the teeth involved have adequate structural integrity and resistance form (sufficient remaining tooth structure under a crown, around a restoration or on an unrestored tooth) to withstand the associated destructive lateral forces (Figure 8.2). Reduction of the height and inclination of non-supporting buccal cusps of teeth with intracoronal restorations involving one or both marginal ridges should be considered as a proactive measure against cusp fracture.

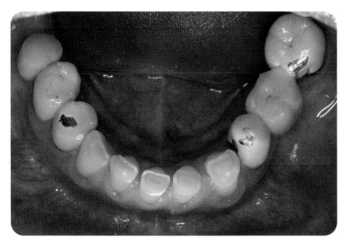

Figure 8.2 A mandibular arch 14 years following partial restoration of the posterior segments. Differential wear has resulted in the initial canine disclusion developing into a group function following extensive parafunction. Note the minimal cusp height and fossa depth and the small cantilevered pontic in the 46 region. Wear of the veneering porcelain has resulted in some exposure of the underlying metal. Veneer chipping has occurred in regions that are not adequately supported by metal.

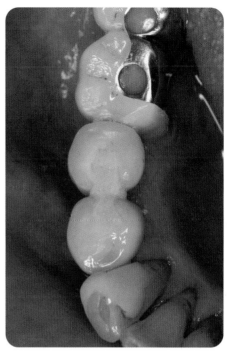

Figure 8.3 Metal rod and composite splinting of lower premolar teeth that developed 'uncomfortable' mobility after 6 years in a patient with periodontal disease susceptibility.

Consideration of differential wear is especially pertinent in the maxillary anterior segment. The maxillary incisors in class I and class II division II occlusal arrangements sustain lateral loading in centric contact (Wiskott & Belser 1995). This often results in the development of ledges in the palatal region or labial flaring of non-restored maxillary incisors and wear of the lower incisors (Figure 8.3). The resistance form of root-filled restored maxillary incisors will be significantly weakened and they will be susceptible to either corono-radicular fracture, if not restored with a post, or vertical root fracture, if restored with a post. Compensatory adjustment of the palatal surfaces of any restorations to ensure clearance of 8–12 μm (Artifoil Shim Stock) in centric contact will reduce the incidence of fracture and wear of lower incisors or unaesthetic development of anterior diastemas (Figure 8.4).

Ongoing loss of attachment in patients who are susceptible to periodontal disease following rehabilitation, even with adequate supportive periodontal therapy, will result in reduced resistance form of the remaining attachment, especially to laterally applied forces. This is likely to cause increased mobility and possible tooth migration. Flattening of cusps and shallowing of fossae will reduce these sequelae, thereby improving comfort and assisting in the ongoing management of the periodontal disease. Splinting teeth that become uncomfortably mobile may also be indicated. This can usually be achieved with composite reinforced with braided archwire or metal rods (Figure 8.3). Minor tooth repositioning may be used to eliminate diastemas prior to splinting.

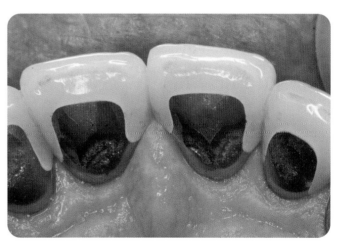

Figure 8.4. Metal–ceramic crowns on maxillary central incisor teeth 3 years after cementation. Note the deep faceting on the palatal surfaces resulting from differential wear and parafunction. Subsequent adjustment ensured shim clearance in intercuspal contact.

There is an ethical dilemma concerning the timing and extent of any radiographic review of prostheses. The development of digital radiography and the wider availability of different techniques, such as the orthopantomogram and computerised tomography, facilitates review and, if used judiciously, exposes the patient to relatively small levels of radiation. However, justification for any radiation exposure is required (the ALARA principle – as low as reasonably achievable). Applying general timetables to every patient cannot be justified. The quality of any radiographic review must be suitable for adequate diagnosis of pathology. Thus, the protocol for radiographic review is complex as it relates to the patient's susceptibility to disease. Changes in general health status, medications and lifestyle will affect this susceptibility.

Caries is often not associated with symptoms. In a patient with high caries susceptibility, bitewing radiographs every 2 years would be indicated, while longer intervals (5 years) would be more appropriate in non-susceptible patients.

Clinical periodontal indicators such as bleeding on probing and increased pocket depths are indicators of the relative activity of periodontal disease. When present, periapical radiographic assessment of bone architecture may also be indicated.

It is well documented that bone levels around implants undergo marked remodelling in the first year after loading (Albrektsson & Zarb 1993). It would seem reasonable to obtain baseline levels after this first year. Further review under 5 years does not seem warranted unless there are clinical signs indicating pathology. Even if detected, there is debate as to the relevance of ongoing bone changes around some osseointegrated implants (Jemt & Albrektsson 2008).

3. The recall visit

3.1 The patient interview

It is important to engage in conversation with the patient before carrying out any examination. Previous notes can be used to reinforce the patient–dentist rapport.

Welcoming the patient into the surgery will allow an assessment that may hint at an altered physical state, especially in the elderly patient. Any documented notification of change in medical condition should be discussed. Onset of diabetes and changes in smoking habits will be particularly relevant to patients susceptible to periodontal disease. Smoking has been associated with an increased risk of implant failure (Heitz-Mayfield & Huynh-Ba, 2009).

Changes in patient demeanour and social circumstances may indicate a changed psychological profile and suggest a state of anxiety or depression. This altered psychological profile may affect the patient's perception of symptoms. Acute pain from a treatable physical cause, such as post-exercise muscle soreness induced by parafunction, may become chronic and less amenable to treatment. Much effort could be wasted and frustration and anxiety increased without recognising this altered patient profile.

The patient's attitude to 'value' for treatment provided will be influenced by the complications experienced. Assessing patient satisfaction with the treatment, addressing concerns in a non-confrontational manner, and offering financial considerations, will minimise the risk of medico-legal consequences. Patient satisfaction with dental prostheses is likely to be significantly influenced by the patient–dentist rapport (Layton & Walton 2009).

3.2 The examination

Extraoral examination should include temporomandibular joint auscultation and jaw and cervical muscle palpation.

A comprehensive examination of periodontal/peri-implant and other soft tissues is indicated. Exudate (with pus) and profuse bleeding on probing around implants would indicate radiographic assessment for signs of peri-implantitis.

Examining the teeth would include:

- evidence of disease (caries);
- loss of seal of retainers (cement failure);
- mechanical failure of teeth (cusp fractures) and materials (chipping, fractures, de-bonding of veneers, looseness or dislodgement of restorations);
- increased tooth mobility;
- altered occlusal contact patterns;
- changes in tooth position (flaring, open interproximal contacts);
- wear facets on the teeth and restorations;
- fremitus between the incisors in centric.

An appropriate radiographic survey would be undertaken.

3.3 Treatment

Recall visits are usually scheduled for 30 minutes, thus there is limited treatment that can be performed. However, any periodic visit should involve:

- elimination of disease (restorations or referrals where indicated);
- smoothing of minor chipping of both teeth and restorations;
- adjustment of centric contacts if indicated to broaden distribution of lateral forces and re-establish the preferred occlusal contact pattern if indicated;
- replacement of lost screw access seals in implant-supported prostheses;
- reactivation of RDP retainers where indicated;
- removal of hard and soft deposits around teeth and implants.

Treatment aimed to prevent further complications could include:

- ensuring shim clearance between the incisor teeth in centric relation and intercuspal contact;
- flattening of cusp inclines and non-supporting cusp tips with compromised resistance form or showing increased mobility;
- splinting of teeth with persistent increased mobility.

4. Documentation

Treatment planning should be based on best evidence. However, irrespective of any published documentation of outcomes of different restorative materials and techniques, each operator will have different capacities, prejudices and experiences. If patients are to be provided with the 'best' treatment, then the likely outcome of the treatment provided by their clinician should be known. It therefore behoves the prosthodontist to consistently document the outcomes of his or her cohort of patients. This information can be used to guide future treatment planning decisions and give the patient realistic expectations of ongoing maintenance costs.

Documentation of complications associated with FDPs has been given minimal consideration in the literature. What is published can be confusing and have little practical relevance in private practice. The same type of complication may have different associated economic and social costs for both clinician and patient.

5. Routine maintenance versus retreatment

Retreatment preformed as part of a planned routine 30-minute recall appointment could be considered part of routine maintenance. This would include smoothing of chipped veneer material that is not an aesthetic concern, tightening of an implant abutment screw, resealing of a screw access hole, adjustment of occlusal contacts or direct splinting of mobile teeth.

Retreatment performed because of a non-planned presentation by the patient would be considered a complication, as it involves an added cost to either the patient or the practice. If the treatment can be completed in 30 minutes then it could be considered a minor complication. Examples would be tightening of a loose screw, smoothing of a chipped veneer material (where again aesthetics is not compromised) or resealing of an implant abutment screw access hole.

Retreatment that takes longer than 30 minutes, requires additional appointments or referral to another discipline would be considered a major complication. It commands a significant economic and personal cost to the patient and possibly to the treating clinician. A chipped or fractured veneer on an implant-supported prosthesis that requires removal and indirect repair to restore acceptable aesthetics would be considered a major complication. A loose screw that results from stripped threads in an implant may require more than just screw replacement and tightening to achieve prosthesis stability.

As indicated above, the one complication type could be considered routine maintenance, a minor or even a major complication. Each circumstance will have different social and economic costs. Effective documentation facilitates realistic discussion of the type, incidence and consequences of maintenance and retreatment requirements.

References

Albrektsson, T. & Zarb, G.A. (1993) Current interpretations of the osseointegrated response: clinical significance. *International Journal of Prosthodontics*, 6 (2), 95–105.

Beyron, H. (1969) Optimal occlusion. *Dental Clinics of North America*, 13 (3), 537–652.

De Boever, A.L., Quirynen, M., Coucke, W. *et al.* (2009) Clinical and radiographic study of implant treatment outcome in periodontally susceptible and non-susceptible patients: a prospective long-term study. *Clinical Oral Implants Research*, 20 (12), 1341–1350.

Fardal, Ø. & Linden, G.J. (2008) Tooth loss and implant outcomes in patients refractory to treatment in a periodontal practice. *Journal of Clinical Periodontology*, 35 (8), 733–738.

Heitz-Mayfield, L.J. & Huynh-Ba, G. (2009) History of treated periodontitis and smoking as risks for implant therapy. *International Journal of Oral & Maxillofacial Implants*, 24 (Suppl.), 39–68.

Jemt, T. & Albrektsson, T. (2008) Do long-term followed-up Branemark implants commonly show evidence of pathological bone breakdown? A review based on recently published data. *Periodontology 2000*, 47, 133–142.

Layton, D. & Walton, T.R. (2009) Profiles of 500 patients who did and 486 patients who did not respond to a prosthodontic treatment questionnaire. *International Journal of Prosthodontics*, 22 (5), 459–465.

Marbach, J.J., Raphael, K.G., Janal, M.N. *et al.* (2003) Reliability of clinician judgements of bruxism. *Journal of Oral Rehabilitation*, 30 (2), 113–118.

Ng, Y.L., Mann, V. & Gulabivala, K. (2010) Tooth survival following non-surgical root canal treatment: a systematic review of the literature. *International Endodontic Journal*, 43 (3), 171–189.

Tan, K., Pjetursson, B.E., Lang, N.P. *et al.* (2004) A systematic review of the survival and complication rates of fixed partial dentures (FPDs) after an observation of at least 5 years. *Clinical Oral Implants Research*, 15 (6), 654–666.

Walton, T.R. (2003) An up to 15-year longitudinal study of 515 metal–ceramic FPDs: Part 2. Modes of failure and influence of various clinical characteristics. *International Journal of Prosthodontics*, 16 (2), 177–182.

Walton, T.R. (2009a) Changes in patient and FDP profiles following the introduction of osseointegrated implant dentistry in a prosthodontic practice. *International Journal of Prosthodontics*, 22 (2), 127–135.

Walton, T.R. (2009b) Changes in the outcome of metal-ceramic tooth-supported single crowns and FDPs following the introduction of osseointegrated implant dentistry into a prosthodontic practice. *International Journal of Prosthodontics*, 22 (3), 260–267.

Wiskott, H.W. & Belser, U.C. (1995) A rationale for a simplified occlusal design in restorative dentistry: historical review and clinical guidelines. *Journal of Prosthetic Dentistry*, 73 (2), 169–183.

Section 4

Cases and Case Presentations

Introduction

Iven Klineberg

Rehabilitation is patient specific (Rivera-Morales & Mohl 1992), as emphasised in Chapter 4. Case management, whether simple or advanced, requires a defined protocol to ensure that the needs of each patient are appropriately addressed and an optimum outcome is more likely to be achieved. This is a requirement to which the clinician becomes committed with the agreed decision to provide oral rehabilitation. In effect, a contract is developed that follows the patients' detailed understanding of what is planned for their management, is clarified through discussion to gain informed consent, and is formalised desirably with a signed agreement to define the commitment by both patient and clinician.

Sequential steps are recommended in a management protocol, which allow clinical decisions to be made within the framework of an appropriate evidence base for informed decision-making:

1. Data acquisition: patient assessment, including medical history and current medical status and medications; social history, including habits of smoking, alcohol intake and diet; dental history and the present condition, which at the outset requires identification of disease, especially dental caries and periodontal disease, which are prioritised in the management plan.

    Patient-specific requests and consideration of treatment options requires imaging, including screening (orthopantomogram), specific dental (periapical) imaging and, where indicated, 3D imaging. The later allows assessment of space-occupying lesions, including bone and periapical pathology, and a determination of bone quality and quantity where dental implants are to be considered, to optimise their location and orientation. Articulated study casts are helpful for occlusal analysis of specific tooth and dental arch orientations and relationships as well as tooth wear, and occlusal vertical dimension assessment.

2. Diagnostic preparations, including diagnostic wax-up of preferred tooth form and occlusal vertical dimension. To maximise the value of diagnostic preparations, their application as a template for clinical temporary and provisional restorations is valuable when applied with adhesive materials to assist patients in appreciating the possibilities and limitations of changes in tooth form and colour. Design of FPDs and/or RDPs requires a vision of the final rehabilitation as a component of informed patient consent, and the preparation of treatment appliances and stabilising splints where required.

3. Informed consent, including preferred treatment options and risk–benefit analysis.

4. Preliminary treatment to eliminate disease and the introduction of an oral health strategy for each patient's sustained oral health; the revision of diagnostic preparations may be required, and the use of longer term provisional restorations may be indicated to assess soft tissue health and patient compliance with oral health maintenance.

5. Definitive treatment must be delivered in an optimum oral environment, with each patient's compliance and understanding to optimise the risks and potential benefits that have been discussed and agreed with the consent process.

6. A maintenance plan is important as a component of the overall oral health care provided and needs to be detailed to each patient's particular medical and personal circumstances within the context of age. Importantly, the maintenance plan needs to acknowledge the ageing process and its variability, as well as the unexpected developments of disease and the specific needs that such changes may bring to the rehabilitation. These considerations need to be discussed as part of the informed consent agreement.

The cases presented in this section have been planned and managed following the protocol indicated. Although the cases are varied and each treatment clinician different, each patient's individual treatment preferences were acknowledged and influenced the desired outcomes.

Oral Rehabilitation: A Case-Based Approach, First Edition. Edited by Iven Klineberg, Diana Kingston.
© 2012 Blackwell Publishing Ltd. Published 2012 by Blackwell Publishing Ltd.

Following a defined protocol ensured that each case was considered comprehensively and each patient's specific expectations provided.

Treatment plans were compiled in acknowledgement of the patient's chief complaint, relevant medical, social and dental history, clinical data and, in most cases, specialist consultations. An evidence-based approach has been used in the development of the treatment plans. In each case, the patient was made aware of the advantages and disadvantages of all available treatment options. Also discussed in detail were: the proposed time involved; the biological costs; and the financial costs of the management plan, including maintenance for the preferred treatment plan. Patients were advised that their treatment was a component of the learning requirements for candidates completing the specialty programme in prosthodontics at the University of Sydney (Appendix 1). Treatment plans follow a standardised protocol as indicated in the cases presented. Variation in display of different stages varied with the candidates' wish to individualise their data.

The sequential steps include:

- medical, social and dental history;
- extraoral examination to assess facial aesthetics, lip posture, smile assessment, occlusal plane orientation, OVD and speaking space, phonetics, TMJ and jaw muscle and regional lymph gland assessment, and jaw movements;
- intraoral examination of soft tissues, palate, tongue, oral hygiene, saliva quality and quantity, gingival biotype, papillae – colour and form, periodontium – probing depth, bleeding on probing (tabled as CPITN); tooth status and presence of dental caries – new or recurrent, occlusal assessment of ICP and RCP, lateral and protrusive guidance, tooth wear and a dental charting;
- alveolar bone level assessment with periapical radiographs and a screening OPG, which are carefully analysed and correlated with the clinical situation; study casts are articulated in RCP for analysis and preliminary diagnostic preparations to simulate the possible rehabilitation;
- a problem list is developed, and treatment options to address the problems are considered and the evidence base and a risk assessment determined;
- discussion of the options with the patient and informed consent obtained to allow treatment to be progressed;
- in each case report, a summary is included of the relevant published data and how it is related to the clinical decisions described.

Following treatment, clinical reviews were completed after 1–2 weeks and after 1 month. Where possible, clinical reviews were also completed at 6 months and on an annual basis. However, not all patients were available for reviews after successful treatment. As a result, in the cases presented in this text, review summaries

are included where possible. The postgraduate prosthodontic clinic is committed to provide ongoing maintenance whenever this is required and successive postgraduates undertake the annual follow-up review or required maintenance. A protocol is followed as shown below.

Already mentioned is the need to determine the evidence base for treatment options and risk assessment with consideration of treatment outcome data. Examples of the information that may be collected is summarised in Appendix 2 (Case 10.2) and Appendix 3 (Case 11.1).

Clinical review of completed clinical cases follow the guidelines below:

1. Oral health status – oral hygiene and plaque control – soft tissue health – note gingival inflammation, colour change – check on home-care programme and advise on frequency of brushing, use of dental floss and mouth rinses; note and record recurrent dental caries associated with restorations or new carious lesions; note periodontal status – check probing depths and record changes; new PA radiographs to check alveolar bone levels (see 4 below).
2. Medical status – change in general health and implications for oral health.
3. Occlusion – check tooth contacts with GHM foil at ICP, RCP, lateral and protrusive excursive contacts – note lateral contact details, especially where there is a fracture of restorative material – record, photograph fracture and contact details with GHM foil and comment on reason for fracture.
4. Radiographs – 1-year review PA views for specific details of the status of crowns on teeth and implants. Check crown margins and alveolar bone levels; measure thread exposure to bone crest around implants and correlate with clinical details as in 1 above; at 2 years an OPG may add global information.
5. Discuss oral health related quality of life – comfort, appearance, function – chewing.
6. Seek any additional comments from the patient about the treatment and whether they would undertake the process again if needed.

Oral rehabilitation and clinical practice are on the brink of a greater change than has been previously possible, notwithstanding the progressive introduction of high-speed instrumentation; supine dental treatment delivery; the use of fluoride; the emphasis on prevention, nutrition and health; and the recognition of patient-centred treatment and quality of life outcomes.

The era of technology advance is already impacting significantly with increasingly sophisticated computer programs that are progressively transforming dental practice, including CAD–CAM technology, already in use for restorations; 3D imaging for detailed treatment planning; and the procedural development of 'teeth-in- an-hour'.

Intraoral scanning of teeth and dental arches and inter-arch relationship to capture the relationship with the jaw and TMJs is in the early stages of development and application. The accurate capture of 3D images of tooth preparations with transfer to a processing centre for ceramic milling of single tooth copings of zirconia for all-ceramic restorations and substructures for FDPs (crown or bridge framework) is already available and proving to be successful by delivering precision fit and appropriate strength and, more recently, a range of ceramic colours where required.

In addition to the format of the case documentation described above, the following will help interpretation of data within each section.

Navigation guide for case templates

The template (see Appendix 4) is divided into the following major sections:

- History.
- Extraoral examination.
- Intraoral examination.
- Special tests.
- Problem list.
- Treatment options.
- Treatment plan.
- Treatment sequence.
- Treatment discussion.
- References.

Within each section, subheadings require information of specific relevance to the section; for example in the first section 'Presenting complaints', the details requested are 'Chief complaint', 'Subsidiary complaints', 'History of complaints' and 'Patient expectations'. Similarly, in all sections specific questions relate to the information needed to assist in informed decision-making. Where a question is listed and there is no relevant information, 'Nil' is listed as the response; this is seen for example in the section on 'Medical history' where there may be little or no relevant information to some questions for a particular case.

Alternatively, where information is listed in table form, as with the section on 'Dental charting', all individual teeth are listed using the two-digit FDI convention, and where there is no relevant information 'Nil' is added to the form. Where a restoration is indicated, such as MOD (mesial-occlusal-distal surfaces restored), or CMC (ceramo-metal crown) and where no comment is added in the adjacent column, the restoration is satisfactory and does not require immediate attention.

As the template was designed as a comprehensive database, sections are removed with particular cases where there is no relevance; for example, the details required for edentulous patients are removed from the template where the patient is dentate. Conversely, for edentulous patients, the sections concerning teeth, occlusion, dental charting and periodontal assessment are removed.

Sections on 'Extraoral examinations' and 'Intraoral examinations' have multiple questions, some or all of which may be relevant for a particular case, and if a response is indicated it is listed briefly. The 'Temporomandibular assessment' provides a shortened version of specific TMJ details of joint sounds with movement, jaw muscle tenderness, and the degree of jaw movement (measured in millimetres). Where there is evidence for further investigation, this would be followed by a comprehensive assessment using the RDC/TMD protocol.

Intraoral examination requires detailed assessment of the teeth, gingival and periodontal tissues and detailed charting. An assessment of the occlusion is indicated with separate odontograms of tooth numbers for specific details of tooth guidance and tooth surface loss – the specific teeth involved are highlighted in each case – and each would require further clinical assessment and management.

Radiographic assessment requires an OPG and periapical radiographs for each case; there may be additional needs for orthodontics requiring cephalometric analysis and implant treatment requiring specific imaging to assess bone volume and suitability for implant placement; this is detailed where required.

Following clinical examination and data collection, a 'Problem list' is developed to identify the explicit case features that need to be addressed.

The analysis of the problem list allows treatment options to be proposed and a risk–benefit analysis considered. The advantages and disadvantages are specified and as part of the informed consent process the cost of each option is detailed and discussed. In the cases presented, costs generally are not included as they are country specific. In addition, as management is generally provided within a teaching hospital facility for public patients rather than a private practice clinic, costs are not relevant. Following informed consent, the treatment selected is indicated and the treatment sequence specified; the latter is important to determine appointment time and frequency and the timeline of laboratory procedures.

Finally the 'Treatment discussion' provides an explanation for the management plan selected and acknowledges relevant publications that support the clinical decisions made for a particular clinical situation to address the patient-specific needs. Clinical reviews are frequent within the first 3 months and then are routine at 6 months. Where possible, annual reviews are carried out; however, patient compliance varies and this is not always possible.

Reference

Rivera-Morales, W.C. & Mohl, N.D. (1992) Restoration of the vertical dimension of occlusion in the severely worn dentition. *Dental Clinics of North America*, 36 (3), 651–664.

9

Single Tooth Restoration

Introduction by Iven Klineberg

Single tooth restoration often presents a challenge in clinical practice. This is particularly so where there is extensive coronal tooth breakdown and uncertainty concerning the sustainability of the residual tooth structure. The question of what treatment is desirable needs consideration given the particular tooth location and the condition of the other teeth in the arch. If the tooth is to be retained but requires further treatment, this needs to be based on the available evidence for long-term outcomes (Schmidlin et al. 2010).

Justification of a proposed course of treatment is important for informed patient consent and may include endodontic therapy followed by post and core to support a full coverage restoration. These considerations would also be based on the strategic importance of the particular tooth. The aesthetic zone may be especially challenging where there is a high smile line and thin gingival biotype. Posterior tooth restoration requires different considerations given the acceptance of the shortened dental arch concept. The data suggest that a dental arch of 20 units, including the anterior segment and all bicuspid teeth in both arches, allows adequate function and does not necessarily predispose to either excessive tooth wear of remaining teeth or TMJ dysfunction (Witter et al. 1999, Wolfart et al. 2005, Walter et al. 2010). It is recognised that retaining molar teeth enhances chewing efficiency, and chewing concerns were reported in a specific population group with loss of posterior teeth (Fueki et al. 2011). This needs further elucidation, but in consideration of replacement of posterior teeth, the evidence base for the shortened dental arch should be discussed with patients. A decision on whether to provide posterior tooth treatment would then be made as a patient-centred decision for which there would be clinician–patient agreement and informed consent.

In consideration of whether to preserve a tooth or replace with an implant-supported crown, the state of the remaining dentition and periodontium is of crucial impor-

tance as it bears directly on the global prognosis of the dentition and the implant-supported restorations (Schmidlin et al. 2010). In addition, the loss of specific sensory features of teeth and their sensorimotor influences in the control of mastication and swallowing needs to be recognised. The following provides an overview of the unique and important sensory mechanisms of teeth and the implications for changed sensory function with tooth loss. It is clear that with loss of one or a few teeth the remaining dentition provides appropriate sensory feedback for function. Greater tooth loss and an unstable occlusion result in functional problems and total edentulism is a state of total dental deafferentation with significant functional impairment and psychosocial dysfunction (Klineberg & Murray 1999).

Teeth provide a uniquely discriminating sense of touch and directional specificity for occlusal awareness, intraoral contact for management of a food bolus, discrimination of food texture and hardness, and control of jaw muscles for mastication and swallowing. These specific features of teeth are closely linked with both periodontal sensitivity (Trulsson 2005, 2006) and pulpal–dentine–enamel sensitivity. Recent evidence on pulpal innervation confirms these implications; for example, an elegant study by Farahani et al. (2011) clarifies the integrated role of the pulp–dentine–enamel complex. These data further confirm the importance of the teeth in the sensorimotor control of jaw function as summarised below.

The neural basis of pulpal sensitivity has been recognised as contributing to the exquisitely discriminatory sensory mechanism of teeth. This feedback system is based on the unique hardness of the enamel surface and its dentinal substructure together with the rich pulpal innervation, vascularity and cellular composition. Of particular importance is the cellular composition of pulpal tissues dominated by odontoblasts with their composite role (Farahani et al. 2011) in which dentinogenesis

Oral Rehabilitation: A Case-Based Approach, First Edition. Edited by Iven Klineberg, Diana Kingston.
© 2012 Blackwell Publishing Ltd. Published 2012 by Blackwell Publishing Ltd.

dominates. Recent data have confirmed that, in addition, odontoblasts have a unique role as sensory cells that contribute to intraoral discrimination as an important component of masticatory function. These sensory cells form a pulpal network (Allard *et al.* 2006, Ikeda & Suda 2006, Farahani *et al.* 2011) and are structurally supported by glial cells in a similar manner to the cellular arrangement in the central nervous system. This cell-rich neurovascular structure provides the matrix of the pulpal neurosensory system, which has the capacity to contribute to function independently but in reality does so in combination with periodontal innervation to provide uniquely sensitive oral mechanosensation for function and discrimination of food types, food texture as well as bite force and force direction.

Periodontal feedback has been identified through human studies using microneurographic recordings that have identified its defining role in proprioceptive discrimination (Trulsson 2006). Anterior teeth, with lower threshold and more rapid response to dynamic loading, match their functional requirements for discrimination of incisal biting and directional controls with incision, while posterior teeth respond more slowly to higher loads as a static response designed to allow sustained bite force for mastication.

With tooth loss, these sensory discriminatory functions are lost and there is no equivalence with implant replacement. The latter is predictable and desirable as a strategy to replace lost teeth, contemporary implants allow rapid osseointegration through contact osteogenesis, and immediate placement and loading are now commonly accepted practices (Salinas & Eckert 2007, Esposito *et al.* 2010). However, the resulting sensory discrimination and contribution to control of masticatory function with implants is no longer provided by the tooth–periodontal complex and is significantly less than that provided by the dentate state (Grigoriadis *et al.* 2011). Nevertheless, function is improved when compared with non-implant rehabilitations.

On the basis of the evidence available, the optimum decision to save teeth is clear and undisputed given the contributions that vital teeth make to the fine controls of jaw function. With the loss of the pulpal–dentinal sensory system, preservation of the enamel surface in conjunction with the periodontal mechanosensitive feedback system will contribute to ongoing tooth contact discrimination and management of food type and texture. However, once a tooth is lost with the complex pulp–dentinal–enamel and periodontal feedback systems, there is an identifiable change in sensory discrimination; in this context sensorimotor cortical changes have been evaluated with functional magnetic resonance imaging as neuroplastic change in response to modification of the dental status (Avivi-Arber *et al.* 2011).

References

Allard, B., Maglore, H., Couble, M.L. *et al.* (2006) Voltage-gated sodium channels confer excitability to human odontoblasts: possible role in tooth pain transmission. *Journal of Biological Chemistry*, 281, 29002–29010.

Avivi-Arber, L., Martin, R., Lee, J.C. *et al.* (2011) Face sensorimotor cortex and its neuroplasticity related to oro-facial sensorimotor function. *Archives of Oral Biology*, available online 2011 May 6 [Epub ahead of print]

Esposito, M., Grusovin, M.G., Polyzos, I.P. *et al.* (2010) Interventions for replacing missing teeth: dental implants in fresh extraction sockets (immediate, immediate-delayed and delayed). *Cochrane Database of Systematic Reviews 2010*: issue 9: CD 005968. DOI: 10.1002/14651858.

Farahani, R.M., Simonian, M. & Hunter N. (2011) Blueprint of an ancestral neurosensory organ revealed in glial networks in human dental pulp. *Journal of Comparative Neurology*, 519(16), 3306–3326.

Fueki, K., Igarashi, Y., Maeda, Y. *et al.* (2011) Factors related to prosthetic restoration in patients with shortened dental arches: a multicentre study. *Journal of Oral Rehabilitation*, 38, 525–532.

Grigoriadis, A., Johansson, R.S. & Trulsson, M. (2011) Adaptability of mastication in people with implant-supported bridges. *Journal of Clinical Periodontology*, 38 (4), 395–404.

Ikeda, H. & Suda, H. (2006) Rapid penetration of Lucifer yellow into vital teeth and dye coupling between odontoblasts and neighbouring pulp cells in the cat. *Archives of Oral Biology*, 51, 123–128.

Klineberg, I. & Murray, G. (1999) Osseoperception: sensory function and proprioception. *Advances in Dental Research*, 13, 120–129.

Salinas, T.J. & Eckert, S. (2007) In patients requiring single-tooth replacement, what are the outcomes of implant- as compared to tooth-supported restorations. *International Journal of Oral & Maxillofacial Implants*, 22(Suppl.), 71–95.

Schmidlin, K., Schnell, N., Steiner, S., *et al.* (2010) Complication and failure rates in patients treated for chronic periodontitis and restored with single crowns on teeth and/or implants. *Clinical Oral Implants Research*, 21 (5), 550–557.

Trulsson, M. (2005) Sensory and motor function of teeth and dental implants: a basis for osseoperception. *Clinical and Experimental Pharmacology & Physiology*, 32 (1–2), 119–122.

Trulsson, M. (2006) Sensory-motor function of human periodontal mechanoreceptors. *Journal of Oral Rehabilitation*, 33, 262–273.

Walter, M.H., Weber, A., Marre, B. *et al.* (2010) The randomized shortened dental arch study: tooth loss. *Journal of Dental Research*, 89, 818–822.

Witter, D.J., van Palenstein Helderman, W.H., Creugers, N.H.J. *et al.* (1999) The shortened dental arch concept and its implications for oral health care. *Community Dentistry and Oral Epidemiology*, 27, 249–258.

Wolfart, S., Heydecke, G., Luthardt, R.G. *et al.* (2005) Effects of prosthetic treatment for shortened dental arches on oral health-related quality of life, self-reports of pain and jaw disability: results from the pilot phase of a randomized multicentre trial. *Journal of Oral Rehabilitation*, 32, 815–822.

Case 9.1 Mrs Kathryn H

Ken Hooi

Patient: Mrs Kathryn H (date of birth 19/06/1960)

Presenting complaints

Date of initial examination	26/04/2007
Chief complaint	'Crown keeps breaking' Recurrent loss of retention of post and crown for right maxillary lateral incisor
Subsidiary complaints	Nil
History of complaints	Referred by regular dentist for assessment of tooth 12, which had loss of retention of its post and crown. This was managed with a prefabricated stainless steel post and direct provisional composite resin restoration. The patient had been comfortable in the interim Prior to 1998, tooth 12 was endodontically treated and restored with a porcelain veneer In 1998, a coronal fracture occurred from the application of a nitrous oxide mask during childbirth. The tooth was definitively restored with a post and CMC Several years later, tooth 12 again sustained a fracture including the post. The post fragment was removed from the canal by an endodontist and the replacement restoration comprised a carbon-fibre post and crown In 2005, there was loss of retention of the crown, while the post was stable *in situ* Between 2005 and March 2007, loss of retention of the crown, often with the post, occurred on several occasions
Patient's expectations	The patient had been advised by her dentist regarding treatment options The patient preferred not to have: • an extraction and partial RDP • an extraction and FDP (tooth-borne) • no treatment The patient had an expectation that extraction and single implant restorations was the best option Retreatment, with a new post and crown, was discounted by the patient, given the history of recurrent loss of retention

History
Medical history

Medical Practitioner	Dr W, General Practice Physician	
Respiratory	Nil	
Cardiovascular	Nil	
Gastrointestinal	Nil	
Neurological	Nil	
Endocrine	Hypercholesterolaemia	
Developmental	Nil	
Musculoskeletal	Nil	
Genitourinary	Nil	
Haematological	Nil	
Other	Allergies	NKA
	Smoking	Ex-smoker (stopped in 1990)
	Infectious diseases	Nil
	Pregnancy	Nil
	Hospitalisation	Childbirth confinement
	Medications	Pravastatin (Pravachol)

Social history

Marital status	Married		
Children	Four sons (ages 14, 13, 9, 8)		
Occupation	Solicitor (private legal firm)		
Smoking	Type	Ex-smoker (tobacco)	
	Frequency	N/A	
	Period:	Until 1990	
Recreational drugs	Nil		
Diet	√	Soft drinks	Diet
		Sports drinks	Nil
		Lemons	Nil
	√	Acidic foods	Tomatoes, balsamic vinegar
	√	Sweet foods	Occasional
	√	Water	Less than 1 L/day
	√	Tea	3 cups/day
	√	Coffee	2 cups/day
	√	Alcohol	10–15 glasses wine/week
		Hard/brittle foods	Nil
	√	Ice crunching	Yes
Habits/hobbies		Musical instrument	Nil
	√	Exercise	Walking, road cycling twice weekly
	√	Oral habits	Fingernails, pens

Dental history

Date of last examination		28/03/2007	Tooth 12 provisional restoration
Oral hygiene	√	Brushing	Twice daily
		Flossing	No
	√	Mouthwash	Once daily
	√	Toothpaste	Fluoridated
Treatment	√	Restorations	Yes
	√	Endodontics	Yes
	√	Periodontics	Yes
		Orthodontics	No
		RDP	No
	√	FDP	Yes
		TMD	No
	√	OMFS	Yes

Extraoral examination (Figures 9.1.1 & 9.1.2)
Aesthetics

Facial symmetry	Symmetrical	
Profile	Mesofacial	
Nasolabial angle	<90°	
Facial folds	Yes	
Midlines	Face/maxillary centrals	Coincident
	Maxillary central alignment	2° counter clockwise rotation
	Maxillary/mandibular centrals	2 mm LHS
Lip posture	Symmetry	Mild asymmetry
	Upper lip	Mild elevation to LHS
	Lower lip	Mild depression to LHS
	Competence	Yes
	Tooth display	Minimal
Occlusal plane	Parallel to ala tragus line	parallel
	Parallel to interpupillary line	2° counter clockwise rotation (between cusp tips of teeth 13 and 23)
	Over-eruption	Nil
Vertical	FWS	Normal
	OVD assessment	Normal
Smile assessment	Symmetry	Mild asymmetry
	Lip line	Minimal prominence of Cupid's bow
	Gingival display	Papillae only
	Tooth display	Complete
	Buccal corridor	RHS minimal, LHS moderate

Phonetics

	Normal	Abnormal
Labial (m)	√	
Labiodental (f/v)	√	
Linguodental (th)	√	
Interdental (s)	√	
Linguopalatal (k/ng)	√	

Temporomandibular assessment

TMJ		Additional information
Click	√	Bilateral, reciprocal, asymptomatic
Crepitus	Nil	
Tenderness	Nil	

Muscle tenderness	Right	Left
Temporalis	Nil	Nil
Masseter	Nil	Nil
Posterior mandible	Nil	Nil
Anterior mandible	Nil	Nil
Glands	Nil	
Nodes	Nil	

Jaw movement	Measurement (mm)	Reference points
Maximal opening	50	Teeth 11–41
Right laterotrusion	5.5	Dental midlines
Left laterotrusion	7.0	Dental midlines
Midline deviation	1.5	Dental midlines
Maximal protrusion	7.0	Teeth 11–41
Opening pathway	Straight	Nose–chin
Overjet	2.5	Teeth 11–41
Overbite	1.5	Teeth 11–41
Further investigation required	Nil	

Intraoral examination (Figure 9.1.3)
Soft tissues

Tissue	Healthy	Abnormal	Additional information
Lips	√		
Labial vestibule	√		
Cheeks	√		
Palate	√		
Oropharynx	√		
Tongue	√		
Floor	√		
Frenal attachments	√		

Ridges	Maxilla	Mandible
Arch shape	U-shaped	U-shaped
Resorption	Not significant	Not significant
Palatal vault	Moderate	N/A
Tori	Nil	Nil
Frenal attachments	Labial frenum continuous with attached mucosa, otherwise average	Average
Mucosa	Normal	Normal
Pathology	Nil	Nil

Oral cleanliness

Condition	Yes	No	
Plaque	√		Sextants 1, 2, 4, 6
Calculus	√		Sextant 5
Food impaction		√	
Stains		√	
Halitosis		√	

Saliva

Daily water intake	Less than 1 L, 3 cups tea, 2 cups coffee
Quality	Within normal limits
Quantity	Within normal limits
Pathology	Nil
Medications affecting	Nil
Further investigation required	No

Periodontium
CPITN

1	1	0
1	2	1

Gingiva	Biotype	Medium
	Colour	Pink
	Contour	Normal
	Consistency	Firm
Papillae	Colour	Pink
	Contour	Normal

Periodontal charting
All gingival tissues healthy and no bleeding on probing. Pocket depths all within the range of 1.00–3.00 mm.

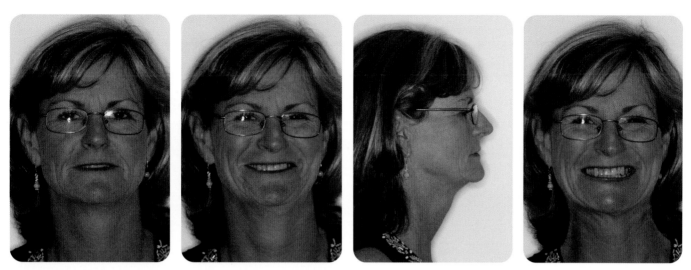

Figure 9.1.1 Extraoral examination.

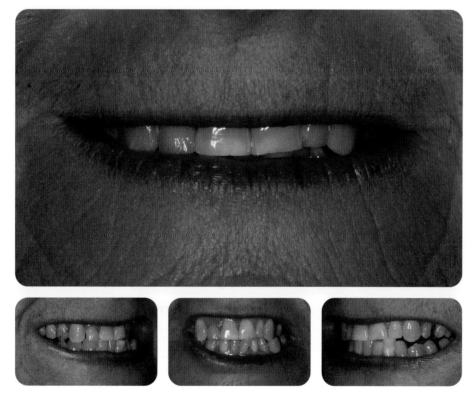

Figure 9.1.2 Smile assessment; note relatively low smile line.

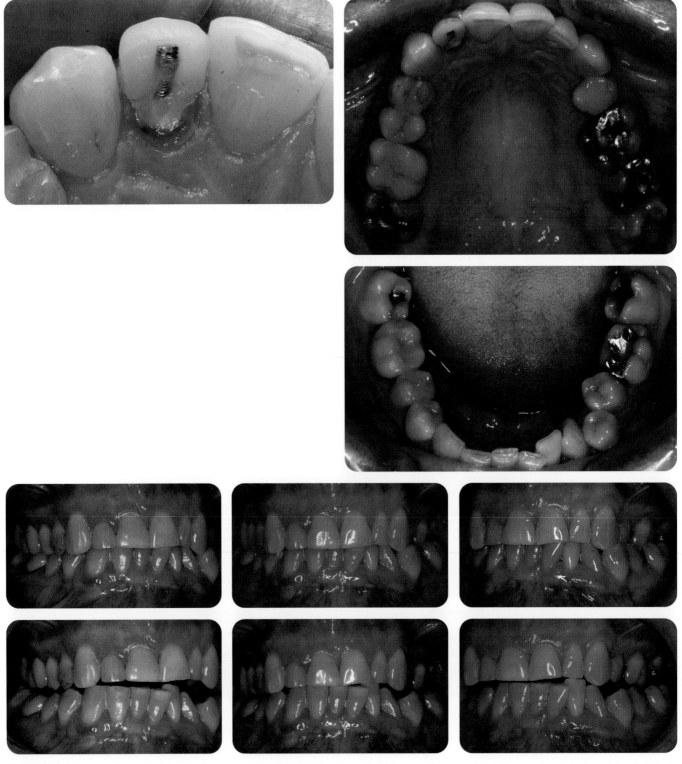

Figure 9.1.3 Intraoral examination indicates tooth relationships, lateral guidance, degree of tooth wear and status of tooth 12 at presentation.

Occlusion (Figure 9.1.3)

Skeletal classification	Type I	
Dental occlusion		
Angle right	Molar	Class I
Angle left	Molar	Class II
Anterior overbite	2.5 mm	
Anterior overjet	1.5 mm	
Cross-bites	23⟺25⟺26/33⟺34⟺35⟺36	
Open-bites	Nil	
Curve of Spee	Average	
Curve of Wilson	Average	
RP to IP slide	Nil	
FWS	Close/M/swallow	4 mm

Tooth guidance

Right laterotrusion

8 7 6 5 4 **3** 2 1 1 2 3 4 5 6 7 8
8 7 6 5 4 **3** 2 1 1 2 3 4 5 6 7 8

Left laterotrusion

8 7 6 5 4 3 2 1 1 2 **3** 4 5 6 7 8
8 7 6 5 4 3 2 1 1 **2 3** 4 5 6 7 8

Protrusion

8 7 6 5 4 **3 2 1 1 2** 3 4 5 6 7 8
8 7 6 5 4 **3 2 1 1 2** 3 4 5 6 7 8

Tooth surface loss

Caries	Nil
Attrition	Nil
Erosion	Nil
Abrasion	Nil
Abfraction	Nil

Dental charting

Tooth no.	Clinical findings	Comments
18	Absent	Removed late 1980s
17	(O) amalgam restoration	
16	CMC	
15	Unrestored, no abnormalities detected	
14	(DO) composite resin restoration	
13	Unrestored, no abnormalities detected	
12	Composite resin complex restoration, recurrent dental caries	
11	(DI) composite resin restoration	
21	Unrestored, no abnormalities detected	
22	Unrestored, no abnormalities detected	
23	Unrestored, no abnormalities detected	
24	Absent	Space closed
25	(MOD) composite resin restoration	
26	(MOD + P groove) amalgam restoration	
27	(MOD + MB + P groove) amalgam restoration	
28	Unrestored, no abnormalities detected	
38	Absent	Removed late 1980s
37	(O) amalgam restoration	
36	(MO) amalgam and (B pit) composite resin restoration	
35	Unrestored, no abnormalities detected	
34	Unrestored, no abnormalities detected	
33	Unrestored, no abnormalities detected	
32	Unrestored, no abnormalities detected	
31	Unrestored, no abnormalities detected	
41	Unrestored, no abnormalities detected	
42	Unrestored, no abnormalities detected	
43	Unrestored, no abnormalities detected	
44	Unrestored, no abnormalities detected	
45	(MOD) amalgam restoration	
46	CMC	
47	(O) amalgam restoration	
48	Absent	Removed late 1980s

Special tests

Test	Performed	Additional information
Percussion	√	Within normal limits
Palpation	√	Within normal limits
Vitality	N/A	
Cusp loading	√	Within normal limits
Transillumination	√	Within normal limits
Selective anaesthesia	N/A	

Radiographs (Figure 9.1.4)
Orthopantomogram (12/04/2007)

Features	Radiographic data
TMJ	Normal
Bone loss	Nil
Sinuses	Normal
Mandibular foramen and canal	Bilateral canal bifurcation or bilateral canalisation of mylohyoid ridges
Mental foramen	Apparent
Retained roots	Nil
Pathology	Multiple calcified nodules bilateral rami

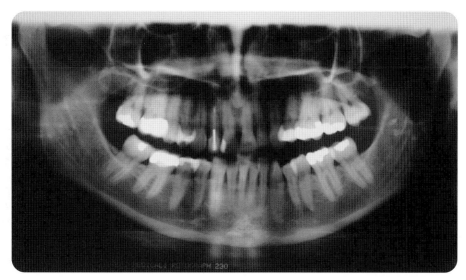

Figure 9.1.4 Radiographic assessment – orthopantomogram (OPG) for screening orofacial structures.

Periapical films (Figure 9.1.5)

Tooth no.	Information	Tooth no.	Information
18		38	
17		37	
16		36	
15		35	
14		34	
13	No abnormality detected	33	
12	Root filling, stainless steel and carbon fibre posts, no periapical pathology	32	
11	No abnormality detected	31	
21		41	
22		42	
23		43	
24		44	
25		45	
26		46	
27		47	
28		48	

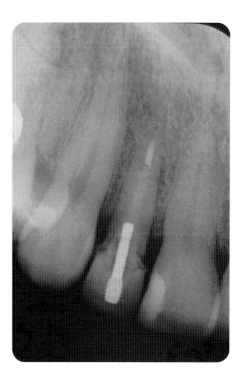

Figure 9.1.5 Radiographic assessment: preoperative periapical image of tooth 12.

Study casts

Articulation	Position	ICP
	Face bow	Yes
Diagnostic wax-up	OVD	Nil
	Occlusal adjustment	Nil
	Crown lengthening	Tooth 12

Problem list

Problem list	Details
Medical condition	Hypercholesterolaemia – controlled; as a metabolic derangement in isolation, there is no direct relevance to dental procedures
Aesthetics	Tooth 12 provisional restoration: • undercontoured • colour • character
Speech	Nil
TMD	Nil
Soft tissue	Nil
Oral hygiene	Recommend supportive periodontal therapy
Saliva	Nil
Periodontal	Nil
Edentulism	Nil
Occlusion	Nil
Tooth surface loss	Mild tooth surface loss of maxillary incisors
Restorative	12 provisional stainless steel post and separated carbon fibre post fragment
Prosthetic	12 provisional composite resin restoration
Endodontic	Nil

Treatment options
Maxilla

Treatment option 1	Treatment time
12 prosthodontic retreatment: • replacement post • replacement core • crown lengthening • replacement crown	8 weeks (minimum)

Treatment option 2	Treatment time
12 single implant restoration: • cross-sectional image (cone-beam or CT scan) • volumetric analysis • surgical prosthodontic protocol prescription • extraction • interim partial RDP • implant insertion under single-stage protocol, possibly immediately following extraction • provisional restoration (implant borne) • definitive restoration (abutment, crown)	12–26 weeks (minimum)

Treatment plan
Maxilla

Treatment option 1 (12 prosthodontic retreatment)
- Replacement post: prefabricated or cast.
- Replacement core: direct or cast.
- Crown lengthening: gingivectomy or apical repositioning.

- Replacement crown: ceramo-metal or all-ceramic with 360° bevel margin.
- Aesthetic references: conformative with existing dentition – tooth/restoration contours, colour and character, and gingival contours.
- Occlusal scheme: conformative with existing dentition.

Treatment sequence (Figure 9.1.6)

Appointment	Procedure
1 (26/4/2007)	Initial examination Periapical and panoramic (OPG) supplied by patient Photographic record Diagnostic cast impressions Treatment plan and consent
2 (3/5/2007)	Initial crown preparation Deconstruction of existing restoration Assessment of residual coronal dentine Provisional core Provisional crown (conformative with original restoration)
3 (28/6/2007)	Crown lengthening (gingivectomy) Refinement of crown margin preparation Provisional crown (aesthetic and emergence profile contours)
4 (26/8/2007)	Aesthetic prescription for definitive crown – colour, character Replacement post (prefabricated) Replacement core (composite resin) Refinement of crown preparation New provisional crown Impression
5 (3/10/2007)	Technical outcome: porcelain–gold crown (360° bevel margin) Crown insertion: resin–modified glass ionomer cement
6 (17/10/2007)	Review
7 (13/12/2010)	Review (Figure 9.1.7)

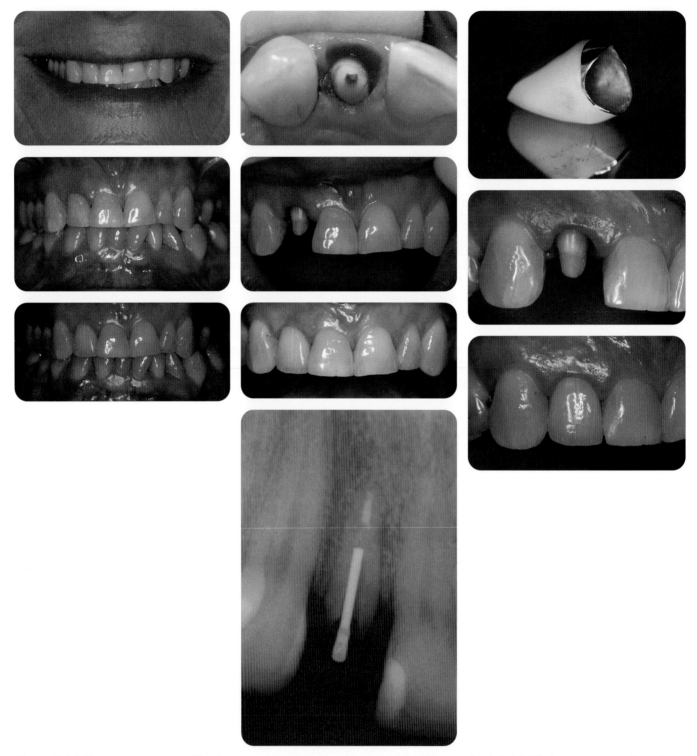

Figure 9.1.6 Treatment progress. Top images: crown insertion (note provisional crown *in situ*). Middle images: crown insertion (note provisional crown *in situ*). Lower images: review at 2 weeks and post-insertion periapical radiograph.

Review at 3 years (Figure 9.1.7)

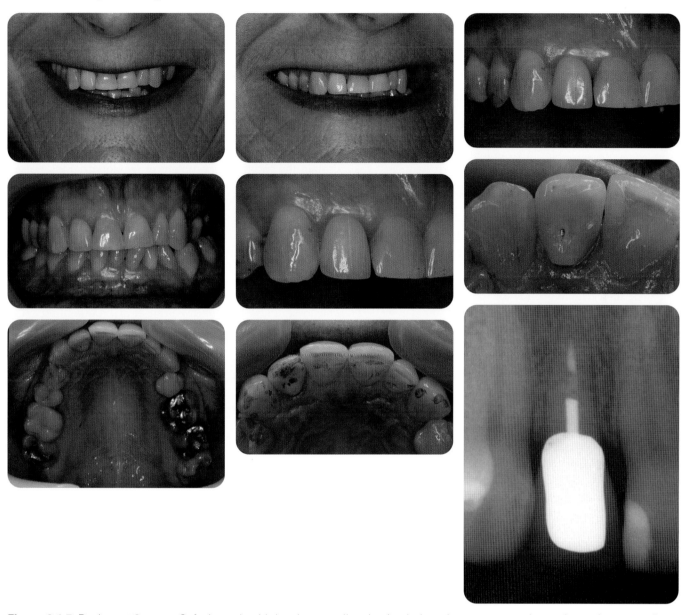

Figure 9.1.7 Review at 3 years. Soft tissue health has been well maintained; there is no apparent change in tooth wear and heavy protrusive contact is seen on the incisal edge of the crown on tooth 12. This was adjusted.

Discussion

The patient was concerned about the prognosis of tooth 12, given its history of recurrent crown loss and the patient's wish for a durable restoration. The retention problem in the absence of a root fracture was related to the structural integrity of the remaining dentine core and ferrule of the crown preparation. Fernandes *et al.* (2003) reported that teeth with carbon-fibre posts have inferior strength compared with those restored with metal posts; however, in this case the failed restoration and separated core were not available for examination.

The important aspects of treatment planning for this case were summarised by Morgano and Brackett (1999):

'The dentist should retain as much coronal tooth structure as possible when preparing pulpless teeth for complete crowns to maximise the ferrule effect. A minimal height of 1.5–2 mm of intact tooth structure above the crown margin for 360° around the circumference of the tooth preparation appears to be a rational guideline for this ferrule effect. Surgical crown lengthening or orthodontic extrusion should be considered with severely damaged teeth to expose additional tooth structure to establish a ferrule. If these provisions for developing a ferrule are impractical, extraction of the tooth and replacement with conventional or implant supported prosthodontics should be considered.'

This approach was followed.

Aesthetic evaluation by Davis (2007) indicated that the existing contours of tooth 12 were inadequate and the gingival display was excessive, compared with other maxillary anterior teeth. As a single unit restoration consideration of the gingival zenith (labial gingival height of contour) was required in relation to smile design. Davis (2007) summarised this situation:

'The gingival contours should be symmetric and the marginal gingival tissues of the maxillary anterior teeth should be located along a horizontal line extending from cuspid to cuspid. Ideally, the laterals reach slightly short of that line. It is also acceptable, although not ideal, to have the gingival height of all six anteriors equal in gingival height on the same plane. In such cases, however, the smile may appear too uniform to be aesthetically pleasing. A gingival height of the laterals that is more apical to the centrals and cuspids is considered unattractive.'

In acknowledgement of these guidelines, tooth 12 required optimising gingival contours and establishing a ferrule – with increasing the axial dimension and elevation of the labial gingival zenith (Davis 2007, Cooper 2008) while retaining the incisal edge position. Bone sounding under local anaesthetic determined the crown lengthening procedure was indicated under type I classification (Lee 2004).

In aesthetic treatment planning for implant restorations, Cooper (2008) noted that the gingival zenith:

'. . . has a remarkable influence on the morphology of the planned restoration . . . affects other objective criteria, including the balance of gingival levels (too inferior or superior), the tooth axis (too distal or mesial), the tooth dimension (too inferior or superior), and the tooth form (triangular becomes ovoid if too inferior). Without the control of the gingival zenith, the clinician's ability to define dental implant esthetics is vastly diminished.'

Although the initial option of extraction of 12 and its replacement with a single implant restoration was feasible, the aesthetic requirements led to the decision to retain the tooth and complete crown lengthening before preparation of a ferrule (Morgano & Brackett 1999) as the essential preliminary requirements to optimise the aesthetic outcome (Lee 2004).

The periodontal tissues and alveolar bone were assessed clinically and radiographically and were healthy. The endodontic prognosis was considered given the existing root filling and carbon fibre post, where orthograde retreatment was possible if the carbon fibre post and root filling could be removed. Ferrari *et al.* (2000a,b) reported a 2% endodontic failure at 4 years for teeth restored with carbon-fibre posts (Composipost) compared with 3% endodontic failure for teeth restored with cast post and core. In a separate, larger study, Ferrari *et al.* (2000b) followed up 1304 non-metallic fibre posts (three different systems) for a period of 1–6 years and recorded an overall incidence of 16 periapical lesions among the 3.2% of failures. An attempt to remove the carbon-fibre post with drill preparation was made, and only the mid-root section was removed successfully. It was decided to leave the most apical carbon-fibre post fragment *in situ*, without any further attempt at endodontic retreatment.

The options for the replacement post and core (for the mid-root and coronal regions) were a single piece (indirect cast gold alloy) and two-piece (direct prefabricated stainless steel post and composite resin core). The latter was preferred and completed after crown lengthening and crown preparation, which resulted in an adequate dentine core and minimal restoration core thickness.

Treatment was completed routinely and without complication.

At the 3-year review, the patient advised she was comfortable with the crown and pleased with her appearance. Clinical evaluation indicated increased protrusive contact and a 0.25 mm diastema between 12 crown and tooth 11. Possible causes include migration of 12 and/or wear of tooth 11. Saliva test confirmed salivary pH within normal range.

Discussion with the patient's dental general practitioner confirmed that there had been no changes to the restoration. Careful removal of the heavy protrusive contact was completed after consulting with the patient, as well as advice that this may need to be repeated.

The use of an occlusal splint was discussed but the patient advised she did not wish to proceed at this time and would consider the need at the next review.

References

Cooper, L.F. (2008) Objective criteria: Guiding and evaluating dental implant esthetics. *Journal of Esthetic and Restorative Dentistry*, 20(3), 195–205.

Davis, N.C. (2007) Smile design. *Dental Clinics of North America*, 51, 299–318.

Fernandes, A.S., Shetty, S. & Coutinho, I. (2003) Factors determining post selection: A literature review. *Journal of Prosthetic Dentistry*, 90, 556–562.

Ferrari, M., Vichi, A. & Garcia-Godoy, F. (2000a) Clinical evaluation of fiber-reinforced epoxy resin posts and cast post and cores. *American Journal of Dentistry*, 13 (Spec No.), 15B–18B.

Ferrari, M., Vichi, A., Mannocci, F. *et al.* (2000b) Retrospective study of the clinical performance of fiber posts. *American Journal of Dentistry*, 13 (Spec No.), 9B–13B.

Lee, E.A. (2004) Aesthetic crown lengthening: Classification, biologic rationale, and treatment planning considerations. *Practical Procedures & Aesthetic Dentistry*, 16(10), 769–778.

Morgano, S. & Brackett, S.E. (1999) Foundation restorations in fixed prosthodontics: Current knowledge and future needs. *Journal of Prosthetic Dentistry*, 82, 643–657.

10

Tooth Wear

Introduction by Iven Klineberg

Tooth wear unrelated to dental caries assessment and management is an integral component of treatment planning and patient care.

The cause is usually multifactorial and difficult to diagnose, which is a concern since without a diagnosis, whatever the restorative treatment selected, a poor prognosis would be expected. Furthermore, the principle of determining a diagnosis as the definitive guide for patient-specific treatment is a fundamental expectation of oral health care as well as general health management.

It is recognised that tooth wear is usually a variable combination of attrition, erosion and abrasion, the diagnosis and management of which is a key element of general restorative and specialist prosthodontic practice. Diagnosis may require interdisciplinary consultation, influence of diet and its assessment ideally from a dietitian, and saliva monitoring. Medical history details may be relevant, particularly prescription medications and their influences. Erosive tooth surface loss may have significant causes linked with gastro-oesophageal reflux disease (GORD), as well as psychological and psychiatric associations. Interdisciplinary involvement of oral medicine and/or interprofessional involvement from a physician or gastroenterologist concerning GORD, and possibly a clinical psychologist or psychiatrist especially for bulimia and anorexia nervosa, is an essential component of management.

The Bartlett group (Moazzez et al. 2004) recognise the prevalence of GORD to be 60% of the population and that in such patients erosive wear is the most significant association with tooth surface loss. Defining the specific erosive pattern was a valuable observation for GORD – greater tooth wear on the palatal surfaces of maxillary anterior teeth and on the occlusal surfaces of posterior teeth.

Monitoring erosive tooth surface loss is confusing given the varied and multiple scoring systems that have been described for evaluation. Bartlett et al. (2008) defined a basic erosive wear examination and scoring system for clinical practice and research and their response to the need for a standardised and internationally recognised evaluation system has significant implications for dentistry.

The interrelationship of attrition and bruxism – awake and sleep bruxism – usually requires interprofessional advice from a clinical psychologist, sleep physician and in some cases a neurologist to determine the aetiology of the habit leading to continual attritional wear. The emphasis on interprofessional clinical management is crucial for successful long-term outcomes.

As a clinical aid to determine the degree of severity and to monitor change over time, Bardsley (2008) has proposed and comprehensively summarised a variety of tooth wear indices. Attritional wear indices have increasing numerical values for increasing severity of tooth surface loss involving enamel alone or enamel and dentine to varying degrees, with minor changes in tooth form to severe breakdown. This latter situation results in reduction in crown height and enamel fracture, with negative impact on aesthetics. The first significant and standardised assessment tool by Smith and Knight (1984) recognised the widespread implications of tooth surface loss and its variable aetiology. Recently the Exact Tooth Wear Index (Fares et al. 2009) graded wear in enamel and dentine as interrelated surface area and depth respectively. A follow-up proposal by Bartlett (2010) described a protocol and screening tool for monitoring tooth wear as a primary role for dental practitioners. The basis for management requires clarification of the key aetiological factors over a period of time to determine an appropriate management strategy.

References

Bardsley, P.F. (2008) The evolution of tooth wear indices. *Clinical Oral Investigations*, 12 (Suppl.1), S15–S19.

Bartlett, D. (2010) A proposed system for screening tooth wear. *British Dental Journal*, 208 (5), 207–209.

Bartlett, D., Ganss, C. & Lussi, A. (2008) Basic Erosive Wear Examination (BEWE): a new scoring system for scientific and clinical needs. *Clinical Oral Investigations*, 12 (Suppl. 1), S65–S68.

Fares, J., Shirodaria, S., Chiu, K. *et al.* (2009) A new index of tooth wear. Reproducibility and application to a sample of 18- to 30-year-old university students. *Caries Research*, 43 (2), 119–125.

Moazzez, R., Bartlett, D.W. & Anggiansah, A. (2004) Dental erosion, gastro-oesophageal reflux disease and saliva: how are they related? *Journal of Dentistry*, 32 (6), 489–494.

Smith, B.G. & Knight, J.K. (1984) An index for measuring the wear of teeth. *British Dental Journal*, 156 (12), 435–438.

Case 10.1 Mr Michael M

Johnson P.Y. Chou

Patient: Mr Michael M (date of birth 16/11/1945)

Presenting complaint

Date	01/08/2007
Chief complaint	Worn teeth
Subsidiary complaints	None
History of complaints	20 years
Patient's expectations	'To stabilise the situation; to eat without problems in the future'

History
Medical history

Medical Practitioner	Dr A	
Respiratory	Nil	
Cardiovascular	Nil	
	Endocarditis	Nil
	High cholesterol	√
Gastrointestinal	Gastrointestinal reflux	√
Neurological	Depression	√
Endocrine	Nil	
Musculoskeletal	Nil	
Genitourinary	Nil	
Haematological	Nil	
	Bleeding nil	
	Immune nil	
Other	Allergies	Nil
	Smoking	Nil
	Infectious diseases	Nil
	Pregnancy	Nil
	Hospitalisation	Nil
	Medications	Dothep 75 mg daily for depression
		Nexium 20 mg daily for gastrointestinal reflux
		Lipitor 10 mg daily for high cholesterol

Social history

Marital status	Single		
Children	0		
Occupation	Landscape gardener		
Smoking	Type	Non-smoker	
Recreational drugs	No		
Diet		Soft drinks	Occasional
		Sports drinks	Nil
		Lemons	Nil
		Acidic foods	Nil
		Sweet foods	Nil
	√	Water	1 glass/day
		Tea	Nil
	√	Coffee	3 cups without sugar
	√	Alcohol	2 glasses red wine/day
		Hard/brittle foods	Nil
		Ice crunching	Nil
Habits/hobbies	√	Musical instrument	Guitar
		Exercise	Minimal
		Oral habits	Not apparent

Dental history

			Further information
Date of last examination		23/03/2007	
Oral hygiene	√	Brushing	Twice daily
	√	Flossing	Once in the morning
		Mouthwash	Nil
	√	Toothpaste	Colgate
Treatment	√	Restorations	
		Endodontics	Nil
		Periodontics	Nil
		Orthodontics	Nil
		RDP	Nil
		FDP	Nil
		TMD	Nil
		OMFS	Nil

Extraoral examination (Figures 10.1.1 & 10.1.2)
Aesthetics

Facial symmetry	Asymmetrical	
Profile	Convex	
Nasolabial angle	<90°	
Facial folds	Nil	
Midlines	Face/maxillary centrals	Coincides
	Maxillary/mandibular centrals	Coincides
Lip posture	Symmetry	Symmetrical
	Upper lip	Average
	Lower lip	Average
	Competence	Yes
	Tooth display	50% mandibular teeth
Occlusal plane	Parallel to ala tragus line	Yes
	Parallel to interpupillary line	No
	Over-eruption	15, 14, 24, 25, 26
Vertical	FWS	4–5 mm
	OVD assessment	Optimal
Smile assessment (Figure 10.1.2)	Symmetry	Yes
	Lip line	Moderate
	Gingival display	None
	Tooth display	50%
	Buccal corridor	Moderate

Phonetics

	Normal	Abnormal
Labial (m)	√	
Labiodental (f/v)	√	
Linguodental (th)	√	
Interdental (s)	√	
Linguopalatal (k/ng)	√	

Temporomandibular assessment

TMJ	Additional information
Click	Nil
Crepitus	Nil
Tenderness	Nil

Muscle tenderness	Right	Left
Temporalis	Nil	Nil
Masseter	Nil	Nil
Posterior mandible	Nil	Nil
Anterior mandible	Nil	Nil
Glands	Nil	
Nodes	Nil	

Jaw movement	Measurement (mm)	Reference points
Maximal opening	56	Tooth 11
Right laterotrusion	7	Maxillary dental midline
Left laterotrusion	10	Maxillary dental midline
Midline deviation	No	
Maximal protrusion	7	
Opening pathway	Straight	
Overjet	1	
Overbite	2	
Further investigation required	No	

Intraoral examination (Figure 10.1.3)
Soft tissues

Tissue	Healthy	Abnormal	Additional information
Lips	√		
Labial vestibule	√		
Cheeks	√		
Palate	√		
Oropharynx	√		
Tongue	√		
Floor	√		
Frenal attachments	√		

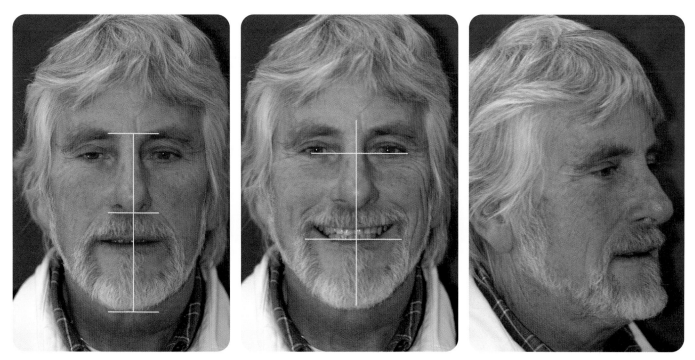

Figure 10.1.1 Extraoral examination.

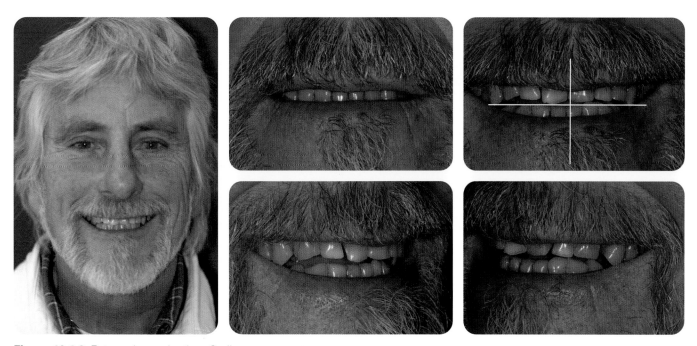

Figure 10.1.2 Extraoral examination. Smile assessment.

Oral cleanliness

Condition	Yes	No			
Plaque	√		Localised	Mild	Supragingival
Calculus	√		Localised	Moderate	Supragingival + subgingival
Food impaction		√			
Stains		√			
Halitosis		√			

Saliva (Figure 10.1.4)

Water intake	1 glass/day
Quality	Moderate
Quantity	Low
Pathology	No
Medications affecting	Dothep (antidepressant)
Further investigation required	No

Periodontium

CPITN

0	0	0
2	2	2

Gingiva	Biotype	Thick
	Colour	Pink
	Contour	Normal
	Consistency	Firm
Papillae	Colour	Pink
	Contour	Normal

Occlusion

Skeletal classification	Class I		
Dental occlusion	Class I		
Angle right	Molar I	Canine	Class I
Angle left	Molar I	Canine	Class I
Anterior overbite	1 mm		
Anterior overjet	2 mm		
Cross-bites	No		
Open-bites	No		
Curve of Spee	RHS+	LHS+	
Curve of Wilson	+		
RP to IP slide	0 mm		
FWS	Close/M/swallow test	4–5 mm	

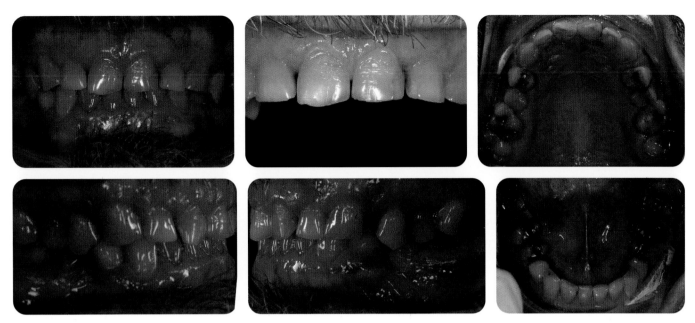

Figure 10.1.3 Intraoral examination. Note generalised mild to moderate tooth wear.

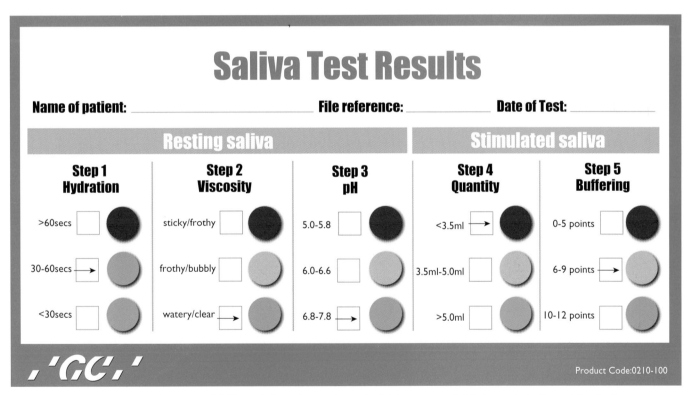

Figure 10.1.4 Saliva test (GC test) and SCL-90-R (psychometric analysis) (courtesy of GC Australasia Dental Pty Ltd).

Tooth guidance

Right laterotrusion

8 7 6 5 4 3 2 1 | 1 2 3 4 5 6 7 8

8 7 6 5 4 3 2 1   1 2 3 4 5 6 7 8

Left laterotrusion

8 7 6 5 4 3 2 1 | 1 2 3 4 5 6 7 8

8 7 6 5 4 3 2 1   1 2 3 4 5 6 7 8

Protrusion

8 7 6 5 4 3 2 1 | 1 2 3 4 5 6 7 8

8 7 6 5 4 3 2 1   1 2 3 4 5 6 7 8

Tooth surface loss

Caries

8 7 6 5 4 3 2 1 | 1 2 3 4 5 6 7 8

8 7 6 5 4 3 2 1   1 2 3 4 5 6 7 8

Attrition

8 7 6 5 4 3 2 1 | 1 2 3 4 5 6 7 8

8 7 6 5 4 3 2 1   1 2 3 4 5 6 7 8

Erosion

8 7 6 5 4 3 2 1 | 1 2 3 4 5 6 7 8

8 7 6 5 4 3 2 1   1 2 3 4 5 6 7 8

Abrasion

8 7 6 5 4 3 2 1 | 1 2 3 4 5 6 7 8

8 7 6 5 4 3 2 1   1 2 3 4 5 6 7 8

Abfraction

8 7 6 5 4 3 2 1 | 1 2 3 4 5 6 7 8

8 7 6 5 4 3 2 1   1 2 3 4 5 6 7 8

Dental charting

Tooth no.	Clinical findings	Comments
18	Missing	
17	Amalgam – small O TSL: mild attrition + mild erosion	Good prognosis
16	Amalgam – small OP TSL: mild attrition + mild erosion	Good prognosis
15	TSL: mild attrition + mild erosion	Good prognosis
14	Amalgam – small O TSL: moderate attrition + mild erosion + mild abrasion	Good prognosis
13	Composite: small I TSL: moderate attrition + moderate erosion + mild abrasion	Good prognosis
12	TSL: moderate attrition + moderate erosion + mild abrasion	Good prognosis
11	Composite: small M TSL: moderate attrition + moderate erosion + mild abrasion	Good prognosis
21	Composite: small D TSL: moderate attrition + moderate erosion + mild abrasion	Good prognosis
22	Composite: small M TSL: moderate attrition + moderate erosion + mild abrasion	Good prognosis

Tooth no.	Clinical findings	Comments
23	Composite: small I TSL: moderate attrition + moderate erosion + mild abrasion	Good prognosis
24	TSL: moderate attrition + moderate erosion + mild abrasion	Good prognosis
25	Amalgam – small MO TSL: moderate attrition + moderate erosion	Good prognosis
26	Amalgam – small O TSL: moderate attrition + moderate erosion	Good prognosis (requires crown lengthening on the distal)
27	Amalgam – medium OB TSL: moderate attrition + moderate erosion	Good prognosis (requires crown lengthening on the mesial + distal)
28	Missing	
38	Missing	
37	Amalgam: medium O + small B TSL: mild attrition	Good prognosis (requires crown lengthening on the distal)
36	Amalgam: medium MO + small B TSL: mild attrition	Good prognosis (Requires crown lengthening on the buccal)
35	Amalgam: medium MOD TSL: mild attrition	Good prognosis (Requires crown lengthening on the buccal)
34	TSL: mild attrition	Good prognosis
33	TSL: mild–moderate attrition	Good prognosis
32	TSL: mild–moderate attrition	Good prognosis
31	TSL: mild–moderate attrition	Good prognosis
41	TSL: mild–moderate attrition	Good prognosis
42	TSL: mild–moderate attrition	Good prognosis
43	TSL: mild–moderate attrition	Good prognosis
44	TSL: attrition + abrasion TSL: mild attrition	Good prognosis
45	Amalgam: medium DO TSL: mild attrition	Good prognosis
46	Amalgam: large MO TSL: moderate attrition + moderate erosion	Good prognosis
47	Amalgam: medium O + small B TSL: attrition	Good prognosis (Requires crown lengthening on the distal)
48	Missing	

Special tests

Test	Performed	Additional information
Percussion	√	All not tender to percussion test
Vitality	√	All positive to cold test

Radiographs (Figure 10.1.5)
Orthopantomogram (06/08/2007)

Features	Radiographic data
TMJ	No pathology
Bone loss	No
Sinuses	No pathology
Mandibular canal	Visualised
Mental foramen	Visualised
Retained roots	No
Pathology	No

Periapical films (06/08/2007 Figure 10.1.6)

Tooth no.	Information	Tooth no.	Information
18	Missing	38	Missing
17	Unrestored	37	Amalgam: small O
16	Amalgam: small O	36	Amalgam: medium MO
15	Unrestored	35	Amalgam: medium DO
14	Amalgam: small O	34	Unrestored
13	Composite: small I	33	Unrestored
12	Unrestored	32	Composite: small I
11	Composite: small M	31	Composite: small I
21	Composite: small D	41	Composite: small I
22	Composite: small M	42	Unrestored
23	Composite: small I	43	Unrestored
24	Unrestored	44	Composite: small B
25	Amalgam: small MO	45	Amalgam: medium MOD encroaching on pulp
26	Amalgam: small O	46	Amalgam: medium MO
27	Amalgam: medium to large OB	47	Amalgam: medium O
28	Missing	48	Missing

Study casts (Figure 10.1.7)

Articulation	Position	RCP
	Face bow	Yes
Diagnostic wax-up	OVD change	+3mm (Figure 10.1.7b)
	Occlusal adjustment	Reduction of 15, 14, 24, 25, 26
	Crown lengthening	26D, 27M + D, 37D, 36B, 35B, 47D

Diagnosis

Medical
- Depression, taking Dothep.
- High cholesterol, taking Lipitor (prescribed June 2009).
- Uncontrolled gastrointestinal reflux (referral to gastro-enterologist was made and Nexium was then prescribed) (Figure 10.1.8).

Biomechanical
- Defective restoration: 37.
- Structural compromises: short clinical crown length on 26 distal, 27 mesial + distal, 37 distal, 36 buccal, 35 buccal and 47 distal.
- Generalised mild to moderate erosion due to GORD.

Functional
- Generalised mild to moderate attrition.
- Decreased occlusal vertical dimension.

Aesthetic
- Incisal length: incisal edge configuration of 13–23 are short of lower lip line and 15, 14, 24, 25, 26 extends over lower lip line.
- Proportions of central incisors: short.
- Tooth to tooth proportions: not ideal.

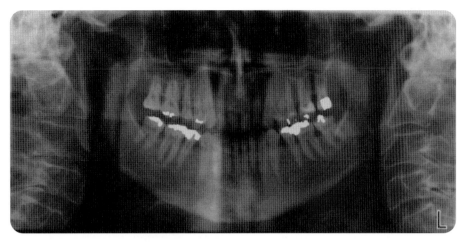

Figure 10.1.5 Preoperative radiograph. Panoramic radiograph.

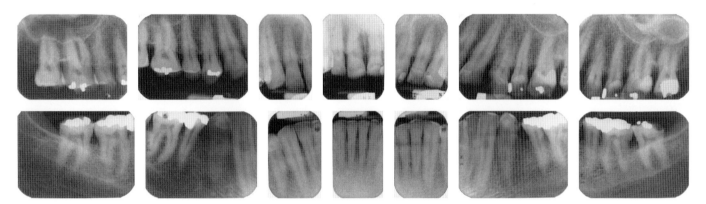

Figure 10.1.6 Preoperative radiographs. Periapical radiographs.

(a)

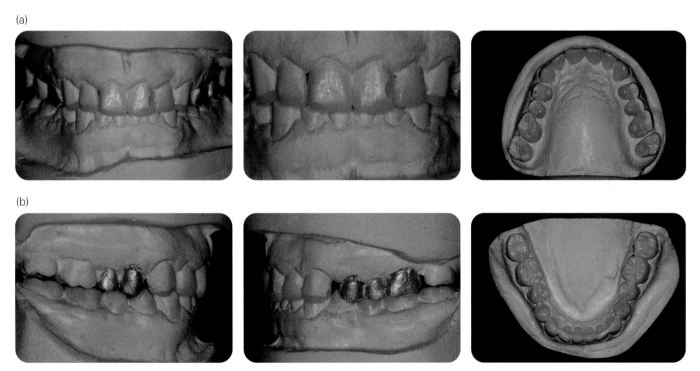

(b)

Figure 10.1.7 (a) Preoperative study casts. (b) Diagnostic wax-up.

PANENDOSCOPY REPORT

23rd October 2007

Endoscopy

Mr Moss presents with damage to his teeth consistent with acid erosion. He reports reflux symptoms since childhood which has not previously been treated.

ENDOSCOPIC FINDINGS

Gastroscopy was performed to the third part of the d. Jenum. There was a short segment of Barrett's oesophagus within the distal oesophagus. There was no active inflammation. The stomach and duodenum appeared otherwise macroscopically normal. There was a very small hiatal hernia formation.

SUMMARY/RECOMMENDATIONS:

I will commence Mr Moss on proton pump inhibitors to suppress his acid. I will give him a booklet on conservative measures to reduce reflux. If Helicobacter is present he should start a course of eradication therapy.

In view of the presence of the Barrett's oesophagus I would recommend follow up gastroscopy in two years.

WARWICK ADAMS MBBS MS FRACS
COLORECTAL SURGEON

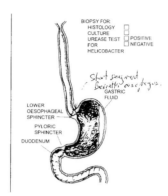

Figure 10.1.8 Uncontrolled gastrointestinal reflux (referral to gastroenterologist and Nexium was prescribed).

Problem list

Problem list	Details
Medical condition	Depression High cholesterol Gastrointestinal reflux
Aesthetics	Incisal edge configuration of 13–23 are short of lower lip line and 15, 14, 24, 25, 26 extend over lower lip line Tooth form not ideal Gingival outline not symmetrical
Speech	None
TMD	None
Soft tissue	None
Oral hygiene	None
Saliva	Low water intake Medications affecting saliva: antidepressant Low quantity and moderate quality of stimulated saliva
Periodontal	None
Edentulism	None
Occlusion	Occlusal plane discrepancy: decreased Spee + increased Wilson Decreased occlusal vertical dimension
Tooth surface loss	Generalised mild to moderate attrition on remaining dentition Localised mild to moderate erosion Localised mild abrasion
Restorative	Defective restoration on tooth 37
Prosthetic	None
Endodontic	None

Treatment goals

Short-term
- Control of disease:
  - behavioural management;
    - diet counselling (increase water intake) + oral hygiene advice;
  - chemical control and protection;
    - bicarbonate rinse straight after reflux;
  - medical: referral to gastroenterologist (see Figure 10.1.8).
- Protect remaining teeth:
  - monitoring: study models and photographs.

Long-term
- Improve facial aesthetics.
- Increase occlusal vertical dimension.
- Correct the occlusal plane: will be part of improving aesthetics.
- Restore function and maintain occlusal stability.
- Protect remaining teeth.

Treatment options

Option 1
Direct restorative materials using composite for anterior teeth and amalgam for posterior teeth to increase occlusal vertical dimension.

Option 2
Direct restorative materials using composite for anterior teeth and amalgam for posterior teeth to increase occlusal vertical dimension and 11 strategic crowns on canines and molars to maintain occlusal stability (gold crowns or onlays on teeth 16, 26, 27, 37, 36, 46, 47; CMCs on teeth 13, 23, 35, 45).

Option 3
Direct restorative materials using composite for mandibular anterior teeth and crowns (gold crowns or onlays on teeth 16, 26, 27, 37, 36, 46, 47; CMCs on teeth 35, 45; all-ceramic crowns [ACCs] on teeth 13, 12, 11, 21, 22, 23] and 2 CEREC onlays (15, 25) to maintain occlusal stability and aesthetics.

Treatment plan and discussion
Patient accepted option 3 for the following reasons:

- maxillary and mandibular dentition have a good prognosis;
- increase in occlusal vertical dimension to increase restorative space;
- composite resin to restore maxillary and mandibular anterior teeth (regular maintenance visits are required);
- crowns to provide key supporting teeth for long-term occlusal and jaw stability.

Tooth prognosis
- Restorability.

Libman and Nicholls (1995), in an *in-vitro* study, showed that a circumferential 1.5 mm ferrule provides 70 times increase in resistance form against crown marginal opening than a 1.0 mm ferrule.

Outcomes of direct restorative material
Posterior teeth
Use of amalgam has better survival compared to composite especially microfill composite. Plasmans *et al.* (1998) conducted a randomised clinical trial of 300 extensive amalgam restorations and reported survival of 88%, with more prone to failure due to oral hygiene, in the older group than in the younger group.

Barlett and Sundaram (2006) conducted a short-term (up to 3 years) survival of 58 direct or indirect microfilled (Heliomolar) composite restorations in patients with severe tooth wear and without tooth wear. They found 50% survival in the severe tooth wear group and 80% survival in the group with no evidence of tooth wear. They concluded that the use of direct/indirect composite for restoring worn posterior teeth is contraindicated.

Anterior teeth
Use of hybrid composite resins in the anterior regions has good short- to medium-term survival; microfill composites have high failure rates.

Poyser *et al.* (2007) conducted a short-term 2.5 year prospective clinical trial on survival of 133 direct Herculite XR restorations in two groups (circumferential preparation versus no preparation) in patients with tooth wear. They found 6% failure and no differences between groups. They concluded that direct composite restorations placed at an increased occlusal vertical dimension are a simple and time-efficient method of managing the worn mandibular teeth.

Redman *et al.* (2003) conducted a short-term retrospective clinical trial on survival of 225 composite restorations (Artglass, Herculite direct/indirect, Durafill) in patients with tooth wear. They found major failure requiring replacement of the restoration was uncommon within the first 5 years. Median survival was 4 years and 9 months. They concluded the placement of resin-based composite restorations at an increased vertical dimension to treat localised anterior tooth wear has good short- to medium-term survival.

Hemmings *et al.* (2000) conducted a short-term 30 month prospective clinical trial on survival of 104 restorations in two groups (Durafill versus Herculite) in patients with tooth wear. They found microfill had 33/52 failures and hybrid 6/52 failures. They concluded direct composite restorations may be a treatment option for localised anterior tooth wear.

Outcomes of single tooth supported indirect restorative materials
Crowns were chosen on the posterior and anterior teeth to stabilise the occlusion and provide guidance in

eccentric jaw movement. ACCs and CMCs have comparable short-term survival rate.

Goodacre *et al.* (2003) conducted a review and found eight studies with a total of 1476 CMCs followed up to an average duration of 6 years (between 1 and 23 years) – a mean complication rate of 11%. The three most common complications were: need for endodontic treatment (3%); porcelain veneer fracture (3%); and loss of retention (2%). There was a mean complication rate of 8% for ACCs from 22 studies of 4277 crowns with a mean follow-up period of 4 years (range 1 month to 14 years). The three most common complications encountered with ACCs were: crown fracture (7%), loss of retention (2%), and need for endodontic treatment (1%).

Pjetursson *et al.* (2007) conducted a systematic review of 34 studies of 5-year survival rates of CMCs and ACCs. They concluded that survival rates at 5 years were comparable for CMCs and ACCs when used for anterior teeth (93.3% and 95.6%, respectively). When used for posterior teeth, densely sintered alumina crowns (94.9%) and reinforced glass–ceramic crowns (93.7%) were similar to those obtained for CMCs. Lower survival rates of 90.4% and 84.4% can be expected for In-Ceram crowns and glass–ceramic crowns.

However, this study did not include zirconia crowns and mean exposure times for CMCs was almost twice as long as for ACCs (9.12 versus 4.9 years).

Conrad *et al.* (2007) conducted a systematic review on current ceramic materials and systems and included 23 studies comprising 19 prospective and four retrospective studies. They found multiple all-ceramic materials and systems are available for clinical use and there is no one single material or system for all clinical situations. These authors concluded that the successful application is dependent upon the clinician matching the materials, manufacturing techniques and cementation or bonding procedures with the individual clinical situation.

Crown lengthening

The principle in crown lengthening for restorative cases is to surgically reduce the bone crest to a more apical position to provide sufficient coronal tooth structure for retention of restoration or to improve aesthetics, while allowing space for re-establishment of a new biological width.

Gargiulo *et al.* (1961) examined 287 individual teeth from 30 autopsy specimens and found a mean biological width of 2.04 mm. This dimension comprised the epithelial attachment of 0.97 mm and connective tissue attachment of 1.07 mm.

Vacek *et al.* (1994) examined 171 individual teeth from 10 autopsy specimens and found a mean biological width dimension of 1.91 mm. Data suggest that the biological width has a range of 0.75–4.33 mm.

With respect to healing time after crown lengthening, of direct clinical importance is the stability of the postoperative position of the gingival margin. In non-aesthetic areas, the patient should be re-evaluated 6 weeks post-surgery prior to continuing with final restorative procedures. In the anterior aesthetic zone, a longer healing period is recommended.

Wise (1985) conducted a prospective study to examine 15 patients with 15 anterior teeth requiring crown lengthening and crowns. The gingival height from the temporary crown was measured postoperatively at intervals of 4, 6 and 8 weeks and every 4 weeks after, up to 24 weeks. They found rapid shrinkage occurred between 6 and 12 weeks. A gradual apical movement followed and reached a mean of 0.9 mm at 20 weeks postoperatively. They concluded that definitive crown preparation should not be made for at least 20 weeks after surgery.

Pontoriero and Carnevale (2001) conducted a prospective study to examine 30 patients with 84 teeth requiring crown lengthening. They followed teeth for 12 months and found that marginal periodontal tissues showed a tendency to grow in a coronal direction from the level defined at surgery and that this pattern of coronal displacement of the gingival margin was more pronounced in patients with thick tissue bio-type.

Treatment sequence

Phase	Procedure
Initial therapy	Preventive advice: • diet counselling: increase water intake + referral to gastroenterologist to investigate gastrointestinal reflux • chemical control and protection: bicarbonate rinse straight after reflux • monitoring: study models and photographs Scaling, root planning, oral hygiene instructions: • mechanical debridement of plaque and calculus deposits adherent to the clinical crowns and roots of teeth or restorative materials both supra- and subgingivally • oral hygiene instruction Direct build-up of anterior and posterior teeth to correct occlusal plane and enhance aesthetics (Figure 10.1.9) Re-evaluation: • establish prognosis of the remaining teeth • function and aesthetics • occlusion • phonetics • mucogingival considerations • emergence profile
Surgical and corrective therapy	Surgical tooth lengthening of tooth 26M, 27M + D, 35B, 36B, 37D and 47D (Figure 10.1.10): • to improve the tooth's biomechanical profile • to enhance retention and resistance form
Prosthetic phase (Figures 10.1.11 & 10.1.12)	11 strategic gold/CMCs/ACCs + gold onlays (16, 13, 23, 26, 27, 37, 36, 35, 45, 46, 47) + 1 CEREC onlay (25) to maintain occlusal stability 4 additional crowns to maintain aesthetics (12, 11, 21, 22)
Maintenance	Maintenance + monitoring + recall

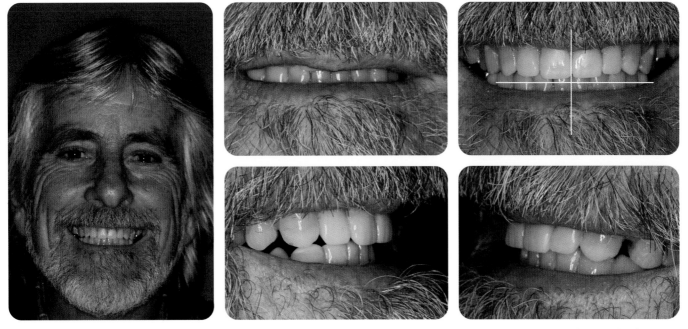

Figure 10.1.9 Operative photographs. Direct build-up of anterior and posterior teeth to correct the occlusal plane and enhance aesthetics.

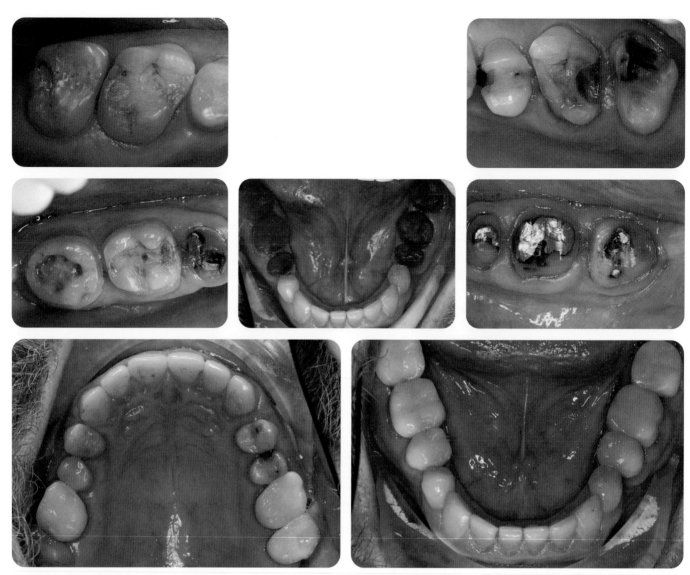

Figure 10.1.10 Operative photographs. Onlay and crown preparations performed on posterior teeth after surgical tooth lengthening of tooth 26M, 27M + D, 35B, 36B, 37D and 47D.

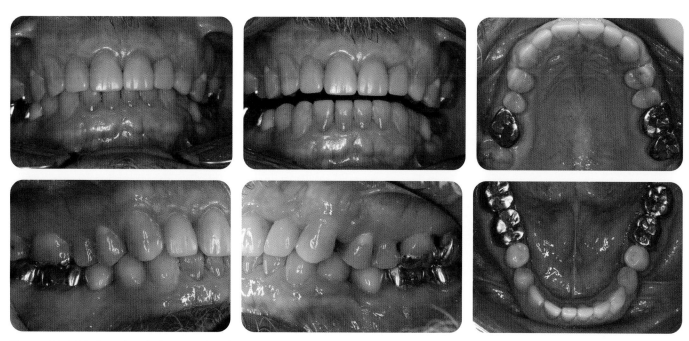

Figure 10.1.11 Completed photographs. Posterior onlays and crowns.

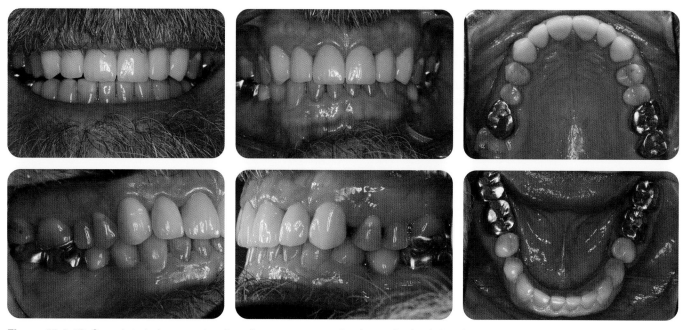

Figure 10.1.12 Completed photographs. Anterior crowns to maintain aesthetics (13–23).

Informed consent

- Benefits:
  - improvement of aesthetics;
  - protect remaining tooth structure .
- Alternatives:
  - no treatment;
  - direct restorative materials using amalgam for posterior teeth and composite for anterior teeth.
- Benefits of treatment:
  - treatment time;
  - provisional restorations will be made during treatment;
  - longevity of the restorations;
  - cost of the treatment.
- Complications:
  - conventional crown and bridges:
    - biological: need for endodontic treatment, caries, periodontal disease, tooth fracture, exposed margin causing poor aesthetics;
    - technical: loss of retention, fracture of materials.
- Maintenance:
  - regular dental visits on a 4–6 monthly basis.

Review at 1 year (Figures 10.1.13, 10.1.14 & 10.1.16)

Oral health status (Figure 10.1.14)
- Oral hygiene and plaque control: *good oral hygiene.*
- Soft tissue health: *no gingival inflammation.*
- Check on home-care programme and advise on frequency of brushing, use of dental floss and mouth rinses: *use of dental floss once a day and brushes twice daily.*
- Note and record recurrent dental caries associated with restorations or new carious lesions: *no new carious lesions.*
- Note periodontal status – check probing depths and record changes; new posterior to anterior (PA) radiographs to check alveolar bone levels (see below): *no changes in periodontal status.*

Occlusion (Figure 10.1.15)
- Check tooth contacts with GHM foil at intercuspal position, retruded contact position, lateral and protrusive excursive contacts – note lateral contact details: *right and left canine guidance.*
- Especially where there is a fracture of restorative material – record, photograph fracture and contact details with GHM foil and comment on reason for fracture.

Radiographs (Figure 10.1.16)
- 1 year review PA views for specific details of the status of crowns on teeth and implants. Check crown margins and alveolar bone levels; measure thread exposure to bone crest around implants and correlate with clinical details as above: *new OPG taken – no radiographic change apparent.*
- At 2 years an OPG may add global information.

Patient discussion
Discuss oral health related quality of life – comfort, appearance; function – chewing and speech; whether there has been a change in confidence, social interaction and relationships. *Patient more confident with this oral reconstruction.*

Feedback
Seek any additional comments from the patient about the treatment and whether they would undertake the process again if needed. *Very pleased with the treatment and the pain control is excellent (very little during the whole treatment). Patient would undertake the process again if needed.*

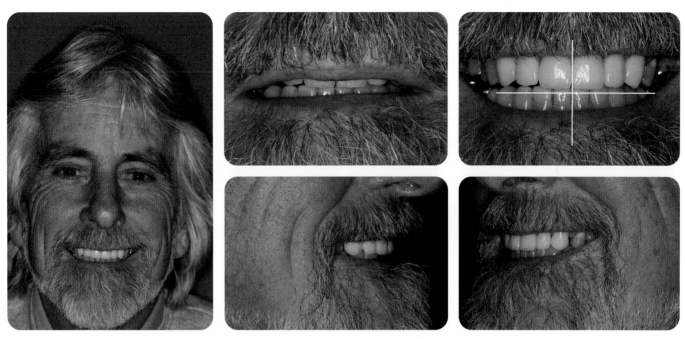

Figure 10.1.13 One-year postoperative extraoral photographs. Smile assessment.

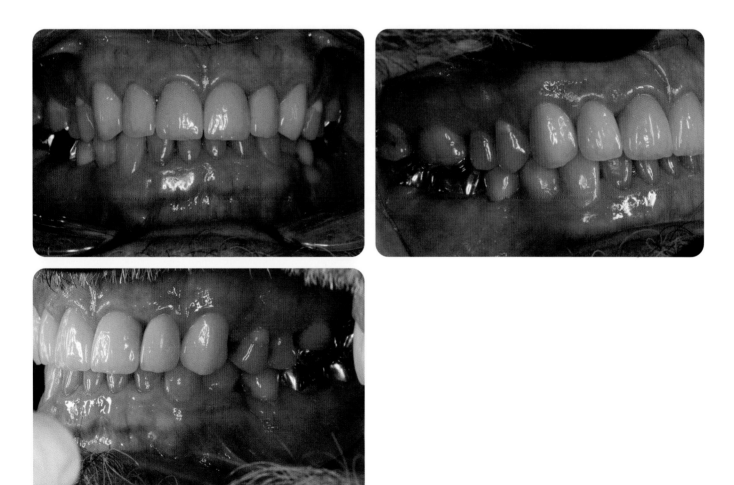

Figure 10.1.14 One-year postoperative intraoral photographs.

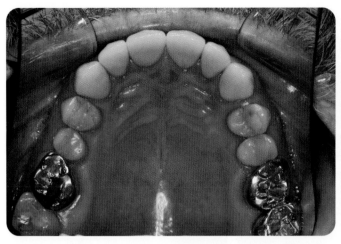 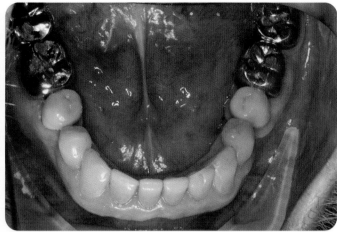

Figure 10.1.15 One-year postoperative intraoral photographs.

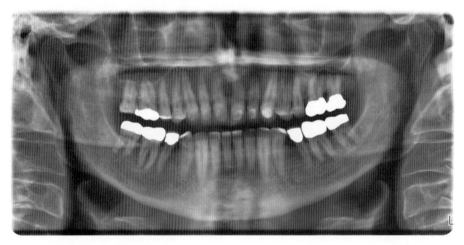

Figure 10.1.16 One-year postoperative radiographs.

References

Barlett, D. & Sundaram, G. (2006) An up to 3-year randomised clinical study comparing indirect and direct resin composites used to restore worn posterior teeth. *International Journal of Prosthodontics*, 19 (6), 613–617.

Conrad, H.J., Seong, W.J. & Pesun, I.J. (2007) Current ceramic materials and systems with clinical recommendations: a systematic review. *Journal of Prosthetic Dentistry*, 98 (5), 389–404.

Gargiulo, A.W., Wentz, F.M. & Orban, B. (1961) Dimensions and relations of the dentogingival junction in humans. *Journal of Periodontology*, 32 (3), 261–267.

Goodacre, C.J., Bernal, G., Rungcharassaeng, K. *et al.* (2003) Clinical complications in fixed prosthodontics. *Journal of Prosthetic Dentistry*, 90 (1), 31–41.

Hemmings, K.W., Darbar, U.R. & Vaughan, S. (2000) Tooth wear treated with direct composite restorations at an increased vertical dimension: results at 30 months. *Journal of Prosthetic Dentistry*, 83 (3), 287–293.

Libman, W.J. & Nicholls, J.I. (1995) Load fatigue of teeth restored with cast posts and cores and complete crown. *International Journal of Prosthodontics*, 8 (2), 155–161.

Pjetursson, B.E., Sailer, I., Zwahlen, M. *et al.* (2007) A systematic review of the survival and complication rates of all-ceramic and metal–ceramic reconstructions after an observation period of at least 3 years. Part I: single crowns. *Clinical Oral Implants Research*, 18 (Suppl. 3), 73–85.

Plasmans, P.J., Creugers, N.H. & Mulder, J. (1998) Long-term survival of extensive amalgam restorations. *Journal of Dental Research*, 77 (3), 453–460.

Pontoriero, R. & Carnevale, G. (2001) Surgical crown lengthening: a 12-month clinical wound healing study. *Journal of Periodontology*, 72 (7), 841–848.

Poyser, N.J., Briggs, P.F., Chana, H.S. *et al.* (2007) The evaluation of direct composite restorations for the worn mandibular anterior dentition – clinical performance and patient satisfaction. *Journal of Oral Rehabilitation*, 34 (5), 361–376.

Redman, C.D., Hemmings, K.W. & Good, J.A. (2003) The survival and clinical performance of resin-based composite restorations used to treat localised anterior tooth wear. *British Dental Journal*, 194 (10), 566–572.

Vacek, J.S., Gher, M.E., Assad, D.A. *et al.* (1994) The dimensions of the human dentogingival junction. *International Journal of Periodontics & Restorative Dentistry*, 14 (2), 154–165.

Wise, M.D. (1985) Stability of gingival crest after surgery and before crown placement. *Journal of Prosthetic Dentistry*, 53 (1), 20–23.

Case 10.2 Mr Graeme S

Max Guazzato

Patient: Mr Graeme S (date of birth 04/08/1952)

Presenting complaint

Description	'. . . with my teeth in general, I find it difficult to chew and eat; I can eat only on one side (right) and only in one position. I can't eat steak, nuts and muesli. I believe that I am grinding a lot and sometimes I wake up and know that I was grinding my teeth'
Onset	'I looked back at old family photos where I could see my teeth in the photos and I think that I started grinding at the age of 20'
Frequency	'Constantly. I got used to having shorter teeth and some missing teeth'
Duration	'For as long as I remember'
Intensity	N/A
Triggering	N/A
Aggravating	N/A
Alleviating	N/A
Treatment received	'I have had only general dentistry treatment. I saw a dentist only if I had a tooth ache. I've had extractions, I've had a number of root canals; most of the teeth that had root canals were then later extracted. I had an implant inserted in 2000 and I never went back to have the crown placed. I went into a dental surgery and had a tooth extracted urgently and an implant was placed at the same time without asking my consent'
Medication	Nil
Allergies	Nil

Other complaints

Function	'Limited chewing, only on one point'
TMD	Grinding
Headaches	Occasionally
Parafunction	NAD
Habits	Grinding
Cervical	Nil
Dental	'Sensitivity in the large posterior fillings, I have to use Sensodyne all the time'
Periodontal	Nil
Dentures	Nil
Splint	Nil
Saliva	Nil
Breathe	Nose breather but through mouth when I have hayfever, depending on season
Cosmetic	'I would like to see my teeth when I smile'

Patient's expectations
- To be able to eat comfortably.
- To have good aesthetic outcome.
- To be able to see more teeth when talking and smiling.
- To be able to smile.

History
Medical history

General Practitioner	I have not seen a doctor for several years. Only for colds and flu
Cardiovascular	Nil
Respiratory	Nil
Gastrointestinal	Nil
Neurological	Nil
Endocrine	Nil
Haematological	Nil
Integumentary	Nil
Genitourinary	Nil
Musculoskeletal	Nil
Immune system	Nil
Allergies	Nil
Operations	Broken bones, a number of skin cancers removed on back and nose
Trauma	Broken arm
Medication	Nil

Social history

Marital status	Married	
Children	2 children and 1 grandchild	
Occupation	Electrician	
Recreational drugs	Nil	
Smoking	Type	Nil
	Frequency	Nil
	Period	N/A
Diet	Not able to chew hard food (nuts, muesli and steak)	
	Soft drinks	Nil
	Sports drinks	Nil
	Lemons	Nil
	Acidic foods	Nil
	√ Sweet foods	Desserts in general
	√ Water	0.75 L/day
	√ Tea	3 cups herbal tea with 1 sugar/day
	√ Coffee	1 cup with 1 sugar/day
	√ Alcohol	Beer and wine socially
	Hard/brittle foods	Nil
	Ice crunching	Nil
Habits/hobbies	Motorbike riding	

Dental history

Date of last examination	2006 'I knew that problems were occurring, especially pain, but I did not want to see a dentist'
Oral hygiene routine	Brushes 1–2 times/day Uses a soft electric brush Floss daily
TMD	Nil
Splint	Nil
OMFS	Nil
Extractions	All teeth in past extracted by a variety of general dentists. Teeth extracted as they were unrestorable
Dentures	Nil
Orthodontics	Nil
Periodontics	Nil
Endodontics	RCT of 12, 26, 42 and 47
Crown and bridge	Nil
Implants	In 2000 during an emergency appointment tooth 24 was extracted and an implant was inserted without consent
Cosmetic	Nil
Other	Nil

Extraoral examination (Figures 10.2.1 & 10.2.2)
Aesthetics

Head and neck	Scar/skin graft on nose due to skin cancer, basal cell carcinomas removed also from the neck and back	
Facial symmetry	Symmetrical	
Profile	Straight	
Nasolabial angle	95° obtuse	
Facial folds	WNL	
Midlines	Face/maxillary centrals	Coincident
	Maxillary/mandibular centrals	Coincident
Lip posture	Symmetry	Symmetrical
	Upper lip	Normal and competent
	Lower lip	Normal
	Competence	Yes
	Tooth display	0 mm
Occlusal plane	Parallel to ala tragus line	Not parallel, inverted curve of Spee
	Parallel to interpupillary line	Lower on LHS due to 44 and 26 over-eruption
	Over-eruption	16, 26, 37, 44
Vertical	FWS	10 mm
	OVD assessment	OVD is in general reduced, with signs of angular cheilitis OVD in CO = 65 mm OVD in CR = 75 mm
Smile assessment	Symmetry	Yes
	Lip line	Low
	Gingival display	Nil
	Tooth display	Only the incisal edge of the maxillary teeth and the occlusal/incisal surface of the mandibular teeth
	Buccal corridor	Normal

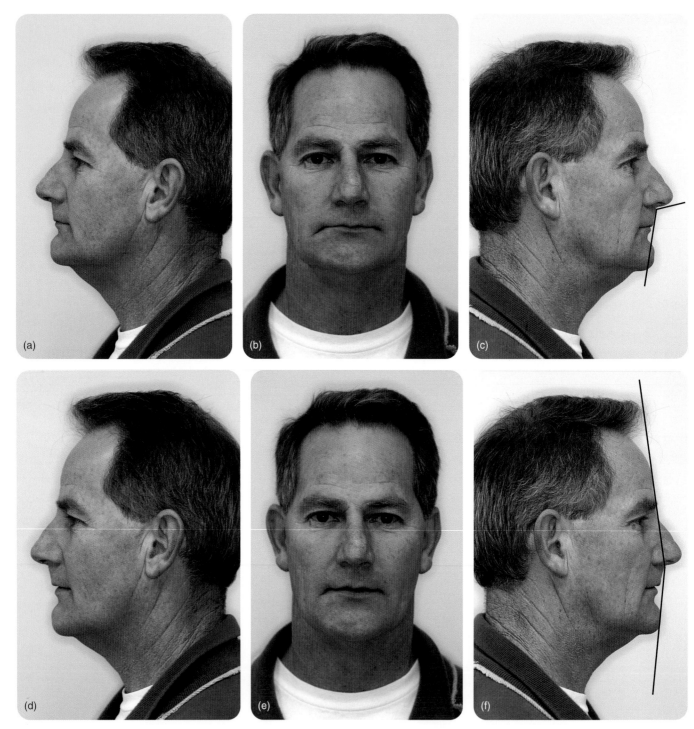

Figure 10.2.1 Extraoral examination: patient in intercuspal position showing reduced occlusal vertical dimension and normal nasolabial curve (a–c); patient in postural position (d–f).

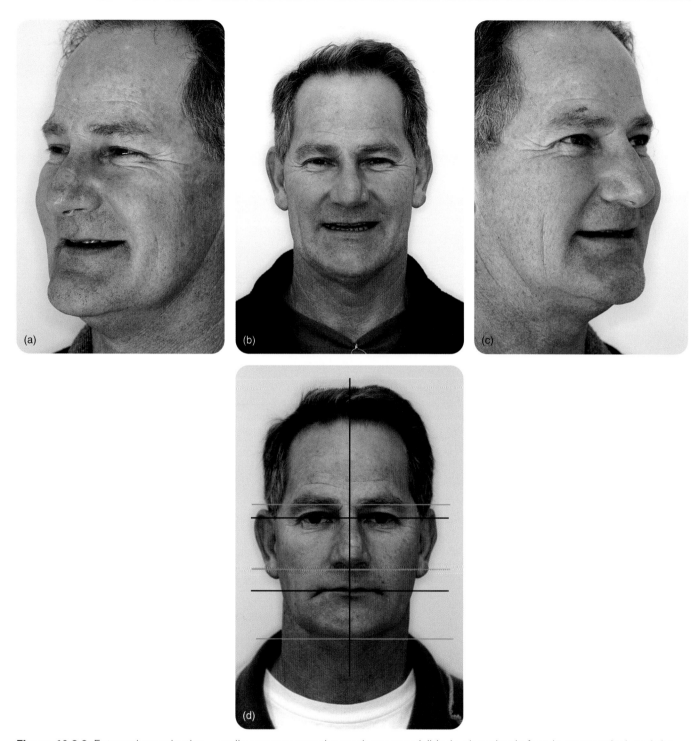

Figure 10.2.2 Extraoral examination – smile assessment: the teeth are not visible (a–c); patient's face is symmetrical; and the lower facial third appeared to be slightly reduced (d).

Phonetics

	Normal	Abnormal
Labial (m)	√	
Labiodental (f/v)	√	
Linguodental (th)	√	
Interdental (s)	√	
Linguopalatal (k/ng)	√	

Temporomandibular assessment

TMJ		Additional information
Click	Nil	
Crepitus	Nil	
Tenderness	Nil	

Muscle tenderness	Right	Left
Temporalis	Nil	Nil
Masseter	Nil	Nil
Posterior mandible	Nil	Nil
Anterior mandible	Nil	Nil
Glands	Nil	Nil
Nodes	Nil	Nil

Jaw movement	Measurement (mm)	Reference points
Maximal opening	55	Tooth 11
Right laterotrusion	18	Maxillary dental midline
Left laterotrusion	15	Maxillary dental midline
Midline deviation	1 mm right	
Maximal protrusion	11	
Opening pathway	Straight	
Overjet	5	
Overbite	3	

Intraoral examination (Figure 10.2.3)
Soft tissues

Tissue	Healthy	Abnormal	Additional information
Lips		√	Angular cheilitis
Labial vestibule	√		
Cheeks	√		
Palate	√		
Oropharynx	√		
Tongue	√		
Floor	√		
Frenal attachments	√		

Ridges	Maxilla	Mandible
Edentulous areas	18, 17, 15, 27, 28	37, 36, 45, 46, 35, 42 45, 46
Arch shape	Moderate V	Moderate V
Resorption	Mild	Mild
Palatal vault	Moderate	
Tori	Nil	Lingual premolar regions
Frenal attachments	Average	Average
Mucosa	Normal	Mild hyperkeratosis
Pathology	Nil	Nil

Oral cleanliness

Condition	Yes	No			
Plaque	√		Generalised	Severe	Supragingival + subgingival
Calculus	√		Localised	Mild	Supragingival + subgingival
Food impaction		√			
Stains	√				
Halitosis	√				

Saliva

Water intake	0.75 L/day; 2–3 cups tea/day; 1 cup coffee/day
Quality	WNL; pH 6.8; buffer test 12; watery
Quantity	WNL; 6 ml in 5 minute test
Pathology	Nil
Medications affecting	Nil

Periodontium
CPITN

2	2	2
2	2	2

Gingiva	Biotype	Medium
	Colour	Pink with localised areas of inflammation and redness
	Contour	Normal
	Consistency	Firm
Papillae	Colour	Pink with localised areas of inflammation and redness
	Contour	Normal

Periodontal charting

A full periodontal charting was carried out and there was no evidence of bleeding on probing or periodontal inflammation; pocket depth was 2–3 mm, presenting a healthy periodontal status.

Occlusal assessment

Arch compatibility	Sufficiently compatible arches with significant posterior and anterior overjet		
Occlusal plane	Curve of Spee	RHS –	LHS –
	Curve of Wilson	RHS –	LHS –
Posterior support	Insufficient		
Skeletal class classification	II (assessed with clinical examination)		
Angle right	Molar	N/A	Canine	Class I
Angle left	Molar	N/A	Canine	Class I
Anterior overbite	4 mm		
Anterior overjet	5 mm		
Cross-bites	Nil		
Open-bites	Nil		
RP to IP	2 mm		
FWS	Close/M/swallow test	6 mm	

Tooth guidance

Right laterotrusion

```
    6   4 3 2 1  1 2 3   5 6

8 7     4 3 2 1  1 2 3 4      8
```

Left laterotrusion

```
    6   4 3 2 1  1 2 3   5 6

8 7     4 3 2 1  1 2 3 4      8
```

Protrusion

```
    6   4 3 2 1  1 2 3   5 6

8 7     4 3 2 1  1 2 3 4      8
```

Tooth surface loss

General tooth surface loss

```
    6   4 3 2 1  1 2 3   5 6

8 7     4 3 2 1  1 2 3 4      8
```

Bruxofacets

```
    6   4 3 2 1  1 2 3   5 6

8 7     4 3 2 1  1 2 3 4      8
```

Erosion

```
    6   4 3 2 1  1 2 3   5 6

8 7     4 3 2 1  1 2 3 4      8
```

Attrition

```
    6   4 3 2 1  1 2 3   5 6

8 7     4 3 2 1  1 2 3 4      8
```

Toothbrush abrasion

```
    6   4 3 2 1  1 2 3   5 6

8 7     4 3 2 1  1 2 3 4      8
```

Dental charting

Tooth no.	Clinical findings	Comments
18	Missing	
17	Missing	
16	MODP amalgam; defected margins	
15	Missing	
14	MO composite; OD amalgam; recurrent caries; abrasion lesion	
13	MPD composite; P amalgam; recurrent caries; abrasion lesion	
12	RCT with access cavity poorly sealed; large MPD composite	Insufficient residual tooth structure, apparently poor RCT although the tooth is asymptomatic
11	MO composite; loss of tooth structure	
21	MO composite; loss of tooth structure	
22	P amalgam; loss of tooth structure	
23	MP composite; loss of tooth structure	
24	Unrestored implant	The patient has no information regarding the brand and type of implant inserted; this is clinically integrated and could be used provided we are able to find the parts
25	MODL composite, defected and stained margins, poor anatomy	
26	MODP amalgam, RCT; defected margins	The lack of cusps capping may expose the tooth to fracture
27	Missing	
28	Missing	
38	Missing	
37	Large MOL composite, defected margins; ML tilting and drifting	The tooth is severely tilted and interferes with the opposing dentition in laterotrusive and protrusive movements
36	Missing	
35	Missing	
34	L composite, severe loss of tooth structure with exposure of incisal dentine	
33	Severe loss of tooth structure with exposure of incisal dentine	
32	Severe loss of tooth structure with exposure of incisal dentine	
31	Severe loss of tooth structure with exposure of incisal dentine	
41	Severe loss of tooth structure with exposure of incisal dentine	
42	RCT, MI composite retained with a post, Severe loss of tooth structure with exposure of incisal dentine	
43	Severe loss of tooth structure with exposure of incisal dentine	
44	Severe loss of tooth structure with exposure of incisal dentine and also severe abrasion lesion; severe distal tilting	The tooth is providing contact during laterotrusive movements and the severity of the abfraction seems to support the theory of the stresses acting on the labial gingival third of the tooth during lateral movements
45	Missing	
46	Missing	
47	RCT and large composite crown, M tilting and drifting	Very poor anatomy
48	Large MO amalgam with M overhang	The patient finds difficult to clean this area due to the overhang

Visualised dental charting

Current Condition

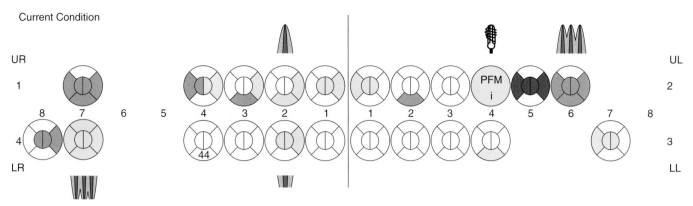

Special tests

Test	Performed	Additional information
Percussion	√	No tenderness
Palpation	√	No tenderness/fremitis
Vitality	√	All teeth are vital apart from 12, 26, 32, 47
Cusp loading	√	No signs/symptoms of cracked tooth syndrome
Other	√	Saliva quality and quantity within normal limits

Aesthetic evaluation (teeth analysis) (Figure 10.2.4)

Criteria	Status	Treatment required
Gingival health	Gingivitis	Oral hygiene instructions, removal of calculus and stains and plaque
Interdental closure	Diastema and gap between 22 and 23	Closure of the spaces
Tooth axis	Normal	
Zenith of the gingival contour	Asymmetric	To be corrected with the definitive prosthesis
Balance of gingival level	Slightly asymmetric	To be corrected with minor crown lengthening and the definitive prosthesis
Level of interdental contact	Asymmetric and missing on the left side	To be corrected with the definitive prosthesis
Relative tooth dimensions	<table><tr><td></td><td>Height</td><td>Width</td><td>Ratio</td></tr><tr><td>Central</td><td>8</td><td>8</td><td>100%</td></tr><tr><td>Lateral</td><td>7</td><td>7</td><td>100%</td></tr><tr><td>Canine</td><td>8</td><td>8</td><td>100%</td></tr></table>	Too short, teeth need to be longer
Tooth form	Short, triangular shape, severe wear and erosion	To be modified with definitive restorations
Tooth characterisation	Opaque	To be modified with definitive restorations
Surface texture	Vertical and horizontal components are missing	To be modified with definitive restorations
Colour	Irregular, low value	To be modified with definitive restorations
Incisal edge configuration	Inverted curve	To be modified with definitive restorations
Lower lip line	Incisal edges are several millimetres away from the lower lip	To be modified with definitive restorations
Smile symmetry	Symmetric	

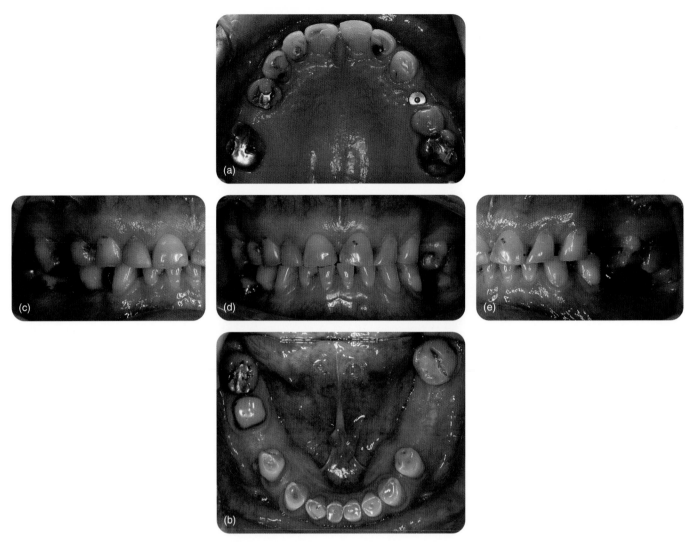

Figure 10.2.3 Intraoral examination – arch form and tooth arrangement: several teeth are missing and the remaining dentition is worn and heavily restored; occlusal views show U-shaped dental arches (a, b); lateral and frontal views show migration and tilting of tooth 44 and Angle's class II tooth relationship (c–e).

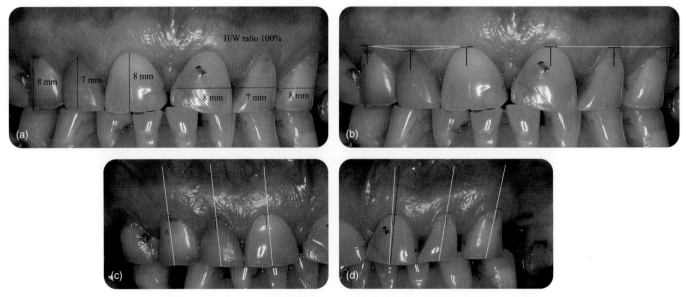

Figure 10.2.4 Intraoral examination – individual tooth analysis: the contour of the soft tissues and the orientation of the axis of the teeth is normal (c, d); the teeth appeared square (height/width ratio is 100%) due to the wear of the incisal edges (a, b).

Radiographs (Figure 10.2.5)
Panoramic radiograph (25/02/07)

Features	Radiographic data
TMJ	Normal
Bone loss	Normal
Sinuses	Normal
Mandibular foramen and canal	Normal
Mental foramen	Normal
Retained roots	No
Pathology	Presence of some endodontic sealer at the apex of 12, with apparently no signs of pathology

Periapical/full mouth radiographs

Periapical radiographs (Figure 10.2.6) were taken after the commencement of the treatment. The initial radiographs were lost when the computer in the practice was stolen.

Study casts (Figures 10.2.7 & 10.2.8)

Articulation	Position	RCP
	Face bow	Yes
Diagnostic wax-up	OVD change	+3 mm
	Occlusal adjustment	Nil
	Crown lengthening	Nil

Clinical and radiographic examinations and prognostic ratings of remaining teeth

good ▮ questionable ▯ poor ▮

Tooth no.	Finding	Prognosis	Tooth no.	Finding	Prognosis
18	Missing	N/A	38	Composite, defected margins, mesial lingual drifting and tilting	questionable
17	Missing	N/A	37	Missing	poor
16	Amalgam, defected margins	good	36	Missing	N/A
15	Missing		35	Missing	N/A
14	Wear, composite, amalgam, caries		34	Wear, composite	good
13	Wear, amalgam		33	Wear, composite	
12	RCT, periapical radiolucency, wear composite		32	Wear, composite	
11	Wear, composite		31	Wear, composite	
21	Wear, composite	questionable	41	Wear, composite	
22	Wear, amalgam	good	42	RCT, post, wear, composite	questionable
23	Wear, composite		43	Wear, composite	good
24	Unrestored implant		44	Wear, severe abrasion/abfraction lesion, severe distal tilting	
25	Wear, composite, caries		45	Missing	N/A
26	RCT, amalgam, lack of cusp cupping		46	Missing	N/A
27	Missing	N/A	47	RCT, composite	good
28	Missing	N/A	48	Amalgam, overhang, caries	

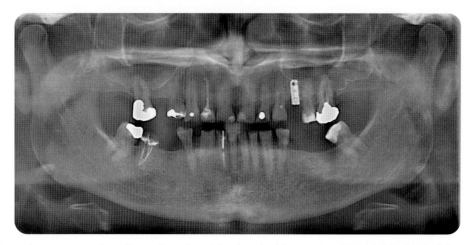

Figure 10.2.5 Radiographs – panoramic radiograph; a dental implant had been placed and left unloaded for 7 years.

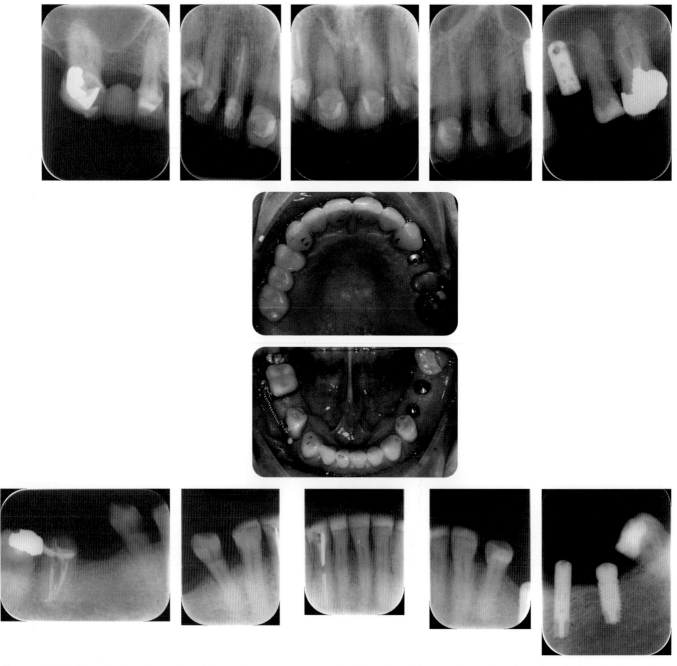

Figure 10.2.6 Periapical radiographs – taken after commencement of treatment (a complete of series of periapicals radiographs was lost due to computer failure). The occlusal view shows the time when the new periapical were taken (immediately before placement of the orthodontic bands).

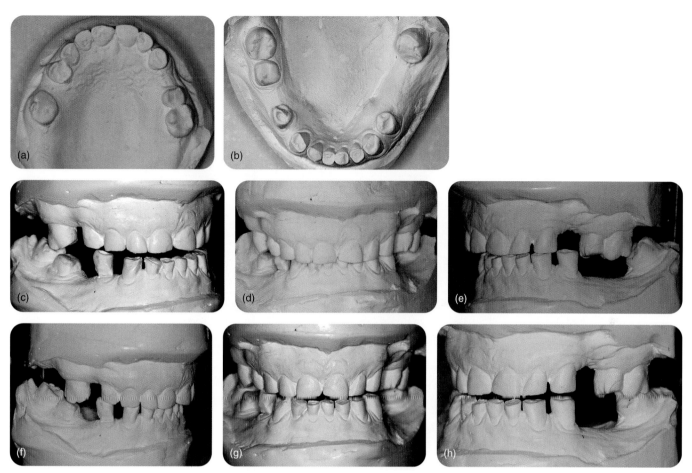

Figure 10.2.7 Study casts – articulated assessment in intercuspal, lateral and protrusive positions: occlusal view (a, b); lateral and frontal view in intercuspal position (c–e); lateral and frontal view lateral and protrusive positions (f–h).

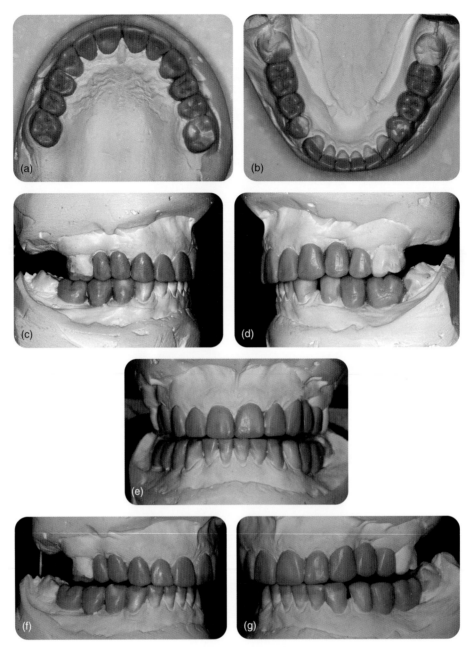

Figure 10.2.8 Study casts – diagnostic preparation: occlusal view (a, b); lateral view in intercuspal position (c, d); views in lateral and protrusive position, a canine and anterior guidance were created (e–g).

Provisional diagnosis

Category	Diagnosis/problem list
Medical conditions	N/A
TMD	History of nocturnal grinding
Orofacial pain	N/A
Aesthetics	Poor teeth display Worn, stained dentition
Phonetics	N/A
Soft tissues	N/A
Oral hygiene	Poor oral hygiene Poor awareness of importance of oral health Poor compliance with professional instructions
Occlusion	Unstable occlusal plane Interference from posterior teeth in protrusion Over-eruption of posterior maxillary teeth Drifting and tilting of mandibular premolars and molars Insufficient posterior support Reduced OVD Negative curve of Spee Anterior deep bite
Saliva	N/A
Tooth surface loss	Severe wear related to all wear mechanisms: attrition, abrasion, abfraction and erosion
Edentulism	Maxillary and mandibular partial edentulism
Restorative	All restorations have defected margins and/or secondary caries
Prosthodontics	Insufficient vertical dimension Irregular occlusal plane Rejection of removable appliances in general, combined with insufficient financial resources and insufficient number of teeth Severe drifting and tilting of some teeth Class II associated to significant overjet
Periodontics	Moderate generalised gingivitis
Endodontics	Poor-quality RCT of several teeth, otherwise asymptomatic

Treatment objectives

Short-term goals
- Diet and oral hygiene advice.
- Preservation existing tooth structure.
- Preservation periodontal tissues.
- Increase patient's awareness of oral health.

Long-term goals
- Restore missing teeth.
- Restore missing tooth structure.
- Improve function.
- Restore occlusal stability.
- Eliminate posterior interferences.
- Restore guidance in anterior and lateral movements.
- Increase OVD.
- Improve aesthetics.

Treatment options

The treatment options for maxillary and mandibular arches are discussed together.

The options include:

- dietary advice;
- oral hygiene instructions;
- non-surgical periodontal treatment;
- occlusal splint.

Treatment option 1: tooth- and implant-supported all-ceramic FDPs; orthodontic up-righting 44; direct composite teeth 44–34
- Direct composite resin restorations 37, 34–44.
- Quartz fibre post and core of 12 and 46.
- Composite core 14–23, 25.
- Amalgam 16, 26.
- Porcelain inlay 47.
- Tooth-supported three-unit FDPs 16–14.
- Tooth-supported single ACCs 13–23, 25, 46.
- Orthodontic up-righting 44.
- Two-stage implants 36, 35, 45.
- Implant-supported all-ceramic FDPs 24, 36, 35, 34.
- Occlusal splint.

Treatment option 2: implant-supported composite FDPs; direct composite build-ups; orthodontic up-righting 44
- Direct composite resin restorations 16, 14–23, 25, 26, 37, 34–44, 47.
- Quartz fibre post and core of 12 and 46.
- Composite crown 46.
- Orthodontic up-righting 44.
- Two-stage implants 36, 35, 45.
- Implant-supported composite crowns 24, 36, 35, 34.
- Occlusal splint.

Treatment option 3: direct composite build-ups; mandibular metal base removable dental prosthesis
- Direct composite resin restorations 16, 14–23, 25, 26, 37, 34–44, 47.
- Quartz fibre post and core of 12 and 46.
- Composite crown 46.
- Mandibular metal base RDP.
- Implant-supported composite crowns 24.
- Occlusal splint.

Treatment plan accepted

Maxilla (option 1)
All-ceramic implant-supported (tooth 24) and tooth-supported FDPs.

Mandible (option 1)
Composite build-up (37, 34–44); all-ceramic implant-supported FDPs (35, 36, 45); ACC 46.

Treatment sequence
Diagnostic phase (Figure 10.2.8)
- Data collection.
- Examination.

- Radiographs (Figure 10.2.9).
- Study casts.
- Articulation.
- Wax-up.
- Mock-up.
- Presentation of treatment options.
- Informed consent.

Surgical phase I (within weeks after the diagnostic phase)
- Oral hygiene instructions.
- Removal of soft and hard deposits.
- Making of a radiographic guide.
- Cone-beam CT scan.
- Stage 1 implants 35, 36.

Restorative phase I (4 weeks after the previous phase) (Figure 10.2.10)
- Composite build-up 38, 34–44, 47.
- Core build-up and provisional 13–23, 25, 26.
- Abutment and provisional 24.
- Core and provisional 46.

Orthodontic phase (2 months after the commencement of the previous phase)
- Upright tooth 44 (see Figure 10.2.11)

Surgical and restorative phase II (4 weeks after the previous phase)
- Stage 2 implants 35, 36.
- Insertion of implant 45.

Surgical and restorative phase III (3 months after the previous phase)
- Stage 2 and provisional 45.

Prosthetic phase IV (weeks after the previous phase)
- Sectional impressions (Figure 10.2.11).
- Copper plating (Figure 10.2.12).
- Positioning impression.
- Maxillomandibular relationship, face bow.
- Master model.
- Zirconia framework try-in.
- Porcelain veneering.

Prosthetic phase V (3 months after the commencement of the previous phase)
- Issue ACC FDP (Figure 10.2.13)
- 2 weeks' review (Figure 10.2.14).

Maintenance
- Review every 6 months (Figure 10.2.15).
- Non-surgical periodontal treatment.
- Radiographs.
- Reinforcement of oral hygiene.
- Examination/occlusion.
- Periodontal probing.
- Issue ACC FDP.

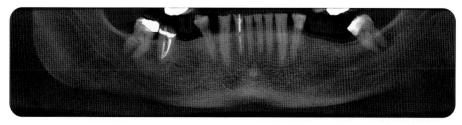

Figure 10.2.9 Radiographic evaluation of edentulous areas with a cone-beam CT scan: cross-sections of the edentulous areas show sufficient bone quantity for the insertion of dental implants as does the panoramic view of the mandible.

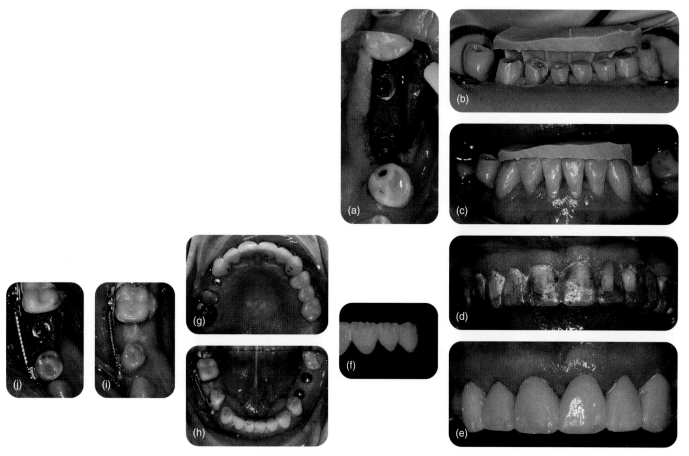

Figure 10.2.10 Treatment phase I – from the wax-up to provisional restorations: insertion of the implant based on the diagnostic wax-up (a); as the implants integrate the occlusal vertical dimension (OVD) was increased with direct composite build up of the mandibular anterior teeth (b, c) and by restoring the maxillary teeth with a provisional fixed acrylic bridge (d–f). The increase in OVD created sufficient interarch space for orthodontic realignment of tooth 44 (g–j); with tooth 44 repositioned, an implant was placed in position 45 (j).

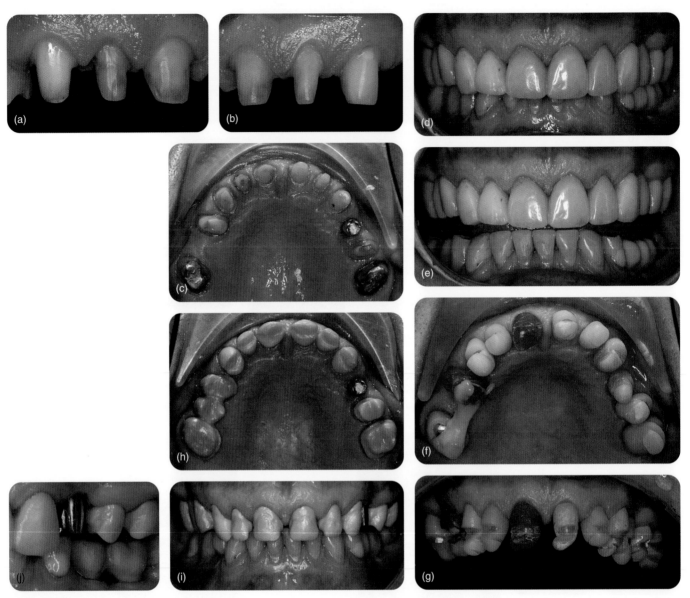

Figure 10.2.11 Treatment phase II – from the provisional restorations to the coping try-in: the preparations were refined and the provisional restorations completed including the implants (a–e); an impression of each abutment to fabricate acrylic copings used for a pick-up impression (f, g); anatomical zirconia copings were fabricated and tried-in (h–j).

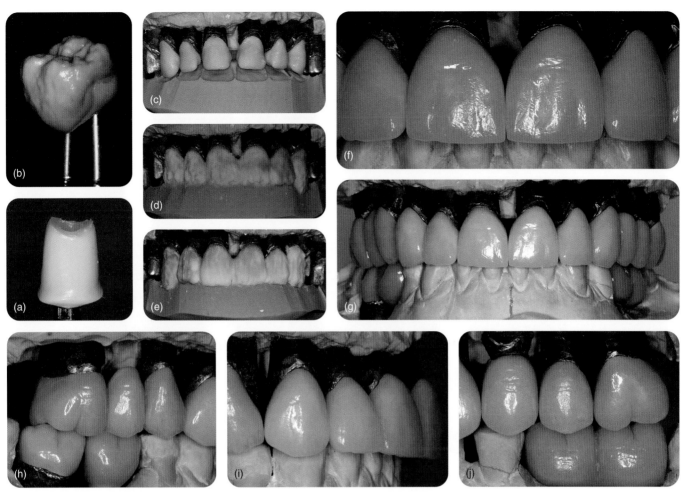

Figure 10.2.12 Treatment phase III – definitive prosthesis, porcelain build-up: details of the wax-up for an implant abutment (a); the anatomical zirconia copings were veneered with a minimal layer of porcelain (b–e); the complete porcelain build-up on the master casts with copper-plated dies.

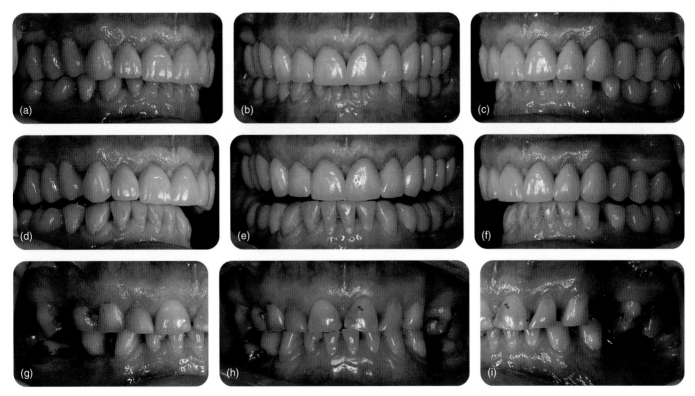

Figure 10.2.13 Issue of definitive all-ceramic restorations: frontal and lateral views in intercuspal position (a–c); views in lateral and protrusive positions show canine and anterior guidance (d–f); intraoral views prior to the treatment (g–i).

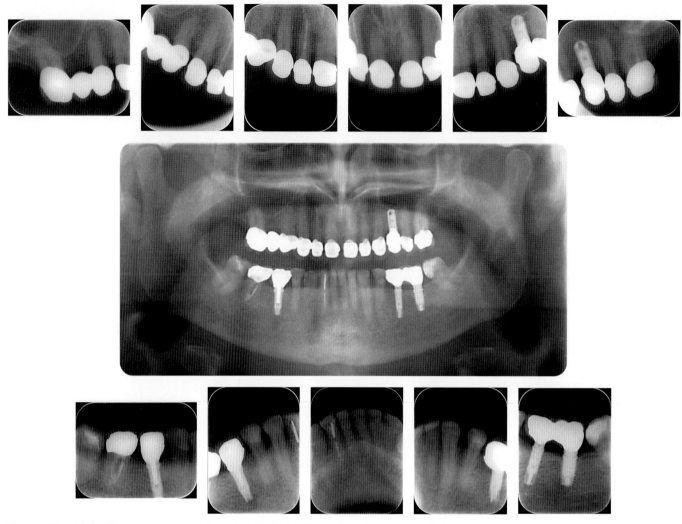

Figure 10.2.14 Radiographs: panoramic and periapical radiographs taken at completion of treatment.

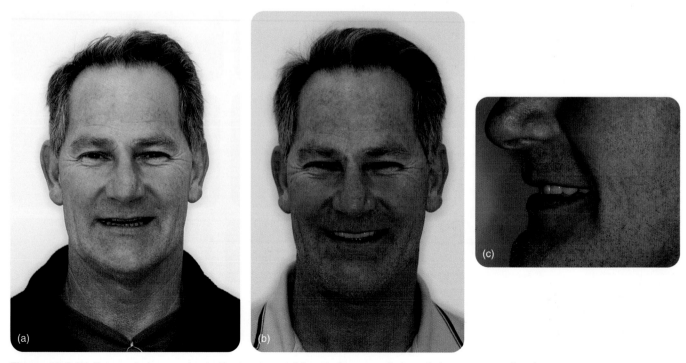

Figure 10.2.15 Extraoral views: prior to the treatment (a) and after completion of the treatment (b, c).

Discussion

Shortened dental arch and worn dentition: treatment or monitoring?

According to van't Spijker *et al.* (2007), the prosthodontist has the responsibility to determine treatment needs, treatment procedures, materials choice and occlusal concepts.

Regarding treatment of the worn dentition, Seligman and Pullinger (1995) showed that tooth wear varies with age and in some patients monitoring rather than early intervention may be advisable. The rate of wear decreases over time due to the increase in occlusal contacts. Seligman and Pullinger noted that the rate of wear recorded in young patients (age range 20–29 years) did not continue at the same rate. As the patient aged, attrition slowed and the authors also noted that canine and anterior tooth integrity played an important role in preventing wear of posterior teeth. For example, mediotrusive wear was delayed until canine wear allowed for contralateral tooth contact. Premature anterior attrition led to functional contacts on posterior teeth that would have otherwise been impossible. Age, patient's concerns and occlusal analysis indicated that the degree of wear of Mr S's dentition was beyond the clinical condition in which Seligman and Pullinger recommended monitoring. However, if the prosthodontist and the patient decide to monitor the degree of tooth wear, a tooth wear index should be recorded in addition to examination and photographs. Five-point tooth wear measurements have been proposed by Lobbezoo and Naeije (2001) and Hooper *et al.* (2004).

Dawson (2007) recommended a less conservative approach and that tooth wear should be diagnosed early and treated to prevent tooth wear progressing beyond a point of acceptable restoration.

Data on when to intervene with tooth and tooth structure loss are indirectly given by studies on the shortened dental arch concept. This was first introduced by Kayser (1981) whose initial study divided 118 patients into six classes according to the degree and symmetry of the shortened arch. It was reported that there was sufficient adaptive capacity in shortened dental arches when at least four posterior occlusal units remained (preferably complete dentition including the second premolars). Patients with less than four posterior occlusal units tended to have a rapid worsening of oral function.

Confirmation of these findings and a better definition of 'oral function' were given in subsequent studies (Witter *et al.* 1994, 2001). Witter *et al.* (1994) compared occlusal stability (number of occlusal contacts, overbite, interdental spacing, alveolar bone support), for a period of 6 years with 55 patients with shortened dental arches (no molar teeth) with 52 subjects with complete dentition. The study showed that shortened dental arches provided occlusal stability, provided the periodontal tissue was healthy. In the study in 2001 the authors added some parameters to the definition of occlusal stability and they compared interdental spacing, occlusal contacts of anterior teeth in ICP, overbite, occlusal tooth wear and alveolar bone support. Subjects with shortened dental arches showed minor differences in interdental spaces in the premolar regions, more anterior teeth in occlusal contact and lower alveolar bone scores. These differences remained constant with time, confirming that occlusal stability is possible in patients with shortened dental arches. Another study conducted on 725 subjects with shortened and extreme shortened dental arches (zero to two pairs of occluding premolars) showed that patients with such extreme shortened dental arches had significantly more interdental spacing, occlusal contact of incisors and vertical overlap (Sarita *et al.* 2003). According to the study, the occlusion in subjects with extreme shortened dental arches was not stable and may deteriorate progressively.

Mr S was classified as presenting with an extreme shortened dental arch. Despite the presence of some posterior teeth, the occlusion presents two asymmetric occlusal units (right side); interdental spacing is evident between 33 and 34 and more severe between 44 and 43 with distal tilting and severe cervical abrasion lesion of 44. Chewing was only possible in the anterior dentition. According to the shortened arch concept, in addition to the loss of tooth structure there is occlusal instability, which is likely to worsen over time, supporting the need for treatment. In addition to this observation, Mr S was concerned about function and aesthetics. The patient reported that he is able to chew only soft food and is also unsatisfied with the appearance of his teeth.

Treatment objective and options

Restoration of aesthetics and function involved three main objectives:

- restoration of missing teeth;
- restoration of missing tooth structure;
- restoration of occlusal stability.

The treatment options for the maxillary and mandibular arches were:

- direct restorations and RDPs;
- direct restorations and implant-supported FDPs;
- indirect tooth-supported FDPs and implant-supported FDPs.

The treatment plan rationale is based on the following:

- comparison of the clinical outcomes of three different approaches: endodontic treatment and restoration of the existing teeth; extraction and implant; or extraction and no treatment;
- clinical outcome of direct restorations;

- clinical outcome of single crowns and FDPs;
- clinical outcome of implant-supported single crowns and FDPs;
- influence of ferrule effect, design and type of post on the prognosis, complications and mode of failure of tooth-supported single CMCs and FDPs of non-vital teeth restored with crowns;
- principles of preparation design in zirconia-based FDPs: accuracy of the margins and factors influencing retention and resistance;
- position of the margins of the restorations: the concept of 'biological width';
- risk analysis and maintenance.

Comparison of the outcomes of the three options: endodontic treatment and restoration of the existing tooth; extraction and implant; or extraction and no treatment

Mr S had several endodontically treated teeth (12, 26, 42 and 46). The clinical question was: 'should non-vital teeth be extracted and replaced with implants or not be restored at all'? Some studies show that the longevity of endodontically treated teeth restored with FDPs is comparable to that of vital teeth restored with FDPs, provided there is sufficient tooth structure (De Backer et al. 2007, Walton 2009). The most important studies have been critically examined in recent systemic reviews. A systematic review by Holm-Pedersen et al. (2007) analysed the longevity of healthy teeth, teeth with compromised tooth structure and dental implants. These data showed that teeth supported by healthy periodontal tissues have a very high longevity (up to 99.5% at 50 years). Patients with controlled periodontitis and treated regularly should expect to maintain 92% of their teeth for a period of 50 years. Oral implants when evaluated after 10 years of service did not surpass the longevity of comparable compromised but successfully treated natural teeth.

A systematic review by Tomasi et al. (2008) described the incidence of tooth and implant loss reported in long-term studies. The authors applied strict inclusion criteria, such as a follow-up period of at least 10 years and drop outs of less than 30%. The incidence of tooth loss among subjects varied from 1.5% to 5%. The percentage of implants reported as lost ranged from 1% to 8%. The loss rate of teeth was lower than that of implants in those patients that were seen regularly for dental care. Despite the consistency with the data of Holm-Pedersen et al., there are several flaws in this study. The most important issue is that due to the strict criteria most of the included studies on implants deal with implant-retained overdentures. The patients' age and medical conditions and also the loading conditions of implants used in overdenture are not comparable with the situation of a fully dentate and healthy patient.

Torabinejad et al. (2007) examined outcomes, benefits and harms of endodontic care and restoration compared with extraction and placement of implant single crowns, FDPs or simply extraction followed by no treatment. The data comparison was difficult because the criteria of each study are heterogeneous. However, where a comparison or analysis was possible, there were interesting observations. The extraction of teeth may not necessarily be followed by replacement with a prosthesis; as seen in the concept of shortened dental arches, the loss of some posterior teeth may not have any impact on the occlusion stability, tooth loading, TMDs, interdental spacing, periodontal disease, patient discomfort or masticatory performance. On the other hand, the loss of visible teeth has a psychosocial impact and patients would reasonably expect replacement.

Torabinejad et al. (2007) stated that the long-term (more than 6-year follow-up period) data on the survival of root canal treated teeth indicated that in patients with healthy periodontal tissues with teeth having pulpal and/or periradicular pathology, RCT resulted in superior survival (97%) to extraction and replacement with an FDP (82%) and resulted in equal outcomes to extraction and replacement of the missing tooth with an implant (97%). However, some data with different definition of success ranked implant therapy (95%) as superior to endodontic treatment (84%), which in turn was ranked as being superior to fixed prosthodontic treatment (80%).

Systematic reviews do not provide guidelines for decision-making. Several factors need to be considered when a decision is made on whether a root canal treated tooth should be retained or replaced with an implant. The important factors influencing treatment planning as indicated by Torabinejad et al. (2007) are:

- Systemic health. Tooth conservation and endodontic treatment are preferred where there are contraindications to surgical procedures (uncontrolled diabetes, uncontrolled bleeding disorders, recent infarction, prolonged administration of intravenous bisphosphonates, immune-suppression, heavy smoker, etc.).
- Periapical lesion are the main preoperative factors associated with less favourable outcomes of endodontic treatment.
- Endodontic treatment is indicated in teeth with irreversible pulpitis, necrotic pulps, restorable crowns, treatable periodontal conditions, salvageable resorptive defects and a favourable crown-to-root ratio.
- Dental implants should be considered when endodontic treatment is contraindicated for mechanical reasons, as with limited remaining tooth structure and the definitive crown is not able to engage at least 1.5–2.0 mm of tooth structure with a cervical ferrule. The studies of De Backer et al. (2007) suggest that it is not clear from a clinical viewpoint whether it is crucial for the ferrule effect to be circumferential.
- The patient's preference is very important. A patient may be willing to accept the risk of failure of the

endodontic treatment and recognise that implant options are still viable.

- The quantity and quality of bone is the major factor affecting the feasibility of implant placement without bone grafting.

Risk analysis

Risk analysis of the dental treatment for Mr S has been divided into:

- risk factors and complications linked to the patients medical conditions, parafunctions and habits;
- risk factors and complications linked to the surgical procedure;
- risk factors and complications linked to the implant-supported single crowns and FDPs;
- risk factors and complications linked to the tooth-supported single crowns and FDPs.

Risk factors and complications linked to the patient's medical conditions, parafunctions and habits

The medical history does not suggest any contraindications to surgical procedures. Parafunctions (diurnal and nocturnal clenching and grinding) has not been reported; however, it cannot be excluded considering the degree of wear of the dentition. The assessment (presence of wear facets) and longevity of the provisional restoration will provide an indication of the presence of parafunctional activity. An occlusal splint has also been planned to protect the definitive restoration and the dentition.

Risk factors and complications linked to the surgical procedure

Infections (3%), implant loss, poor healing, bleeding, neurosensory disturbance related to damage of the mental or mandibular nerves and increased bone loss have been reported in most studies on clinical outcomes of dental implants and the corresponding literature reviews (Adell et al. 1990, Goodacre et al. 2003, Herrmann et al. 2005).

Such complications are best prevented by using a sterile protocol during implant insertion in addition to the administration antibiotics and antiseptic mouthwashes. A CT scan and a surgical guide are used to increase the accuracy of the procedure and prevent damage of the nerves.

Risk factors and complications linked to the implant-supported single crowns and fixed dental prostheses

Complications with dental implants supporting partial FDPs can be biological and technical (Brägger et al. 2005, Pjetursson et al. 2007). The most common biological complications are: peri-implant mucosal lesions (peri-implantitis, gingivitis, hyperplasia), increased rate of bone loss, and loss of integration. The most common technical complications are: loose abutments or screws, loss of retention, aesthetic complications, and ceramic chipping or fracture.

To prevent biological and technical complications reported, the implant-supported FDP for Mr S has been fabricated with an innovative design. The design is the result of the data from in vitro studies and for zirconia-based restorations (Guazzato et al. 2004a,b,c,d, 2005, 2010). Mr S's missing dentition will be restored with implant-supported ACCs for teeth 45 and 24. Two implants will be used to retain two splinted crowns restoring teeth 35 and 36. Crowns will be screw-retained on to multi-unit abutments. Advantages of this prosthesis design:

- Titanium multi-unit abutments are placed immediately after stage two surgery and will favour the attachment of epithelium which is undisturbed during all subsequent phases.
- The two ACCs are splinted to minimise the transmission of rotational movements to the implants.
- Thickness of the crowns is optimised, which helps reduce mechanical fractures.
- Crowns are screw-retained on the multi-unit abutments. The screws are the weakest link; their premature or frequent loosening is an indication of excessive masticatory load or parafunction and will warn the operator that the occlusion and prosthesis design need to be modified.
- The screws can be easily retrieved in case of fracture.
- The design of the prosthesis can be easily modified should mechanical problems become unusually frequent.
- The thickness of the zirconia core is optimised to support and strengthen the veneering porcelain.
- The firing schedule for the veneering porcelain has been modified to minimise the development of thermal stresses and the onset of porcelain chipping.

Risk factors linked to the tooth-supported single crowns and fixed dental prostheses

Clinical studies reporting outcomes and complications of zirconia-based FDPs have been discussed. The most common complication of zirconia-based FDPs is the chipping of veneering porcelain that has been consistently reported in clinical studies (Raigrodski et al. 2006, Sailer et al. 2007, Tinschert et al. 2008). Sailer et al. (2007) also reported a high incidence of dental caries; 12 of 57 FDPs were replaced due to development of caries. This unusually high incidence of caries was explained in the fact that the computer-aided design and computer-aided manufacturing (CAD/CAM) system used for the fabrication was in a development phase and restoration accuracy was poor. In addition, supervised undergraduate students carried out the treatment and some technical mistakes were accidentally made, contributing to premature restoration failure.

Tinschert et al. (2008) investigated the clinical outcome of 65 FDPs monitored over a mean period of 38 months and reported de-bonding of two. In addition, three teeth required endodontic treatment after cementation.

Maintenance and definition of clinical success

Treatment will be reviewed after 6 months and then annually. At review, the following parameters will be assessed (Salvi & Lang 2004):

- plaque accumulation;
- mucosal condition;
- presence of bleeding/pus;
- peri-implant probing depth;
- width of keratinised mucosa;
- implant mobility/discomfort;
- bone loss;
- loosening of the gold screws;
- integrity of the prostheses;
- occlusion.

Clinical implant success is defined by Testori *et al.* (2003) as:

- no clinically detectable mobility;
- no evidence of peri-implant radiolucency;
- no peri-implant infection;
- no pain;
- no paraesthesia;
- no crestal bone loss exceeding 1.5 mm at the end of the first year and 0.2 mm/year in subsequent years.

Rationale for the treatment plan

The treatment option selected with Mr S was based on implant-supported and tooth-supported single ACCs and FDPs. The rationale for the treatment is supported in previous sections and the most important points are summarised as follows:

- Occlusion, degree of wear and interdental spacing indicate that there is no occlusal stability and the clinical situation of Mr S is likely to progressively worsen. This observation and the patient's concerns support the need for treatment.
- The patient wishes to preserve his own teeth and does not accept RDPs.
- The patient initially decided on option 3 – implant-supported provisional composite crowns and direct composite for the remaining dentition.
- The zirconia-based indirect restorations were then offered free of charge. They would be fabricated by the clinician with materials and copings being donated.
- Ceramo-metal restorations are indicated for Mr S. The choice of zirconia-based ceramic was financially affordable and was prepared by the operator.
- An innovative design and manufacturing of the prostheses should minimise the risk of complication.
- Option 3 consisted of direct composite restorations which would perform poorly in the long term and thus must be considered as a medium-term solution.

- In vital teeth, failure rate and need for maintenance of direct restorations (amalgams) is double compared with that of crowns.
- In endodontically treated teeth, the use of direct restorations instead of crowns is more likely to lead to catastrophic failure and even tooth fracture.
- The longevity of dental implants is not superior to that of endodontically treated teeth restored with a crown or an FDP, provided the quantity of tooth structure is sufficient to achieve a ferrule effect.
- The ferrule effect does not need to be circumferential.
- The criteria to define 'sufficient tooth structure' are clinical, not mathematical. The literature provides clear indications but no mathematical equation that can be applied to each specific situation.
- The presence of a periapical lesion is the main preoperative factor associated with less favourable outcomes of endodontic treatment.
- The preparation of the canal to allocate the post follows the principles of minimal length (half length of the canal) and maximum diameter (no more than one third of the tooth diameter).
- The material used for the post does not appear to affect the outcome.
- The post must be passive.
- In order to preserve soft tissues, the margins are located equigingival wherever possible.
- Appropriate cervical–occlusal dimension may be achieved by increasing the OVD.

Review at 18 months

1. Oral hygiene and plaque control: *excellent oral hygiene, minimal deposit of plaque and calculus.*
2. Soft tissue health: *no gingival inflammation, no bleeding on probing, and peri-implant tissue is healthy.*
3. Check on home-care programme and advise on frequency of brushing, use of dental floss and mouth rinses: *patient brushes and flosses regularly twice a day; Superfloss and interproximal toothbrushes are used daily to clean underneath the maxillary FDP and the mandibular implant-supported FDP.*
4. Note and record recurrent dental caries associated with restorations or new carious lesions; note periodontal status – check probing depths and record changes; new PA radiographs to check alveolar bone levels (see 7): *the soft tissue is firm and pale; an update periodontal charting shows periodontal sulcus probing depth with a range of 0.5–1.5 mm; no bleeding on probing; however, gingival recession was recorded in several sites and related to aggressive brushing with a hard bristle toothbrush; no PA radiographs were taken at the 18-month review.*
5. Medical status – change in general health and implications for oral health: *the medical history is unchanged.*
6. Occlusion – check tooth contacts with GHM foil at intercuspal position, retruded contact position, lateral and protrusive excursive contacts; note lateral contact

details, especially where there is a fracture of restorative material – record, photograph fracture and contact details with GHM foil and comment on reason for fracture: *the occlusion is stable; no wear of the occlusal surface or chipping of the porcelain was visible; the patient wears an occlusal splint at night.*

7. Radiographs – 1-year review PA views for specific details of the status of crowns on teeth and implants. Check crown margins and alveolar bone levels; measure thread exposure to bone crest around implants and correlate with clinical details as above: *a panoramic radiograph was taken showing that the bone level has been maintained and no bone loss has occurred at tooth and implant regions.*

8. Discuss oral health related quality of life – comfort, appearance, function – chewing and speech; whether there has been a change in confidence, social interaction and relationships: *the patient ranked comfort, appearance, function, chewing and speech as very satisfactory; the treatment improved the patient's confidence and social interaction from 5 to 9 on a visual analogue scale (graded from 0 to 10).*

9. Seek any additional comments from the patient about the treatment and whether they would undertake the process again if needed: *the patient was satisfied with the treatment and would undertake the procedure again if required.*

References

Adell, R., Ericksson, B., Lekholm, U. *et al.* (1990) A long-term follow-up study of osseointegrated implants in the treatment of totally edentulous jaws. *International Journal of Oral & Maxillofacial Implants*, 5 (4), 347–359.

Brägger, U., Karoussis, I., Person, R. *et al.* (2005) Technical and biological complications/failures with single crowns and fixed partial dentures on implants: a 10 year prospective cohort study. *Clinical Oral Implants Research*, 16 (3), 326–334.

Dawson, P.E. (2007) *Functional Occlusion: From TMJ to Smile Design.* Mosby, St Louis.

De Backer, H., Van Maele, G., Decock, V. *et al.* (2007) Long-term survival of complete crowns, fixed dental prostheses and cantilever fixed dental prostheses with posts and cores on root canal-treated teeth. *International Journal of Prosthodontics*, 20 (3), 229–334.

Goodacre, C.J., Bernal, G., Rungcharassaeng, K. *et al.* (2003) Clinical complications with implants and implant prostheses. *Journal of Prosthetic Dentistry*, 90 (2), 121–132.

Guazzato, M., Albakry, M., Ringer, S.P. *et al.* (2004a) Strength, fracture toughness and microstructure of a selection of all-ceramic materials. Part I: pressable and alumina glass-infiltrated ceramics. *Dental Materials*, 20 (5), 441–448.

Guazzato, M., Albakry, M., Ringer, S.P. *et al.* (2004b) Strength, fracture toughness and microstructure of a selection of all-ceramic materials. Part II: Zirconia-based dental ceramics. *Dental Materials*, 20 (5), 449–456.

Guazzato, M., Albakry, M., Quach, L. *et al.* (2004c) Influence of grinding, sandblasting, polishing and heat treatment on the flexural strength of a glass-infiltrated alumina-reinforced dental ceramic. *Biomaterials*, 25 (11), 2153–2160.

Guazzato, M., Proos, K., Quach, L. *et al.* (2004d) Strength, reliability and mode of fracture of bilayered porcelain/zirconia (Y-TZP) dental ceramics. *Biomaterials*, 25 (20), 5045–5052.

Guazzato, M., Quach, L., Albakry, M. *et al.* (2005) Influence of surface and heat treatments on the flexural strength of Y-TZP dental ceramics. *Journal of Dentistry*, 33 (1), 9–18.

Guazzato, M., Walton, T.R., Franklin, W. *et al.* (2010) Influence of thickness and cooling rate on the development of spontaneous cracks in porcelain fused to zirconia structures. *Australian Dental Journal*, 55 (3), 306–310.

Herrmann, I., Lekholm, U. Holm, S. *et al.* (2005) Evaluation of patient and implant characteristics as potential prognostic factors for oral implant failures. *International Journal of Oral & Maxillofacial Implants*, 20 (2), 220–230.

Holm-Pedersen, P., Lang, N.P. & Muller, F. (2007) What are the longevities of teeth and oral implants? *Clinical Oral Implants Research* 18 (Suppl. 3), 15–19.

Hooper, S.M., Meredith, N. & Jagger, D.C. (2004) The development of a new index for measurement of incisal/occlusal tooth wear. *Journal of Oral Rehabilitation*, 31 (3), 206–212.

Kayser, A.F. (1981) Shortened dental arches and oral function. *Journal of Oral Rehabilitation*, 8 (5), 457–462.

Lobbezoo, F. & Naeije, M. (2001) A reliability study of clinical tooth wear measurements. *Journal of Prosthetic Dentistry*, 86 (6), 597–602.

Pjetursson, B.E., Sailer, I., Zwahlen, M. *et al.* (2007) A systematic review of the survival and complication rates of all-ceramic and metal–ceramic reconstructions after an observation period of at least 3 years. Part I: single crowns. *Clinical Oral Implants Research*, 18 (Suppl. 3), 73–85.

Raigrodski, A.J., Chiche, G.J., Potiket, N. *et al.* (2006) The efficacy of posterior three-unit zirconium-oxide-based ceramic fixed partial dental prostheses: A prospective clinical pilot study. *Journal of Prosthetic Dentistry*, 96 (4), 237–244.

Sailer, I., Feher, A., Filser, F. *et al.* (2007) Five-year clinical results of zirconia frameworks for posterior fixed partial dentures. *International Journal of Prosthodontics*, 20 (4), 383–388.

Salvi, G.E. & Lang, N.P. (2004). Diagnostic parameters for monitoring peri-implant conditions. *International Journal of Oral & Maxillofacial Implants*, 19 (Suppl.), 116–127.

Sarita, P.T., Kreulen, C.M., Witter, D.J. *et al.* (2003) A study on occlusal stability in shortened dental arches. *International Journal of Prosthodontics*, 16 (4), 375–380.

Seligman, D.A. & Pullinger, A.G. (1995) The degree to which dental attrition in modern society is a function of age and of canine contact. *Journal of Orofacial Pain*, 9 (3), 266–275.

Testori, T., Del Fabbro, M., Szmukler-Moncler, S. *et al.* (2003) Immediate occlusal loading of Osseotite implants in the completely edentulous mandible. *International Journal of Oral & Maxillofacial Implants*, 18 (4), 544–551.

Tinschert, J., Schulze, K.A., Natt, G. *et al.* (2008) Clinical behaviour of zirconia based fixed-partial dentures made of DC-Zirkon: 3 year results. *International Journal of Prosthodontics*, 21 (3), 217–222.

Tomasi, C., Wennstrom, J.L. & Berglundh, T. (2008) Longevity of teeth and implants – a systematic review. *Journal of Oral Rehabilitation*, 35 (Suppl. 1), 23–32.

Torabinejad, M., Anderson, P., Bader, J. *et al.* (2007) Outcomes of root canal treatment and restoration, implant-supported single crowns, fixed partial dentures, and extraction without replacement: a systematic review. *Journal of Prosthetic Dentistry*, 98 (4), 285–311.

van't Spijker, A., Kreulen, C.M. & Creugers, N.H. (2007) Attrition, occlusion, (dys)function, and intervention: a systematic review. *Clinical Oral Implants Research*, 18 (Suppl. 3), 117–126.

Walton, T.R. (2009) Changes in the outcome of metal-ceramic tooth-supported single crowns and FDPs following the introduction of osseointegrated implant dentistry into a prostho-

dontic practice. *International Journal of Prosthodontics*, 22 (3), 260–267.

Witter, D.J., de Haan, A.F., Kayser, A.F. *et al.* (1994). A 6-year follow-up study of oral function in shortened dental arches. Part I: occlusal stability. *Journal of Oral Rehabilitation*, 21 (2), 113–125.

Witter, D.J., Creugers, N.H., Kreulen, C.M. *et al.* (2001) Occlusal stability in shortened dental arches. *Journal of Dental Research*, 80 (2), 432–436.

Case 10.3 Mr Nicholas H

Agnes Lai

Patient: Mr Nicholas H (date of birth 26/07/1971)

Presenting complaints

Chief complaint	Moderate to severe tooth loss from dental erosion Aesthetic concerns – teeth are shorter and smaller
Subsidiary complaints	Sensitivity
History of complaints	Tooth wear has occurred progressively over the past 6 years
Patient's expectations	Prevent erosion; 'look reasonable' – in proportion Not concerned about midline or missing 15

History
Medical history

Gastrointestinal	GORD Endoscopy indicated no ulcer/oesophagitis/GORD
Hospitalisation	Zygomatic fracture
Medications	Nil

Social history

Marital status	Married
Children	Twin daughter and son and a new born daughter
Occupation	Carpenter
Smoking	Frequency: social
Diet	5 meals a day Soft drinks (bourbon and coke 3–4/day, ginger beer) Sports drinks (Stemanade – hot day/training) Acidic foods (olives) Water (3–4 L) Tea (2 cups/day with milk and 1 tsp sugar) Alcohol (beer) Hard/brittle foods (nuts, toast)
Habits/hobbies	Oral habits (holding pencils between teeth)

Dental history

Date of last examination	April 2008
Oral hygiene	Brushes: twice/day Flosses: occasionally Mouthwash: use of Listerine recently Toothpaste: Colgate sensitive/Pronamel
Treatment	Restorations (amalgam and composites) TMD (nil) OMFS (removal of 15, 28, 18)

Extraoral examination (Figures 10.3.1 & 10.3.2)
Aesthetics

Facial form	Dolicofacial	
Facial symmetry	Nose tip is right of facial midline – history of fracture Left facial tone is more depressed	
Profile	Straight	
Nasolabial angle	90°	
Facial folds	Moderate	
Midlines	Maxillary central incisors alignment to the left of facial midline Maxillary/mandible centrals not coincident Mandible midline 2 mm to the right	
Lip posture	Symmetry	Left side open – potentially from a pencil-holding habit
	Upper lip	Moderate
	Lower lip	Moderate
	Competence	Good
	Tooth display	Mild
Occlusal plane	Parallel to ala-tragus line Not parallel to interpupillary line; is reversed Over-eruption of 42–32	
Vertical	FWS	3 mm
	OVD assessment	Compensated
Smile assessment	Symmetry	Good at maximum smile, left side delay (Figure 10.3.2)
	Lip line	High
	Gingival display	>2 mm on maxillary laterals and canines
	Tooth display	100% in maxilla, 35% in mandible
	Buccal corridor	Narrow

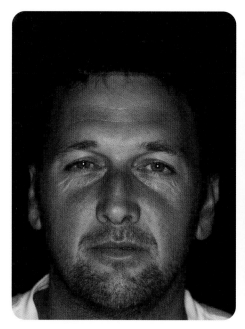
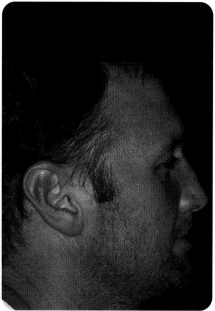

Figure 10.3.1 Extraoral examination.

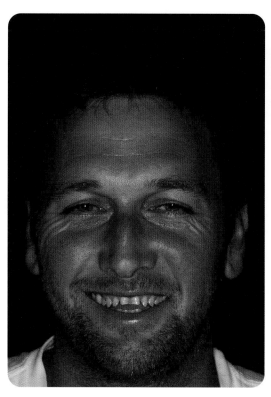

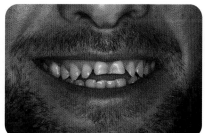
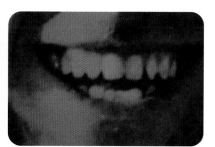

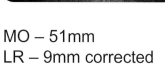

MO – 51mm   Straight
LR – 9mm corrected   Tooth contact – 47

LL – 13mm corrected   Tooth contact – 38
P – 12mm   Tooth contact – 38, 47
Over jet: 0.5mm
Over bite: –3mm
TM and phonetics assessment – NAD

Figure 10.3.2 Extraoral examination – smile assessment; note incisor tooth wear and compare with right smile view 6 years before.

Temporomandibular assessment

No TMJ sounds or tenderness
No muscle tenderness
No signs or symptoms from glands and lymph node
    assessments

Jaw movement	Measurement	Reference points
Maximal opening	51 mm corrected	11 and 41
Right laterotrusion	9 mm corrected	
Left laterotrusion	13 mm corrected	
Midline deviation	Maxillary midline 2 mm to the left	
Maximal protrusion	12 mm corrected	
Opening pathway	Straight	
Overjet	0.5 mm	
Overbite	–3 mm	
Further investigation required	No	

Phonetics

	Normal	Abnormal
Labial (m)	√	
Labiodental (f/v)	√	
Linguodental (th)	√	
Interdental (s)		√ Some lisping, compensate with tongue
Linguopalatal (k/ng)	√	

Intraoral examination (Figure 10.3.3)
Oral cleanliness

Condition	Yes	No			
Plaque	√		General	Mild	Supragingival
Calculus		√			
Food impaction		√			
Stains		√			
Halitosis		√			

Saliva

Water intake	3–4 L/day
Quality	Good, watery, pH7, buffering capacity 10–12 points
Quantity	Good, >1 ml/minute stimulated
Pathology	Nil
Medications affecting	Nil
Further investigation required	No

Soft tissues

	Healthy	Abnormal	Additional information
Lips	√		
Labial vestibule	√		
Cheeks	√		
Palate	√		
Oropharynx	√		
Tongue	√		
Floor	√		
Frenal attachments	√		

Ridges	Maxilla	Mandible
Arch shape	V	V
Resorption	15 saddle mild	Dentate
Palatal vault	High	
Tori	Nil	Nil
Frenal attachments	NAD	NAD
Mucosa	NAD	NAD
Pathology	Nil	Nil

Dental assessment

Skeletal classification	Class I			
Dental occlusion	Class I open bite			
Angle right	Molar	Class II	Canine	Class I
Angle left	Molar	Class I	Canine	Class I
Anterior overbite	3 mm open-bite			
Anterior overjet	0.5 mm			
Cross-bites	Nil			
Open-bites	Anterior			
Curve of Spee	RHS +		LHS +	
Curve of Wilson	RHS −		LHS −	
RP to IP slide	0 mm			
FWS	Close/M/ swallow test		3 mm	
Tooth guidance	Molar			

Tooth guidance

Right laterotrusion

```
 7 6   4 3 2 1 | 1 2 3 4 5 6 7
 8 7 6 5 4 3 2 1   1 2 3 4 5 6 7 8
```

Left laterotrusion

```
 7 6   4 3 2 1 | 1 2 3 4 5 6 7
 8 7 6 5 4 3 2 1   1 2 3 4 5 6 7 8
```

Protrusion

```
 7 6   4 3 2 1 | 1 2 3 4 5 6 7
 8 7 6 5 4 3 2 1   1 2 3 4 5 6 7 8
```

Tooth surface loss

General

```
 7 6   4 3 2 1   1 2 3 4 5 6 7
 8 7 6 5 4 3 2 1   1 2 3 4 5 6 7 8
```

Attrition

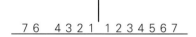

```
 7 6   4 3 2 1   1 2 3 4 5 6 7
 8 7 6 5 4 3 2 1   1 2 3 4 5 6 7 8
```

Erosion

```
 7 6   4 3 2 1   1 2 3 4 5 6 7
 8 7 6 5 4 3 2 1   1 2 3 4 5 6 7 8
```

Abrasion

```
          |
 7 6   4 3 2 1   1 2 3 4 5 6 7
 8 7 6 5 4 3 2 1   1 2 3 4 5 6 7 8
```

Bruxofacets

```
          |
 7 6   4 3 2 1   1 2 3 4 5 6 7
 8 7 6 5 4 3 2 1   1 2 3 4 5 6 7 8
```

Aetiology: predominantly erosion

Periodontium

Gingiva	Biotype	Medium
	Colour	Pink
	Contour	Normal
	Consistency	Normal
Papillae	Colour	Pink
	Contour	Normal
Symmetry	Asymmetry in zenith	

Periodontal examination

	03	04	05
CPITN	0	1	0
	1	0	1
	08	07	06

Facial upper

Tooth no.	17	16	14	13	12	11	21	22	23	24	25	26	27
Recession													
Pocket	213	222	214	323	222	211	223	323	323	423	322	213	322
Bleeding				√		√							
Suppuration													
Buccal furcation													
Distal furcation													
Vitality	+	+	+	+	+	+	+	+	+	+	+	+	+

Palatal upper

Tooth no.	17	16	14	13	12	11	21	22	23	24	25	26	27
Recession													
Pocket	213	212	222	222	321	213	212	211	111	111	212	112	211
Bleeding						√		√					
Suppuration													
Mesial furcation													
Mobility													

Lingual lower

Tooth no.	48	47	46	45	44	43	42	41	31	32	33	34	35	36	37	38
Recession																
Pocket	333	323	323	323	312	311	111	111	111	111	111	112	211	323	322	313
Bleeding												√	√			
Suppuration																
Furcation																
Mobility																

Facial lower

Tooth no.	48	47	46	45	44	43	42	41	31	32	33	34	35	36	37	38
Recession																
Pocket	323	313	322	213	223	322	113	311	111	312	312	323	313	322	323	322
Bleeding		√														
Suppuration																
Furcation																
Vitality	+	+	+	+	+	+	+	+	+	+	+	+	+	+	+	+

Mobility	Grade I = ≤1 mm; II = >1 mm; III = >1 mm including vertical component
Furcation	Class I = ≤3 mm; II = >3 mm; (horizontal probing, e.g. 3H, 4H, 5H); III = through and through
Recession	Distance (mm) from CEJ to FGM. If not clear, CEJ from restorative margin

Dental charting

Tooth no.	Clinical findings	Comments
18	Absent	Nil
17	Present and clear	Mesial drift
16	Present and clear	Mesial drift
15	Absent	Nil
14	Moderate wear, composite restoration	Vital and sensitive – erosion, over-eruption
13	Moderate wear, composite restoration	Vital and sensitive – erosion, over-eruption
12	Moderate wear, composite restoration	Vital and sensitive – erosion, over-eruption
11	Moderate wear	Vital and sensitive – erosion
21	Moderate wear	Vital and sensitive – erosion
22	Moderate wear	Vital and sensitive – erosion
23	Moderate wear	Vital and sensitive – erosion
24	Moderate wear	Vital and sensitive – erosion
25	Moderate wear	Vital and sensitive – erosion
26	Amalgam restoration	Nil
27	Present and clear	Nil
28	Absent	Nil
38	Present and clear	Nil
37	Occlusal wear	Erosion and attrition
36	Occlusal wear	Erosion and attrition
35	Occlusal wear	Erosion and attrition
34	Occlusal wear	Erosion and attrition
33	Erosion	Buccal surface – sensitive
32	Present and clear	Over-eruption
31	Present and clear	Over-eruption
41	Present and clear	Over-eruption
42	Present and clear	Over-eruption
43	Erosion, buccal abrasion	Sensitive
44	Erosion, buccal abrasion	Sensitive
45	Erosion, buccal abrasion	Sensitive
46	Occlusal wear, buccal abrasion	Nil
47	Occlusal wear	Nil
48	Present and clear	Nil

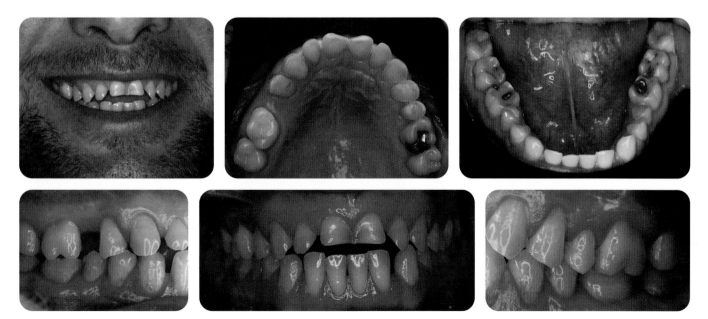

Figure 10.3.3 Intraoral examination – buccal views show incisal wear and occlusal views indicate erosion and attrition contributions to tooth wear.

Special tests

	Performed	Additional information	
Percussion	√	NAD	
Palpation	√	NAD	
Vitality	√	All vital	
Cusp loading	√	No signs/symptoms of cracked tooth syndrome	
Transillumination			
Selective anaesthesia			
Other	√	Saliva test	NAD
		Endoscopy	NAD

Radiographs
Panoramic radiograph

General bone loss	Minimal
Sinuses	Clear
Retained roots	Nil
Pathology	Nil
Caries	Nil
Restorations	Composite and amalgam
Other	Nil

Orthopantomogram
An OPG was done on 20/10/2008 (Figure 10.3.4).

Periapical films
Periapical films were taken on 20/10/2008 – nothing abnormal was detected (Figures 10.3.5 & 10.3.6).

Study casts and diagnostic wax-up

Articulation	Position	ICP
	Face bow	Yes
Diagnostic	OVD change	0 mm
wax-up	Occlusal adjustment	Need to assess further
	Crown lengthening	Required

Provisional diagnosis
- Moderate erosion of maxillary 14–25.
- Combined erosion–attrition mandibular posterior dentition.

- Tooth surface loss associated with extrinsic acids in lifestyle.
- Anterior open bite with passive eruption.
- Missing 15.
- Mild generalised gingivitis.
- Over-erupted 38 and 48.
- Dental class I canine; molar class I L, class II R.

Problem list
Patient perceived
- Tooth surface loss associated with erosion and lifestyle.
- Anterior open-bite.

Dentist perceived
- Small and short teeth.
- Anterior open-bite, difficult to eat.
- Wear of teeth over time.
- Patient lives 4 hours away.
- Cost.

Treatment goals
Short term
- Improve aesthetics.
- Improve function.
- Identify aetiology for tooth wear, education and monitor.

Long term
- Maintainable prosthesis that provides reasonable longevity, catering for patient's lifestyle, eating pattern, general health and oral hygiene ability.
- Increase patient knowledge and awareness of oral health and regular dental visits, as well as ongoing maintenance.

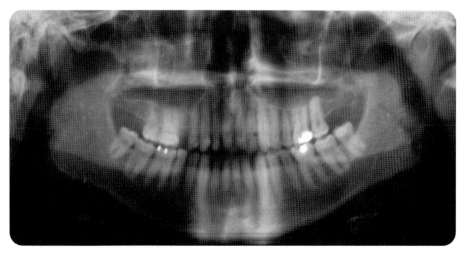

Figure 10.3.4 Radiograph – orthopantomogram.

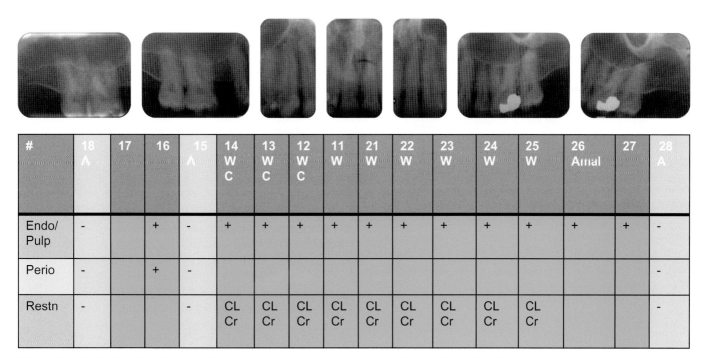

#	18 A	17	16	15 A	14 W C	13 W C	12 W C	11 W	21 W	22 W	23 W	24 W	25 W	26 Amal	27	28 A
Endo/Pulp	-		+	-	+	+	+	+	+	+	+	+	+	+	+	-
Perio	-		+	-												-
Restn	-			-	CL Cr	CL Cr	CL Cr	CL Cr	CL Cr	CL Cr	CL Cr	CL Cr	CL Cr			-

Figure 10.3.5 Periapical radiographs for preoperative assessment of maxilla confirming healthy periodontal status and optimal dental status (green code) with the exception of tooth wear.

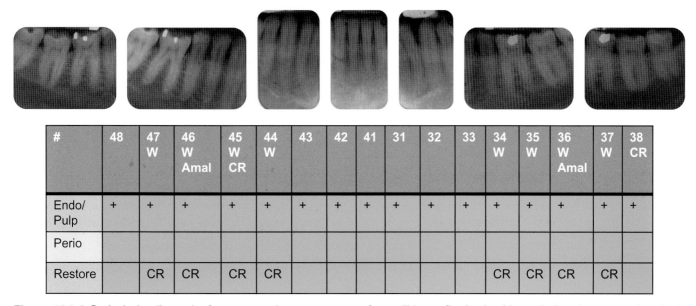

#	48	47 W	46 W Amal	45 W CR	44 W	43	42	41	31	32	33	34 W	35 W	36 W Amal	37 W	38 CR
Endo/Pulp	+	+	+	+	+	+	+	+	+	+	+	+	+	+	+	+
Perio																
Restore		CR	CR	CR	CR							CR	CR	CR	CR	

Figure 10.3.6 Periapical radiographs for preoperative assessment of mandible confirming healthy periodontal status and optimal dental status (green code) with the exception of tooth wear.

Treatment options

Maxilla

- Full coverage crowns from 14 to 25, crown lengthening in the palatal aspect required for resistance form in preparation:
  - ○ options: ceramo-metal or all-ceramic;
  - ○ monitor 6 monthly.

Mandible

- No treatment and monitor:
  - ○ composite resin restorations;
  - ○ monitor 6 monthly.

Adjunctive management: fluoride toothpaste and tooth mousse with trays.

Treatment discussion

After discussion, the patient understood that tooth surface loss has an underlying cause that requires time to ascertain and to monitor its management. A provisional phase of 6–9 months is preferred prior to reassessment for the definitive treatment (Ibbetson 1999, Chu *et al.* 2002).

Depending on the assessment of parafunction and amount of forces generated with function at the end of provisional phase treatment, a decision on ceramo-metal or all-ceramic crowns would be made for the maxillary dentition. Full-coverage restorations offer improved aesthetics and function; however, the patient is aware that tooth surface loss is still possible below the margins of these crowns and an ongoing commitment for prevention is required (Ibbetson 1999, Chu *et al.* 2002, Spear & Holloway 2008).

Mandibular dentition will be assessed. If restoration is required and the acid environment is controlled, composite restorations offer an easy-to-maintain option. These restorations have a good success for up to 5 years, require frequent monitoring of margins and polishing, but are readily maintained at low cost and may be carried out without change (Ibbetsen 1999, Chu *et al.* 2002, Manhart *et al.* 2004).

In the maxilla, the patient wishes to improve gingival aesthetics, requiring crown lengthening, which will also involve labial gingivectomy with a surgical guide to improve zenith symmetry.

The patient understands that 6-monthly recall prophylaxis is an important part of ongoing oral health maintenance. Lifestyle adjustments must be maintained to prevent progression of tooth surface erosion. Adjunctive management with tooth mousse and fluoride agents can help prevent future erosion and sensitivity but therapy relies on a change of lifestyle (Ibbetson 1999).

Complications with crowns include porcelain chipping and decementation, and routine check-up is important to reduce risk of dental caries and need of endodontic treatment. As the patient's parafunctional activity is low, the risk for this is minimal depending on food choice and

nocturnal wear of an occlusal splint will help to prevent ceramic fracture (Goodacre *et al.* 2003, Pjetursson *et al.* 2007, Tinschert *et al.* 2008).

Composite resin restorations are subject to marginal leakage and a risk of secondary dental caries. Routine check-up will help to reduce these complications as it can assist timely intervention with repair and polishing (Manhart *et al.* 2004). Johansson *et al.* (2008) is another useful reference on the rehabilitation of worn dentition.

Treatment sequence

Hygiene phase

- Dietary advice.
- Oral hygiene instructions.
- Acid control regime.
- Prophylaxis.

Provisional phase (Figures 10.3.7–10.3.9)

- Provisional crowns from 14 to 25.
- Tooth mousse with trays.
- Splint.

Reassessment phase

- No significant parafunction elicited.
- Only one provisional crown decemented over 6 months.
- Some attritional facets on crowns.
- Sensitivity under control.
- Restricted finance.

Definitive phase (Figures 10.3.10–10.3.12)

- Composite resin 34–37, 44–47 occlusal only.
- 14–25 single zirconia crowns.
- Soft splint in maxilla – for night-time protection of crowns and serve also as a tray for tooth mousse.
- Tray in mandible for tooth mousse.

Maintenance

- Initial 3-month follow-up (Figures 10.3.13 & 10.3.14).
- Regular 6-monthly prophylaxis and check-up for life.
- Model taking for tooth wear assessment in the first year.

Review at 3 months

1. Oral health status: oral hygiene and plaque control; soft tissue health; check home-care programme and advise on frequency of brushing, use of dental floss and mouth rinses; note and record recurrent dental caries associated with restorations or new carious lesions; note periodontal status – check probing depths and record changes; new PA radiographs to check alveolar bone levels. *Excellent oral hygiene and prosthesis hygiene.*
2. Medical status: change in general health and implications for oral health. *More aware of signs of oral reflux and ongoing acid erosion has been prevented and*

controlled by this increase in patient's awareness of his restored oral situation.

3. Occlusion: check tooth contacts with GHM foil at ICP, RCP, lateral and protrusive excursive contacts.
4. Radiographs: 1-year review PA views for specific details of the status of crowns on teeth and implants. Check crown margins and alveolar bone levels; measure thread exposure to bone crest around implants and correlate with clinical details as above.
5. Discuss oral health related quality of life – comfort, appearance, function – chewing and speech; whether there has been a change in confidence, social interaction and relationships. *Patient observed that the*

rehabilitation provided a major improvement with speech and general health, as well as the ability to relax and sleep. Social life and ability to work were improved and he was very satisfied with his appearance, eating/enjoyment of food, smiling/laughing and self confidence.

6. Additional comments about the treatment and whether they would undertake the process again. *Patient was very happy with the aesthetic result and improved speech and self confidence. He also appreciated the early rectification of acid erosion impact on his dentition and oral health and is now more dentally aware. He would undertake the treatment again if needed.*

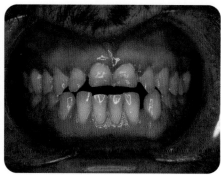

Figure 10.3.7 The left image illustrates the aesthetic evaluation with a stent in place as a guide for crown lengthening. The right image shows the result of crown-lengthening after 2 weeks.

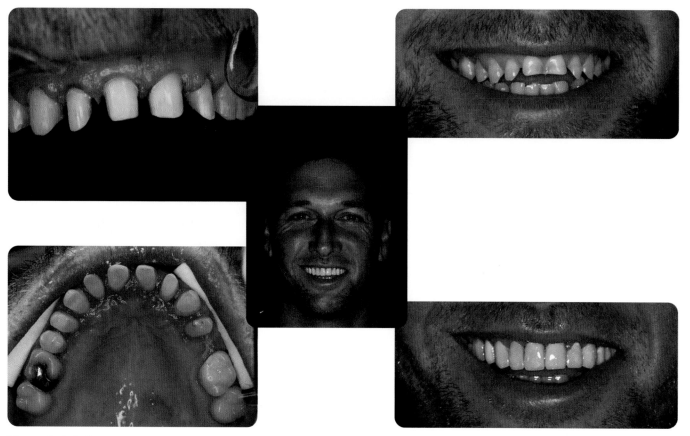

Figure 10.3.8 Crown preparations and immediate provisionalisation; immediate provisional crowns constructed in acrylic resin.

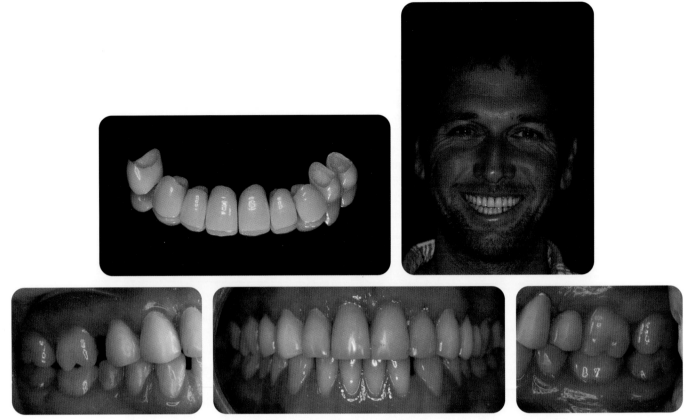

Figure 10.3.9 The provisional phase was maintained for 6–12 months to monitor the patient's tooth wear status. Art Glass crowns were fitted at 12 months and were in place for a further 6 months to continue the monitoring of tooth wear. After that time final preparations were planned as it appeared that the tooth wear was under control.

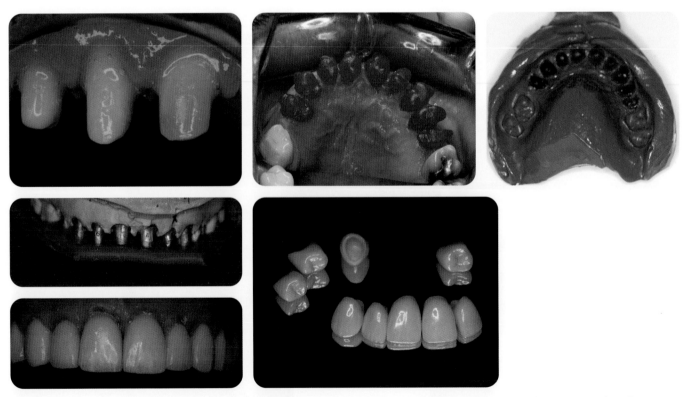

Figure 10.3.10 From left to right, top to bottom: final tooth refinement and definitive crown preparation at 9 months after immediate provisionalisation – the gingival response and stability achieved during the provisional phase; bonnet pick-up impression; Moyco wax verification of cast accuracy; and final single all-ceramic crown restorations in zirconia.

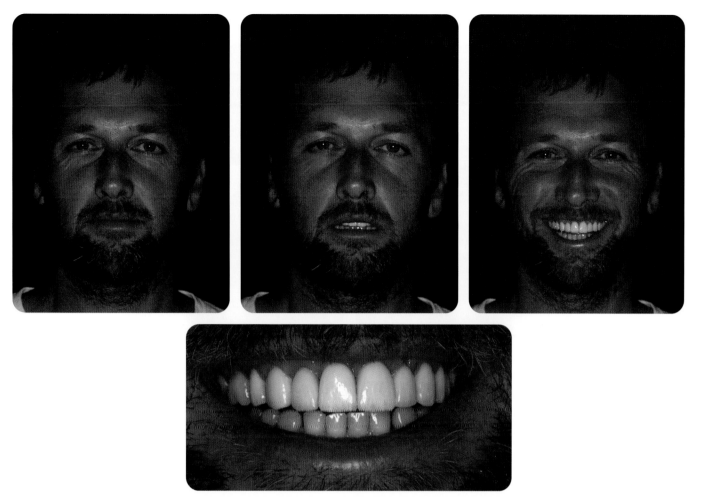

Figure 10.3.11 Definitive maxillary zirconia anterior crowns at trial fitting at the biscuit-bake stage.

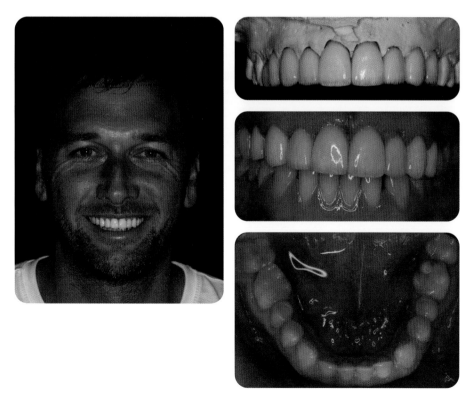

Figure 10.3.12 Final rehabilitation with 15–24 zirconia single crowns following crown lengthening; also addition of composite resin on the occlusal surfaces of 34–37 and 44–47.

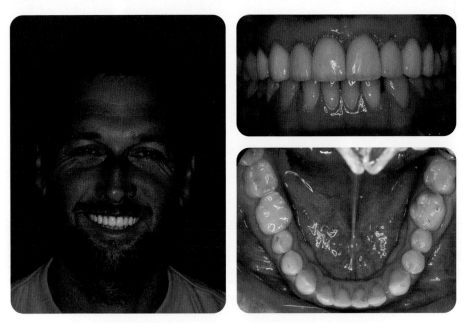

Figure 10.3.13 Initial 3-month follow-up.

Satisfaction on his new teeth	
Eating or enjoyment of food	Very good
Appearance	Very good
Speech	Good
General health	Good
Ability to relax or sleep	Good
Social life	Good
Romantic relationship	Good
Smiling or laughing	Very good
Confidence	Very good
Carefree manner (lack of worry)	Very good
Mood	Very good
Work or ability to do your usual job	Good
Finances	Good
Personality	Very good
Comfort	Very good
Breath odour	None

Figure 10.3.14 Review at 3 months – Patient satisfaction table.

References

Chu, F.C., Yip, H.K., Newsome, P.R. *et al.* (2002) Restorative management of the worn dentition: I. Aetiology and diagnosis. *Dental Update*, 29(4), 162–168.

Goodacre, C.J., Bernal, G., Rungcharassaeng, K. *et al.* (2003) Clinical complications in fixed prosthodontics. *Journal of Prosthetic Dentistry*, 90 (1), 31–41.

Ibbetson, R. (1999) Tooth surface loss. 9. Treatment planning. *British Dental Journal*, 186 (11), 552–558.

Johansson, A., Johansson, A.K., Omar, R. *et al.* (2008) Rehabilitation of the worn dentition. *Journal of Oral Rehabilitation*, 35 (7), 548–566.

Manhart, J., Chen, H.Y., Hamm, G. *et al.* (2004) Buonocore Memorial Lecture. Review of clinical survival of direct and indirect restorations in posterior teeth of permanent dentition. *Operative Dentistry*, 29(5), 481–508.

Pjetursson, B.E., Sailer, I., Zwahlen, M. *et al.* (2007) A systematic review of the survival and complication rates of all-ceramic and metal–ceramic reconstructions after an observation period of at least 3 years. Part I: single crowns. *Clinical Oral Implants Research*, 18 (Suppl. 3), 73–85.

Spear, F. & Holloway, J. (2008) Which all-ceramic system is optimal for anterior aesthetics? *Journal of the American Dental Association*, 139 (Suppl.), 19S–24S.

Tinschert, J., Schulze, K.A., Natt, G. *et al.* (2008) Clinical behaviour of zirconia based fixed-partial dentures made of DC-Zirkon: 3 year results. *International Journal of Prosthodontics*, 21 (3), 217–222.

Case 10.4 Ms Carmen P

Glen Liddelow

Patient: Ms Carmen P (date of birth 5/04/1971)

Presenting complaints

Chief complaint	Teeth 'wearing out'
Subsidiary complaints	Reduced display of teeth when smiling and talking Aesthetics of anterior teeth Sensitivity of retained 85 and discoloured 41
History of complaints	Aware of clenching and grinding, wears an occlusal splint nightly
Patient's expectations	To have her teeth restored to improve aesthetics with a long-lasting aesthetic and functional result

History
Medical history

Medical Practitioner	Dr B	
Respiratory	NAD	
Cardiovascular	NAD	
Gastrointestinal	NAD	
Neurological	NAD	
Endocrine	Partial thyroidectomy May 2007 for a benign tumour; no ongoing medication as thyroid-stimulating hormone levels were normal	
Developmental	NAD	
Musculoskeletal	NAD	
Genitourinary	NAD	
Haematological	NAD	
Other	Allergies	NKA
	Smoking	10 cigarettes/day for 16 years
	Infectious diseases	Nil
	Pregnancy	Nil
	Hospitalisation	Partial thyroidectomy May 2007, nasal trauma, pregnancy
	Medications	Zinc, ginseng, vitamin C and multivitamins

Social history

Marital status	Single		
Children	1 teenage daughter		
Occupation	Dental practice manager		
Smoking	Type	Cigarettes	
	Frequency	10/day	
	Period	16 years	
Recreational drugs	Nil		
Diet	√	Soft drinks	1 every 2 days
		Sports drinks	Nil
		Lemons	Nil
		Acidic foods	Nil
	√	Sweet foods	1 chocolate/day
	√	Water	1.5 L/day
	√	Tea	1 cup/day
		Coffee	Nil
	√	Alcohol	2 glasses white wine/day
		Hard/brittle foods	Nil
		Ice crunching	Nil
Habits/hobbies		Musical instrument	Nil
		Exercise	Nil
	√	Oral habits	Nail biting

Dental history

			Further information
Date of last examination	6 months previously		
Oral hygiene	√	Brushing	3 times/day
	√	Flossing	Once every 2 days
		Mouthwash	Nil
	√	Toothpaste	Sensodyne, Colgate
Treatment	√	Restorations	Nil
	√	Endodontics	41
		Periodontics	Nil
	√	Orthodontics	16 years ago
		RDP	Nil
		FDP	Nil
		TMD	Nil
	√	OMFS	38 extraction

Extraoral examination (Figures 10.4.1 & 10.4.2) Aesthetics

Facial symmetry	Deviation to left	
Profile	Straight	
Nasolabial angle	Obtuse	
Facial folds	Nil	
Midlines	Face/maxillary centrals	Coincident
	Maxillary central alignment	Parallel to facial midline
	Maxillary/mandibular centrals	Deviated 2 mm to left
Lip posture	Symmetry	Symmetrical
	Upper lip	Moderate
	Lower lip	Moderate
	Competence	Yes
	Tooth display	90%
Occlusal plane	Parallel to ala-tragus line	Yes
	Parallel to interpupillary line	Yes
	Over-eruption	Nil
Vertical	FWS	4 mm
	OVD assessment	Optimal
Smile assessment	Symmetry	Yes
	Lip line	Moderate
	Gingival display	Minimal
	Tooth display	70%
	Buccal corridor	moderate

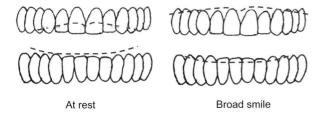

At rest   Broad smile

Phonetics (Figure 10.4.3)

	Normal	Abnormal
Labial (m)	√	
Labiodental (f/v)	√	
Linguodental (th)	√	
Interdental (s)	√	
Linguopalatal (k/ng)	√	

Temporomandibular assessment

TMJ		Additional information
Click	Nil	NAD
Crepitus	Nil	
Tenderness	Nil	

Muscle tenderness	Right	Left
Temporalis	Nil	Nil
Masseter	Nil	Nil
Posterior mandible	Nil	Nil
Anterior mandible	Nil	Nil
Glands	NAD	
Nodes	NAD	

Jaw movement	Measurement (mm)	Reference points
Maximal opening	45	11
Right laterotrusion	15	
Left laterotrusion	15	
Midline deviation	2 mm to left	
Maximal protrusion	10	
Opening pathway	Straight	
Overjet	2	
Overbite	2	
Further investigation required		No

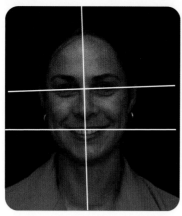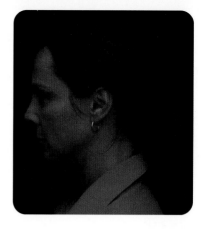

Interpupillary line vs horizon | Slanted right
Commisural line vs horizon | Parallel
Facial midline | Deviated left

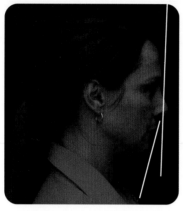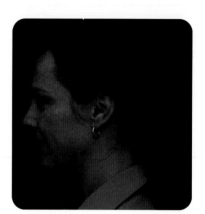

Profile | Normal
E-line | Mx 2mm Mn 2mm
Lips | Medium

Figure 10.4.1 Extraoral examination.

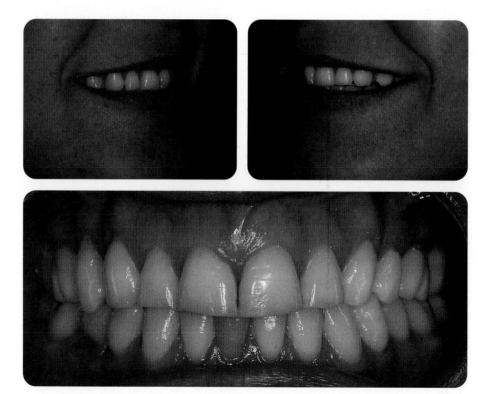

Figure 10.4.2 Extraoral examination. Smile assessment: incisal edge to lower lip convex; smile line – average exposure; labial contour average; interincisal to midline – coincident; occlusal plane to commissures is oriented to the right.

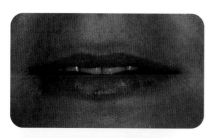

M
Interocclusal rest
space 4 mm
Dental exposure Mx
2–3 mm

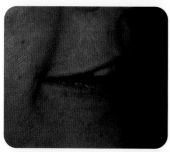

F,V
Vermillion
1 mm lingual

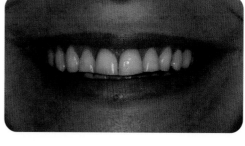

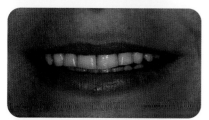

E
Interlabial space
occupied by Mx
teeth 72%

Incisal curve vs lower lip	Convex-flat
Smile line	Average
Smile width	10 teeth visible
Labial corridor	Normal
Interincisal line vs midline	Coincident
Occlusal plane vs commissural line	Slanted right slightly

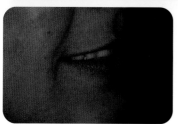

S
Mandibular
movement
Horiz 2 mm

Figure 10.4.3 Phonetic assessment. 'M' interocclusal rest space 4 mm; maxillary anterior teeth exposure of 2–3 mm; 'F', 'V' vermillion border 1 mm lingual; 'E' labial space show of 70% of maxillary anterior teeth; 'S' mandibular movement of 2 mm.

Intraoral examination (Figures 10.4.4 & 10.4.5)
Soft tissues

Tissue	Healthy	Abnormal	Additional information
Lips	√		Nil
Labial vestibule	√		Nil
Cheeks		√	Buccal ridging
Palate	√		Nil
Oropharynx	√		Nil
Tongue		√	Lateral scalloping
Floor	√		Nil
Frenal attachments	√		Nil

Oral cleanliness

Condition	Yes	No			
Plaque	√		Localised	Mild	Supragingival
Calculus	√		Localised	Mild	Supragingival
Food impaction		√			
Stains	√		Nicotine		
Halitosis		√			

Saliva

Water intake	1.5 L/day
Quality	Watery/clear resting saliva with pH 6.8–7.8, stimulated saliva has pH of 6.8–7.8, with 10–12 points of buffering capacity
Quantity	Hydration from rest <30 s, 3.5–5.0 ml stimulated salivary flow over 5 minutes
Pathology	NAD
Medications affecting	NAD
Further investigation required	No

Periodontium

CPITN	2	1	2
	2	2	2

Gingiva	Biotype	Normal to thin
	Colour	Pink
	Contour	Normal
	Consistency	Firm
Papillae	Colour	Normal
	Contour	Normal with localised recession

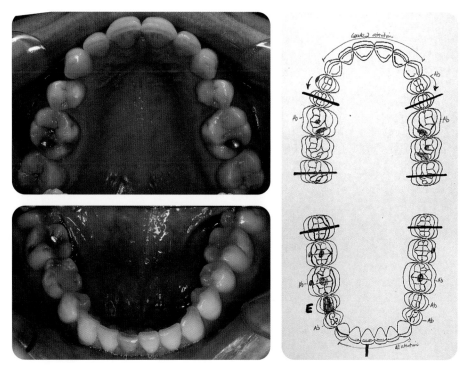

Figure 10.4.4 Intraoral examination – occlusal view diagram specifies tooth positions.

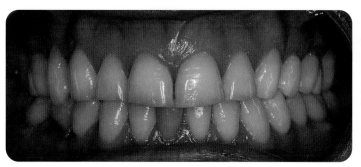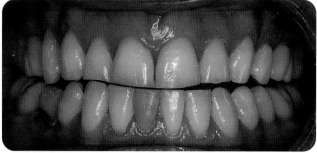

Max vs Mn interincisal line	Deviated Lt 2mm
Tooth type	Square tapering
Texture	Macro slight, Micro slight
Mx central incisors	W/H ratio 92%
Profile	Slightly palatal

Maxillary 6 anterior teeth

Contour	Adormal	Gingival margins	Symmetric (ex 13)
Proportion	Abormal	Zeniths	Regular
Interincisal angles	Normal	Papillae	Good
Tooth axes	Normal	Biotype	Medium to thin
Tooth arrangement	Normal		

Mandibular 6 anterior teeth

Contour	Sl Wear	Gingival margins	Symmetric
Proportion	Normal	Papillae	Good
Tooth axes	Normal	Biotype	Medium
Tooth arrangement	Regular	Alterations	Colour variation
Incisal edge	Slanted Lt		

Figure 10.4.5 Intraoral examination – labial view specifies tooth and gingival positions.

Periodontal charting

Maxillary buccal

Tooth no.	18	17	16	15	14	13	12	11	21	22	23	24	25	26	27	28
Pocket		222	223	313		222	222	222	222	322	322		222	222	332	
Bleeding																
Suppuration																
Recession		4		4		2							2		023	
Buccal furcation																
Distal furcation																
Mobility																

Maxillary palatal

Tooth no.	18	17	16	15	14	13	12	11	21	22	23	24	25	26	27	28
Pocket		223	323	222		222	223	324	222	222	223		322	322	322	
Bleeding																
Suppuration																
Recession																
Mesial furcation																

Mandibular lingual

Tooth no.	48	47	46	85	44	43	42	41	31	32	33	34	35	36	37	38
Pocket		223	323	322	422	222	222	212	222	222	223	323	323	323	322	
Bleeding																
Suppuration																
Recession																
Furcation																

Mandibular buccal

Tooth no.	48	47	46	85	44	43	42	41	31	32	33	34	35	36	37	38
Pocket		223	322	312	122	122	212	213	312	212	222	222	222	222	222	
Bleeding					0											
Suppurations																
Recession					4	3			1	1		1	1			
Furcation																
Mobility					1											

Occlusion

Skeletal classification	Class II				
Dental occlusion	Class I				
Angle right	Molar	Class II		Canine	Class I
Angle left	Molar	Class II		Canine	Class I
Anterior overbite	2 mm				
Anterior overjet	2 mm				
Cross-bites	Nil				
Open-bites	Nil				
Curve of Spee	Flat				
Curve of Wilson	++				
RP to IP slide	0 mm				
FWS	4 mm				

Tooth guidance

Right laterotrusion

8 **7** 6 5 4 **3** 2 1 | 1 2 3 4 5 6 7 8

8 7 **6** 5 4 **3** 2 1 1 2 3 4 5 6 7 8

Left laterotrusion

8 7 6 5 4 3 2 1 | 1 2 **3 4 5 6 7** 8

8 7 6 5 4 3 2 1 1 2 **3 4 5 6 7** 8

Protrusion

8 7 6 5 4 3 **2 1 1 2** 3 4 5 6 7 8

8 7 6 5 4 3 **2 1 1 2** 3 4 5 6 7 8

Tooth surface loss

Caries

8 7 6 5 4 3 2 1 | 1 2 3 4 5 6 7 8

8 7 6 5 4 3 2 1 1 2 3 4 5 6 7 8

Attrition

8 7 6 5 4 **3 2 1 1 2 3** 4 5 6 7 8

8 7 6 5 4 **3 2 1 1 2 3** 4 5 6 7 8

Erosion (specify surface)

8 7 6 5 4 3 2 1 | 1 2 3 4 5 6 7 8

8 7 6 5 4 3 2 1 1 2 3 4 5 6 7 8

Abrasion (specify surface)

8 7 6 5 4 3 2 1 | 1 2 3 4 5 6 7 8

8 7 6 5 4 3 2 1 1 2 3 4 5 6 7 8

Abfraction (specify surface)

8 **7** 6 **5** 4 **3** 2 1 | 1 2 3 4 **5** 6 **7** 8

8 7 **6 E 4** 3 2 1 1 2 3 4 5 6 7 8

Dental charting

Tooth no.	Clinical findings	Comments
18	Not present	Nil
17	Unrestored	Nil
16	Satisfactory occlusal amalgam	Nil
15	Unsatisfactory buccal restoration, grade 1 attrition	Nil
14	Not present	Nil
13	Unrestored, grade 2 attrition	Nil
12	Unrestored, grade 2 attrition	Nil
11	Unrestored, grade 2 attrition	Nil
21	Unrestored, grade 2 attrition	Nil
22	Unrestored, grade 2 attrition	Nil
23	Unrestored, grade 2 attrition	Nil
24	Not present	Nil
25	Unrestored	Nil
26	Satisfactory occlusal amalgam	Nil
27	Satisfactory occlusal composite	Nil
28	Not present	Nil
38	Not present	Nil
37	Satisfactory buccal composite resin	Nil
36	Satisfactory occlusal composite resin	Nil
35	Unrestored, small abfraction	Nil
34	Unrestored, small abfraction	Nil
33	Unrestored grade 1–2 attrition	Nil
32	Unrestored grade 1–2 attrition	Nil
31	Unrestored grade 1–2 attrition	Nil
41	Unsatisfactory silver point endodontic treatment	Nil
42	Unrestored grade 1–2 attrition	Nil
43	Unrestored grade 1–2 attrition	Nil
44	Unrestored small abfraction	Nil
45	Unsatisfactory MO composite	Root resorption and thermal sensitivity
46	Satisfactory occlusal and buccal amalgams	Nil
47	Satisfactory occlusal and buccal amalgams	Nil
48	Not present	Nil

Special tests

	Performed	Additional information
Percussion	√	NAD
Palpation	√	NAD
Vitality	√	All +ve, except 41

Radiographs (Figure 10.4.6)
Orthopantomogram (12/7/2007)

Features	Radiographic data
TMJ	NAD
Bone loss	NAD
Sinuses	NAD
Mandibular canal	Visualised
Mental foramen	Visualised
Retained roots	Nil
Pathology	41 silver point, widened PDL minor root resorption
Other	85 advanced root resorption and furcation involvement

Periapical films

Tooth no.	Information	Tooth no.	Information
18	Nil	38	Nil
17	Nil	37	Nil
16	Nil	36	Nil
15	Nil	35	Nil
14	Nil	34	Nil
13	Nil	33	Nil
12	Nil	32	Nil
11	Nil	31	Nil
21	Nil	41	Nil
22	Nil	42	Nil
23	Nil	43	Nil
24	Nil	44	Nil
25	Nil	45	Ag point endodontic widened PDL, minor root resorption
26	Nil	46	Nil
27	Nil	47	Nil
28	Nil	48	Nil

Other radiographs (Figure 10.4.7)

	Date	Radiographic data
Lat ceph	30/8/2007	For orthodontic/prosthetic tracing (Figure 10.4.6)

Study casts (Figure 10.4.8)

Articulation	Position	ICP
	Face bow	Recorded
Diagnostic wax-up	OVD change	Not required
	Occlusal adjustment	Not required
	Crown lengthening	Orthodontic intrusion 11, 21
	Orthodontic/prosthodontic diagnostic wax-up	Flare and intrude 11, 21 by 1 mm, flatten curve of Wilson, reduce 85 to premolar space, de-rotate, close spaces and consolidate buccal segments, 33–43 to remain as is, veneers 14–24

Problem list

Problem list	Details
Tooth surface loss	Attrition of anterior segment
Parafunction	Sleep bruxism and possibly awake bruxism
Aesthetics compromised due to tooth wear	Compromised due to tooth wear
Restorative	Sensitive, retained 85 – 5-year longevity poor, strategic value in overall plan negligible
Endodontics	Silver point RCT on 41, tooth discoloured
Psychological	High aesthetic demand
Malocclusion	Posterior interferences, lack of adequate anterior guidance, excessive curve of Wilson

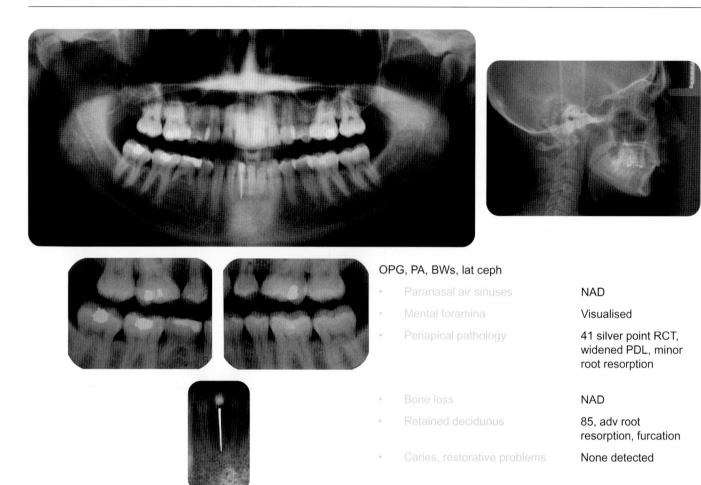

OPG, PA, BWs, lat ceph

• Paranasal air sinuses	NAD
• Mental foramina	Visualised
• Periapical pathology	41 silver point RCT, widened PDL, minor root resorption
• Bone loss	NAD
• Retained deciduous	85, adv root resorption, furcation
• Caries, restorative problems	None detected

Figure 10.4.6 Radiographs – orthopantomogram, bite wings, periapical of 4.1, lateral cephalometric views.

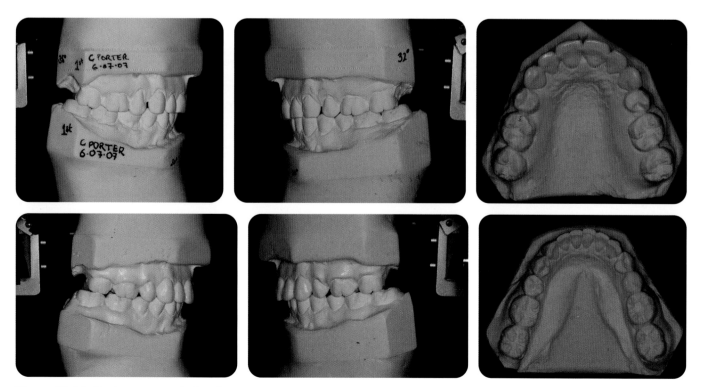

- SNA   77.5   (82)
- SNB   74   (80)
- ANB   3.5   (2)
- A-NPerp   -4mm   (1mm)
- Po-NPerp   -11mm   (0)
- I-I angle   139   (130)
- MxI-pal pl   103   (109)
- MnI-Mn pl   93   (93)

Relative to cranial base, maxilla is retrusive. Mandible is mildly retrusive to maxilla. Dentally maxillary incisors are mildly retroclined and lower incisors are ideal to mandibular base.

Curve of Wilson

- Initial thoughts were problematic
- – Increased tooth contact posteriorly, greater chance of mediotrusive interferences
- – Orthodontic literature suggest link with midline shift
- – Not conforming to flat occlusal plane and anterior guidance for age group
- More recent studies show no correlation with occlusal scheme and attrition
- Will be improved as part of finishing of posterior segments in combination with orthodontics for other reasons

Spijker A, Kreulen C, Creugers N. Attrition, occlusion, (dys)function and intervention: a systematic review. Clin Oral Impl Res 2007;18:117-126.
Klineberg I, Kingston D. Murray G. The bases for using a particular occlusal design in tooth and implant borne reconstructions and complete dentures. Clin Oral Impl Res 2007;18:151-167.

Figure 10.4.7 Cephalometric analysis (values measured with mean values in brackets) – SNA 77.5 (82); SNB 74 (80); ANB 3.5 (2); A–N Perp – 4.0 mm; Po–N Perp -11 (0); incisor angle 139 (130); Mxi–pal pi 103 (109); Mni–Mn pi 93 (93). The values suggest the following – relative to the cranial base the maxilla is retrusive; the mandible is mildly retrusive to the maxilla. Maxillary incisors are mildly retroclined and lower incisors are in an ideal position to the mandibular base (Klineberg *et al.* 2007, Spijker *et al.* 2007).

Figure 10.4.8 Study casts – articulated.

Treatment options

The dentition could be maintained in its present condition with:

- periodontal maintenance;
- replacement of the 45 with a single tooth implant;
- endodontic retreatment for 41 and internal bleaching;
- continual occlusal splint compliance;
- conservative restorative care as required.

These treatment options were supported by data from Holm-Pedersen *et al.* (2007) and Mordohai *et al.* (2007).

Improvement in aesthetics could be achieved with:

- composite or porcelain veneers 13–23;
- full coverage ACC or CMC;
- orthodontics to increase space for restorative material and minimise tooth reduction prior to the options above.

Discussion

The patient preferred as optimal an aesthetic result as possible with minimal tooth preparation and did not object to orthodontic treatment; she also preferred porcelain rather than composite resin veneers.

The compliance with occlusal splint wearing had 2 years of positive outcome, therefore it was assumed that this would continue. Dental awareness and understanding of the limitations in strength of restorative replacement was high, resulting in comprehensive informed consent.

Aesthetics improvement may be achieved with veneering of teeth 13–23 only; however, the increase in length and size requested would result in long thin teeth (Magne & Belser 2003, Fradeani & Barducci 2004–2008). In addition, further tooth structure would need to be removed and an unfavourable interincisal angle may place more strain on the veneers.

Prerestorative orthodontics would:

- allow improved space for restorative material and minimal tooth reduction;
- provide consolidation of teeth within the arch;
- reduce mesiodistal space for 45 in preparation for implant placement;
- improve buccal occlusion.

The considerations above are supported by data from Johansson et al. (1993), Magne and Belser (2003), Fradeani and Barducci (2004–2008), Spear *et al.* (2006), Cohen *et al.* (2008) and Kokich (2008).

The reduced requirement for tooth reduction results in more enamel for bonding increasing the potential longevity of porcelain-bonded restorations (Magne & Belser, 2003, Layton & Walton 2007). Reduction of the single tooth space (45) results in less cantilever forces from a large occlusal surface and concomitant screw loosening (Goodacre *et al.* 2003).

The patient has committed to smoking cessation. The effects on general and dental health in addition to osseointegration and maintenance of integration will be improved (Moy *et al.* 2005, DeLuca *et al.* 2006, Strietzel *et al.* 2007). The effect on the dentition of increased stress and associated bruxism, especially during waking hours, may be reduced with stress reduction strategies such as exercise, yoga and meditation. Such strategies have been instigated in an effort to reduce bruxism. Nocturnal bruxism is recognised as a centrally generated sleep disorder, therefore it may be modulated with stress-reduction efforts; however, the local effects of tooth surface loss are best prevented with the use of an occlusal splint (Lavigne *et al.* 2007).

Interdisciplinary treatment planning and provision requires close collaboration between specialties and regular review during treatment delivery; therefore patient compliance and availability, as well as a designated treatment coordinator, is necessary to ensure that the treatment goals from each specialty are achieved (Smalley 1995, Spear *et al.* 2006, Cohen *et al.* 2008).

Treatment sequence

Control phase

The treatment plan details were discussed to ensure that all procedures were understood and based on the evidence to achieve patient consent.

- Dental prophylaxis and reinforcement of the importance of plaque control as a key element of oral hygiene.
- Remove unsatisfactory tooth restorations and determine:
  - individual tooth restorability;
  - their strategic value in the overall treatment plan.
- Reassess and re-evaluate the dentition and oral health.

Holding phase

- Lateral cephalometric imaging and orthodontic/prosthodontic diagnostic wax-up was required.
- Extraction of 45 and allow at least 6 weeks of soft tissue healing before implant placement at the site.
- Endodontic retreatment for 41 and internal bleaching to proceed.

Orthodontics to include:

- Intrusion (by 1 mm) and slight flaring of maxillary incisor teeth.
- Reduction of premolar space of 45, which will require implant anchorage. The implant will be placed according to diagnostic preparation and is to be provisionalised after 3 months. Mesial movement of 46 with implant anchorage estimated at 0.75 mm/month (see data from Roberts, 2004).
- Consolidation of posterior segments with space closure.
- Reduction of the curve of Wilson

Following further discussion with the patient, her response to the treatment proposal allowed the treatment to commence (Figure 10.4.9).

Reconstructive phase

- A revised diagnostic preparation of the veneers for teeth 13–23 was required.
- An intraoral diagnostic mock-up followed for patient information and clinician confirmation of the appropriateness of the plan (Figure 10.4.10).
- Aesthetics and phonetics assessed and modified as required.
- Preparations to teeth for feldspathic veneers with use of silicone preparation guides from finalised diagnostic wax-up (Figure 10.4.11).
- Provisionals were assessed for aesthetics, phonetics and modified as required.
- Definitive feldspathic veneers constructed from cast and index of the provisional restorations (Figure 10.4.12).
- Definitive implant restoration for 45 as screw-retained Procera zirconia crown.
- A new occlusal splint was designed and fitted (maxillary full-arch).
- Reassessment and re-evaluation (Figure 10.4.13).

Maintenance and monitoring phase

- Ongoing preventive strategies were followed.
- Plaque control as defined by Hirschfield and Wassermann (1978) and Holm-Pederson *et al.* (2007) and reviews tailored to patient needs.
- Prosthodontic review 6 monthly, as recommended by Mordohai *et al.* (2007).

Review at 1 year (Figure 10.4.14)

- Oral health status: oral hygiene and plaque control. *Patient excellent, brushes 2–3 times per day, flosses once a day.*
  - Soft tissues – healthy, pink, firm. No carious lesions.
  - All probing depths of 1–3 mm with no change from previous charting.
  - Bone levels around single tooth implant restoration on 45 were similar to marginal bone level at prosthetic connection.
  - No change in periapical appearance of endodontically treated 41.
  - All margins of restorations sound with no sign of microleakage.
  - OPG: no apparent abnormality.
- Occlusion. *No change in occlusion. Patient wearing maxillary occlusal splint and thermoplastic retainer for mandibular arch nightly.*
- Radiographs. *No change noted.*
- Oral health related quality of life. *Comfort and appearance have changed significantly with self-reported improvement; enjoys many comments on 'my lovely smile'; is more confident, general well-being and in social settings. Has ceased smoking for over 1 year. General improvement in overall health with fitness regime and diet.*
- Additional comments. *'Would absolutely do it all again if I had to!' 'I couldn't handle going back to my previous teeth so I look after these as much as I can.'*

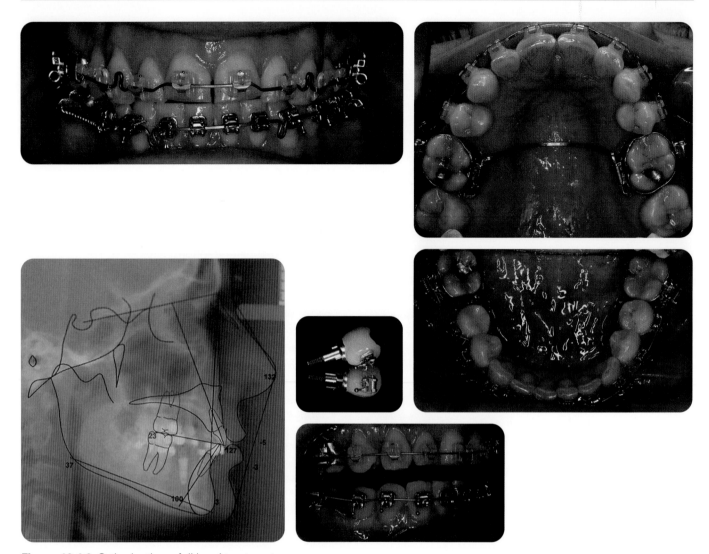

Figure 10.4.9 Orthodontics – full-band treatment.

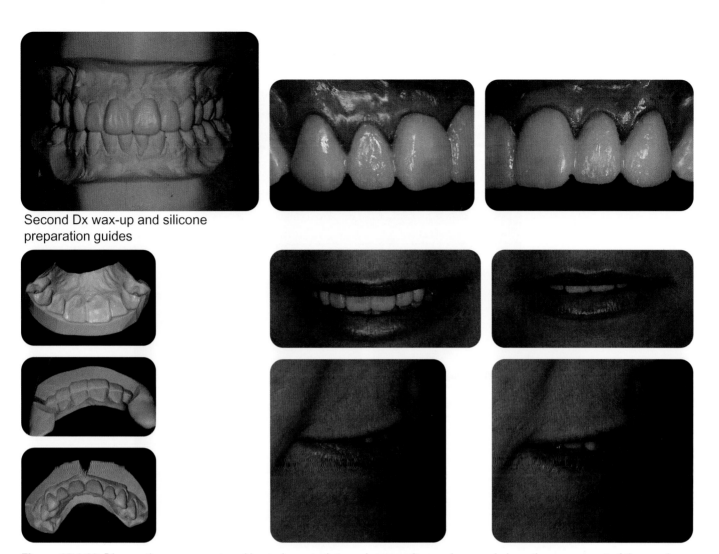

Second Dx wax-up and silicone
preparation guides

Figure 10.4.10 Diagnostic wax-up captured in study casts; intraoral composite mock-up, and phonetic assessment of the mock-up.

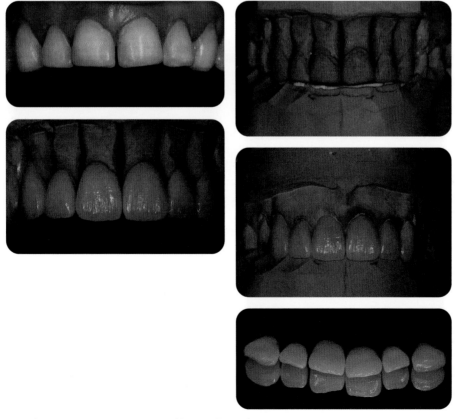

Figure 10.4.11 Direct provisional veneers constructed in acrylic resin.

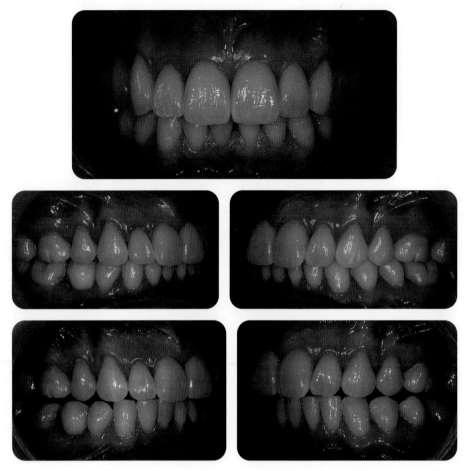

Figure 10.4.12 Definitive feldspathic veneers that were accurately modelled on the provisional restorations.

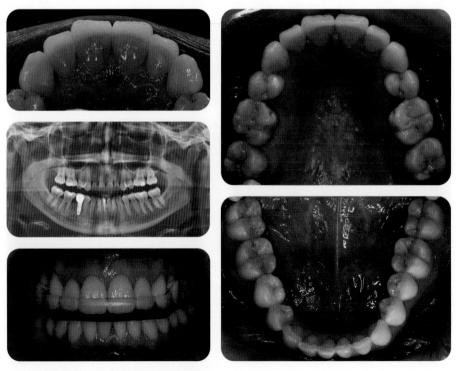

Figure 10.4.13 Reassessment and re-evaluation at 1 month.

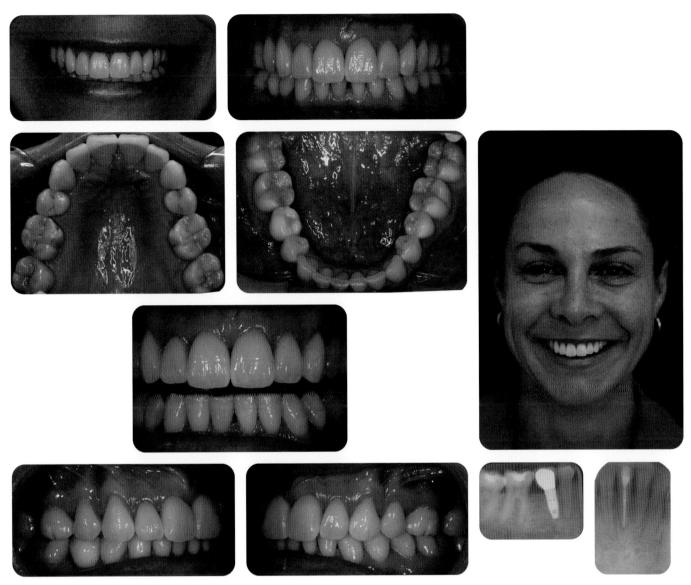

Figure 10.4.14 Review at 1 year.

References

Cohen, M. (ed.) (2008) *Interdisciplinary Treatment Planning: Principles, Design, Implementation.* Quintessence, Chicago.

DeLuca, S., Habsha, E. & Zarb, G.A. (2006) The effect of smoking on osseointegrated dental implants. Part 1: implant survival. *International Journal of Prosthodontics*, 19 (5), 491–498.

Fradeani, M. & Barducci, G. (2004–2008) *Esthetic rehabilitation in fixed Prosthodontics.* 2 vols. Quintessence, Chicago.

Goodacre, C.J., Bernal, G., Rungcharassaeng, K. *et al.* (2003) Clinical complications in fixed prosthodontics. *Journal of Prosthetic Dentistry*, 90 (1), 31–41.

Hirschfield, L. & Wassermann, B. (1978) A long term survey of tooth loss in 600 treated periodontal patients. *Journal of Periodontology*, 49 (5), 225–237.

Holm-Pedersen, P., Lang, N.P. & Müller, F. (2007) What are the longevities of teeth and oral implants? *Clinical Oral Implants Research*, 18 (Suppl. 3), 15–19.

Johansson, A., Kiliaridis, S., Haraldson, T. *et al.* (1993) Covariation of some factors associated with occlusal tooth wear in a selected high-wear sample. *Scandinavian Journal of Dental Research*, 101 (6), 398–406.

Klineberg, I., Kingston, D. & Murray G. (2007) The bases for using a particular occlusal design in tooth and implant borne reconstructions and complete dentures. *Clinical Oral Implants Research*, 18, 151–167.

Kokich, V. (2008) Altering vertical dimension in the perio-restorative patient: the orthodontic possibilities. In: *Interdisciplinary Treatment Planning: Principles, Design, Implementation* (ed. M. Cohen), pp. 49–80. Quintessence, Chicago.

Lavigne, G. J., Huynh, N., Kato, T. *et al.* (2007) Genesis of sleep bruxism: motor and autonomic-cardiac interactions. *Archives of Oral Biology*, 52 (4), 381–384.

Layton, D. & Walton, T. (2007) An up to 16-year prospective study of 304 porcelain veneers. *International Journal of Prosthodontics*, 20 (4), 389–396.

Magne, P. & Belser, U. (2003) *Bonded Porcelain Restorations in the Anterior Dentition: a biomimetic Approach.* Quintessence, Chicago.

Mordohai, N., Reshad, M., Jivraj, S. *et al.* (2007) Factors that affect individual tooth prognosis and choices in contemporary treatment planning. *British Dental Journal*, 202 (2), 63–72.

Moy, P.K., Medina, D., Shetty, V. *et al.* (2005) Dental implant failures and associated risk factors. *International Journal of Oral & Maxillofacial Implants*, 20 (4), 569–577.

Roberts, W.E., Engen, D.W., Schneider, P.M. *et al.* (2004) Implant-anchored orthodontics for partially edentulous malocclusions in children and adults. *American Journal of Orthodontics and Dentofacial Orthopedics*, 126 (3), 302–304.

Smalley, W.M. (1995) Implants for tooth movement: determining implant location and orientation. *Journal of Esthetic Dentistry*, 7 (2), 62–72.

Spear, F.M., Kokich, V.G. & Mathews, D. (2006) Interdisciplinary management of anterior dental esthetics. *Journal of the American Dental Association*, 137 (2), 160–169.

Spijker, A., Kreulen, C. & Creugers, N. (2007) Attrition, occlusion, (dys)function and intervention: a systematic review. *Clinical Oral Implants Research*, 18, 117–126.

Strietzel, F.P., Reichart, P.A., Kale, A. *et al.* (2007) Smoking interferes with the prognosis of dental implant treatment: a systematic review and meta analysis. *Journal of Clinical Periodontology*, 34 (6), 523–544.

11

The Broken Down Dentition

Introduction by Iven Klineberg

The progressive deterioration of the dental status has a complex multifactorial aetiology, usually involving a variety of behavioural, medical and local factors.

Attrition, erosion and abrasion may be a catalyst, and less than optimal general dental care is generally a contributor, with undercontoured restorations, periodic extractions, and extrusion and migration of teeth adjacent to and opposing edentulous spaces. Loss of harmony of occlusal plane orientation follows progressively and, in association with bruxism (awake and/or sleep), progressive reduction in anterior tooth length leads to an aesthetically compromised appearance. A reduced OVD may also develop.

Adaptation within the stomatognathic system (Sessle 2005) is a continuous biological expectation throughout life, and is triggered within the orofacial complex by continual changes in tooth form, number, orientation and interarch relationship, which may influence lower face height and facial appearance. Attritional wear has been reported by Lambrechts et al. (1984) to be of the order of 68 µm per year. Seligman and Pullinger (1995) reported non-linear progression over time with slower tooth wear with increasing age, up to 1000 µm per year in non-bruxers and of the order of 400–500 µm per year in bruxers. These authors also reported on canine guidance providing a limit to posterior tooth wear and that canine form should be evaluated in clinical assessment.

Given the average enamel thickness at the incisal and occlusal surfaces is 2.0–2.6 mm, contributing factors to tooth breakdown include the following:

- parafunction (nail biting, chewing pencils/pens, chewing abrasive foods);
- abrasion (abrasive diet, airborne abrasive/acidic particles from industrial pollution);
- erosion (low intraoral pH linked with a diet high in acidic foods and fruits, acidic drinks, as well as gastric reflux from gastro-oesophageal disease or anorexia nervosa and/or bulimia, as well as gastrointestinal disorders);
- presence of missing teeth leading to increased loading of remaining teeth and bone.

Within the complexity of the system, occlusal and incisal tooth wear is compensated by progressive tooth eruption to maintain a consistent spatial interarch dental relationship. As a result, clinical perceptions of loss of OVD may be incorrect in relation to lower face height; however, as a restorative and prosthodontic requirement, an increase in OVD may be essential to provide adequate crown height for aesthetic rehabilitation. The need for an increase in OVD is a biologically accepted prosthodontic necessity. The adaptive process for an increase in OVD was first described by Goldspink (1976) in an animal study involving the masseter muscle, with the addition of sarcomeres in series with increased OVD to re-establish a biologically acceptable occlusal plane and functional interdental space. Any perceived uncertainty by clinicians was further discounted by Carlsson et al. (1979) with an electromyogram study on the masseter muscle indicating adaptation to an increase in OVD. Subsequently, studies by Sessle (2006), Svensson et al. (2006) and Sessle et al. (2009) confirmed neuroplastic changes at the sensorimotor cortex followed small and large changes to tooth shape and occlusal form. Klineberg et al. (2007) proposed a new paradigm for occlusal rehabilitation in acknowledgement of central neuroplasticity. More recently, human studies by Lai et al. (unpublished data) with comprehensive data including functional magnetic resonance imaging analyses have confirmed that neuroplasticity at the sensorimotor cortex occurred as an immediate response to an increase in OVD.

References

Carlsson, G.E., Ingervall, B. & Kocak, G. (1979) Effect of increasing vertical dimension on the masticatory system in subjects with natural teeth. *Journal of Prosthetic Dentistry*, 41 (3), 284–289.

Goldspink, G. (1976) The adaptation of muscle to a new functional length. In: *Mastication: Proceedings of a Symposium on the Clinical and Physiological Aspects of Mastication held at the Medical School, University of Bristol on 14–16 April 1975* (eds D.J. Anderson & B. Mathews), pp. 90–99. John Wright, Bristol.

Klineberg, I., Kingston, D. & Murray, G. (2007) The bases for using a particular occlusal design in tooth and implant-borne reconstructions and complete dentures. *Clinical Oral Implants Research*, 18 (Suppl. 3), 151–167.

Lambrechts, P., Vanherle, G., Vuylsteke, M. *et al.* (1984) Quantitative evaluation of the wear resistance of posterior dental restorations: a new three dimensional measuring technique. *Journal of Dentistry*, 12 (3), 252–267.

Seligman, D.A. & Pullinger, A.G. (1995) The degree to which dental attrition in a modern society is a function of age and canine contact. *Journal of Orofacial Pain*, 9 (3), 266–275.

Sessle, B.J. (2005) Biological adaptation and normative values. *International Journal of Prosthodontics*, 18 (4), 280–282.

Sessle, B.J. (2006) Mechanisms of oral somatosensory and motor functions and their clinical correlates. *Journal of Oral Rehabilitation*, 33 (4), 243–261.

Sessle, B.J., Klineberg, I. & Svensson, P. (2009) A neurophysiologic perspective on rehabilitation with oral implants and their potential side effects. In: *Osseointergration and Dental Implants* (ed. A. Jokstad), pp. 333–344. Wiley-Blackwell, Ames, Iowa.

Svensson, P., Romaniello, A., Wang, K. *et al.* (2006) One hour of tongue-task training is associated with plasticity in corticomotor control of the human tongue musculature. *Experimental Brain Research*, 173 (1), 165–173.

Case 11.1 Mr Divo C

Max Guazzato

Patient: Mr Divo C (date of birth 09/08/1948)

Presenting complaints

Description	'I find it difficult to chew and eat, the bottom denture moves and food gets underneath and I have to continually clean it. I seldom have problems with the top denture. Pain only when biting on natural teeth. I cannot eat foods such as biscuits, almond biscuits, pepper. My dentures are not stable, I have infections associated with the remaining teeth and I would like a long term solution'
Onset	'I had periodontal disease . . . my teeth loosened over a period of 25 years. I have had surgical periodontal therapy and cleaning every 1–3 months for 25 years'
Frequency	Constantly
Duration	'Constantly I have had a abscess going up and down'
Intensity	N/A
Triggering	N/A
Aggravating	N/A
Alleviating	N/A
Treatment received	General dentist every 1–3 months for 25 years
Medication	Nil
Allergies	Nil

Other complaints

Function	'I have limited chewing ability; at the moment I feel aware of the dentures'
TMD	Nil
Headaches	Nil
Parafunction	Nil
Habits	Nil
Cervical	Nil
Dental	No restorations in the existing teeth
Periodontal	All existing teeth are mobile (grade III mobility)
Dentures	Upper and lower partial acrylic prostheses
Splint	Nil
Saliva	pH 7.8; 20 ml of saliva for 5 minute test. Buffer test: 12. Saliva watery Drinks 1.5 L water/day, 3–4 cups coffee/day
Breathe	Nose breather
Cosmetic	Nil

Patient's expectations

- To be able to eat comfortably.
- To have a denture that is stable.
- To have good aesthetic outcome.
- No more infections.
- 'Preferably I do not want to find food stuck under the denture.'

History
Medical history

General Practitioner	Once a year. Moderately high cholesterol, low blood pressure/normal no problems. No regular doctor
Cardiovascular	Nil
Respiratory	Nil
Gastrointestinal	Nil
Neurological	Nil
Endocrine	Nil
Haematological	Nil
Integumentary	Nil
Genitourinary	Nil
Musculoskeletal	Nil
Immune system	Nil
Allergies	Nil
Operations	Appendix 40 years ago
Trauma	Car accident, nil to teeth. Tore muscles/tendon
Medication	Nil

Social history

Marital status	Married		
Children	3		
Occupation	Salesman – tape drives to back up computers		
Recreational drugs	Nil		
Smoking	Type		Nil
	Frequency		N/A
	Period		N/A
Diet	Only soft food		
		Soft drinks	Nil
		Sports drinks	Nil
		Lemons	Nil
	√	Acidic foods	Vinegar
	√	Sweet foods	Rarely
	√	Water	1.5 L/day
	√	Tea	Rarely
	√	Coffee	3–4 cups coffee/day
	√	Alcohol	Beer and wine with moderation
		Hard/brittle foods	Nil
		Ice crunching	Nil
Habits/hobbies	Walking		

Dental history

Date of last examination	6-monthly check-ups
Oral hygiene routine	Brushes twice a day with manual brush Flossing never; occasionally using interdental brushes No mouthwashes
TMD	Nil
Splint	Nil
OMFS	Nil
Extractions	Several extractions over time; the last time was 4 years ago when four teeth were extracted
Dentures	A few upper and lower partial acrylic dentures
Orthodontics	Nil
Periodontics	Surgical and non-surgical periodontal therapy over 25 years
Endodontics	Nil
Crown and bridge	Nil
Implants	Nil
Cosmetic	Nil
Other	Nil

Extraoral examination (Figures 11.1.1 & 11.1.2)
Aesthetics

Head and neck	NAD	
Facial symmetry	Within normal limits	
Profile	Convex	
Nasolabial angle	120°	
Facial folds	Shallow nasolabial folds	
Midlines	Face/maxillary centrals	Midline coincident
	Maxillary/mandibular centrals	Mandibular midline deviated on the right side by 3 mm
Lip posture	Symmetry	Symmetrical
	Upper lip	Medium to long with asymmetric pull to the right when smiling
	Lower lip	Normal and competent
	Competence	Yes
	Tooth display	From 15 to 25, normal lip line
Occlusal plane	Parallel to ala tragus line	Not assessable
	Parallel to interpupillary line	Not assessable
	Over-eruption	All remaining teeth
Vertical	FWS	4 mm
	OVD assessment	OVD normal OVD in CO = 80 mm OVD in rest position = 84 mm
Smile assessment	Symmetry	No
	Lip line	Normal
	Gingival display	In the right side, not in the left side
	Tooth display	From 15 to 25
	Buccal corridor	Normal

Phonetic

	Normal	Abnormal
Labial (m)	√	
Labiodental (f/v)	√	
Linguodental (th)	√	
Interdental (s)		√
Linguopalatal (k/ng)	√	

Temporomandibular assessment

TMJ	Additional information
Click	Nil
Crepitus	Nil
Tenderness	Nil

Muscle tenderness	Right	Left
Temporalis	Nil	Nil
Masseter	Nil	Nil
Posterior mandible	Nil	Nil
Anterior mandible	Nil	Nil
Glands	Normal	
Nodes	Normal	

Jaw movement	Measurement (mm)	Reference points
Maximal opening	42	Tooth 11
Right laterotrusion	15	Maxillary dental midline
Left laterotrusion	15	Maxillary dental midline
Midline deviation	Right (3)	
Maximal protrusion	6	
Opening pathway	S-shaped as the existing teeth interfere then mandible shifts to the left for maximum occlusal contact	
Overjet	0	
Overbite	0	

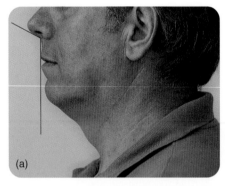
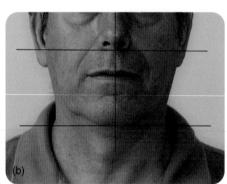
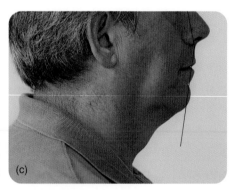

Figure 11.1.1 Extraoral examination. Patient in intercuspal position showing an open nasolabial angle and a convex profile (a, b). Vertical dimension is normal (c).

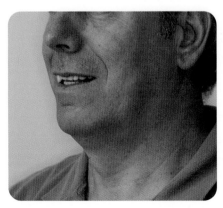
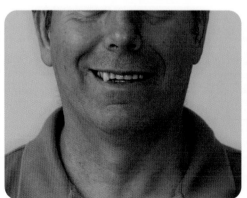
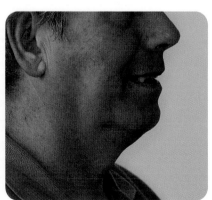

Figure 11.1.2 Extraoral examination – aesthetic evaluation. The upper right canine is over-erupted and contacts the lower lip. The incisal edges of the other teeth are short and do not follow the lip curvature. Patient's lack of confidence is associated with poor tooth display.

Intraoral examination (Figure 11.1.3)
Soft tissues

Tissue	Healthy	Abnormal	Additional information
Lips	√		
Labial vestibule		√	Swelling and pus in the region of 13
Cheeks	√		
Palate	√		
Oropharynx	√		
Tongue	√		
Floor	√		
Frenal attachments	√		

Ridges	Maxilla	Mandible
Edentulous areas	Only 13, 15 present	Only 44, 45 present
Arch shape	U	U
Resorption	Not significant	Thin anterior ridge
Palatal vault	Moderate	
Tori	Nil	Nil
Frenal attachments	Average	Average
Mucosa	Normal	Normal
Pathology	Nil	Nil

Oral cleanliness

Condition	Yes	No			
Plaque	√		Generalised	Severe	Supragingival + subgingival
Calculus	√		Localised	Severe	Supragingival + subgingival
Food impaction	√		Under the existing dentures		
Stains	√		Generalised		
Halitosis	√				

Saliva

Water intake	1.5 L/day; 3–4 cups coffee/day
Quality	WNL
Quantity	WNL
Pathology	Nil
Medications affecting	Nil

Periodontium

CPITN			
	4	–	–
	4	–	–

Gingiva	Biotype	Medium
	Colour	Pink with localised areas of inflammation and redness
	Contour	Normal
	Consistency	Firm
Papillae	Colour	Pink with localised areas of inflammation and redness
	Contour	Normal

Periodontal charting

Irrelevant as the teeth are terminal.

Occlusal assessment

Existing dentures.

Arch compatibility	Medium compatible arches in skeletal class II	
Occlusal plane	Curve of Spee	N/A
	Curve of Wilson	N/A
Posterior support	Non-existent	
Skeletal class classification	II (assessed with clinical examination)	
Angle right	Molar N/A	Canine N/A
Angle left	Molar N/A	Canine N/A
Anterior overbite	0 mm	
Anterior overjet	0 mm	
Cross-bites	Nil	
Open-bites	Dentures have limited contact points in IP	
RP to IP slide	0 mm	
FWS	Close/M/swallow test	4 mm

Tooth guidance

Irrelevant as there is no guidance.

Tooth surface loss

Not applicable.

Dental charting

Tooth no.	Clinical findings	Prognosis	Comments
18	Missing	Nil	
17	Missing	Nil	
16	Missing	Nil	
15	Unrestored	Hopeless	Mobility grade III, deep periodontal pocket
14	Missing	Nil	
13	Unrestored	Hopeless	Mobility grade III, deep periodontal pocket, pus and bleeding, large periapical radiolucency
12	Missing	Nil	
11	Missing	Nil	
21	Missing	Nil	
22	Missing	Nil	
23	Missing	Nil	
24	Missing	Nil	
25	Missing	Nil	
26	Missing	Nil	
27	Missing	Nil	
28	Missing	Nil	
38	Missing	Nil	
37	Missing	Nil	
36	Missing	Nil	
35	Missing	Nil	
34	Missing	Nil	
33	Missing	Nil	
32	Missing	Nil	
31	Missing	Nil	
41	Missing	Nil	
42	Missing	Nil	
43	Missing	Nil	
44	Unrestored	Hopeless	Mobility grade III, deep periodontal pocket
45	Unrestored	Hopeless	Mobility grade III, deep periodontal pocket
46	Missing	Nil	
47	Missing	Nil	
48	Missing	Nil	

Previous prosthesis – N/A

Teeth replaced

8 7 6 5 4 3 2 1 1 2 3 4 5 6 7 8

8 7 6 5 4 3 2 1 1 2 3 4 5 6 7 8

	Mandible	Maxilla
Age	5 years old	5 years old
Type	Acrylic base partial	Acrylic base partial
Kennedy classification	Class I	Class I
Appearance	Unsatisfactory	Unsatisfactory
OVD	Poor	Poor
Stability	Poor	Poor
Support	Poor	Poor
Retention	Poor	Poor
Hygiene	Poor	Poor
Patient opinion	Totally unsatisfactory	Totally unsatisfactory

Radiographs (Figure 11.1.4)
Orthopantomogram (12/11/08)

Features	Radiographic data
TMJ	Normal
Bone loss	Mild
Sinuses	Normal
Mandibular foramen and canal	Normal
Mental foramen	Normal
Retained roots	No
Pathology	Large cystic-like lesion surrounding the tooth 13 extending to the nasal–palatal canal and tooth 15 Calcified sternohyoid ligament

Periapical/full mouth series radiographs (Figure 11.1.5)

Computed tomography scan analysis (Figure 11.1.6)

Study casts (Figure 11.1.7)

Articulation	Position	RCP
	Face bow	Yes
Diagnostic wax-up	OVD change	+2 mm
	Occlusal adjustment	Nil
	Crown lengthening	Nil

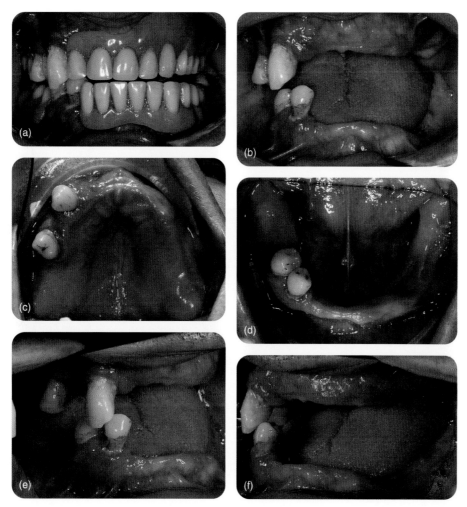

Figure 11.1.3 Intraoral examination. Frontal view with the existing partial removable prosthesis (a) Frontal, occlusal and lateral views without prostheses show healthy alveolar ridge tissues and some dental plaque and gingival inflammation associated with the teeth (b–f).

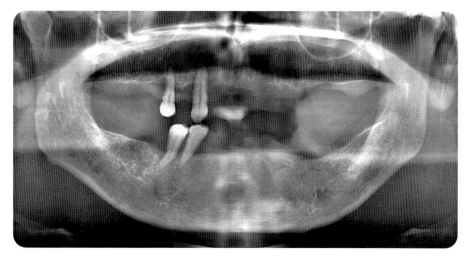

Figure 11.1.4 Panoramic radiograph. The alveolar ridge is well preserved. Tooth 13 presents with a large periapical radiolucency that clinically manifested with discharge. There is significant bone loss around the remaining teeth.

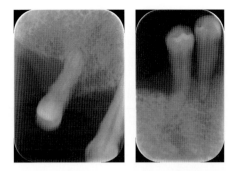

Figure 11.1.5 Periapical radiographs. Details of bone levels with remaining teeth and potential periodontal pocket depth.

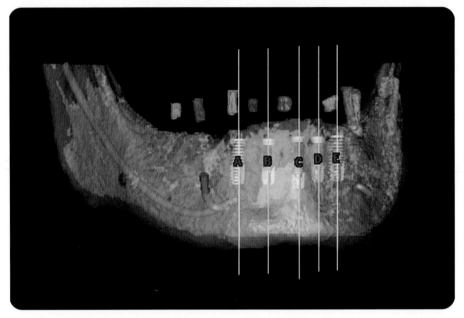

Figure 11.1.6 Treatment planning. The treatment simulated on the 3D model consists of an osteotomy of the thin alveolar ridge crest and the insertion of 5 implants in the interforaminal region of the mandible.

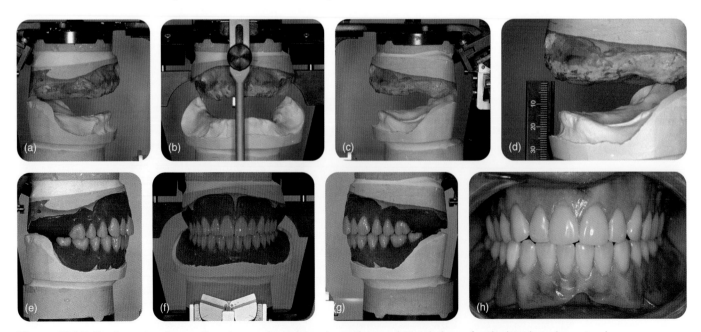

Figure 11.1.7 Study casts, diagnostic set-up and provisional prostheses. Lateral view of articulated study casts shows insufficient interarch space and the thin mandibular alveolar ridge (d). Owing to the limited interarch space the teeth were set slightly labial to the ridge for the provisional removable dental prostheses (e–g). Intraoral view of the provisional prostheses (h).

Clinical and radiographic examination findings

Tooth no.	Clinical findings	Prognosis	Comments
18	Missing		Nil
17	Missing		Nil
16	Missing		Nil
15	Unrestored	Hopeless	Mobility grade III, deep periodontal pocket
14	Missing		Nil
13	Unrestored	Hopeless	Mobility grade III, deep periodontal pocket, pus and bleeding, large periapical radiolucency
12	Missing		Nil
11	Missing		Nil
21	Missing		Nil
22	Missing		Nil
23	Missing		Nil
24	Missing		Nil
25	Missing		Nil
26	Missing		Nil
27	Missing		Nil
28	Missing		Nil
38	Missing		Nil
37	Missing		Nil
36	Missing		Nil
35	Missing		Nil
34	Missing		Nil
33	Missing		Nil
32	Missing		Nil
31	Missing		Nil
41	Missing		Nil
42	Missing		Nil
43	Missing		Nil
44	Unrestored	Hopeless	Mobility grade III, deep periodontal pocket
45	Unrestored	Hopeless	Mobility grade III, deep periodontal pocket
46	Missing		Nil
47	Missing		Nil
48	Missing		Nil

Provisional diagnosis

Category	Diagnosis/problem list
Medical conditions	Nil
TMD	Nil
Orofacial pain	Nil
Aesthetics	Poor retention and stability of partial dentures particularly on eating and talking Poor position/angle/colour/shape/size of the dentures teeth
Phonetics	Difficulty with some words and letter 'S'
Soft tissues	Bleeding and pus gingival tooth 13
Oral hygiene	Lost interest in oral hygiene
Occlusion	Existing occlusion is unacceptable Skeletal class II
Saliva	Nil
Tooth surface loss	Nil
Edentulism	Total edentulism is inevitable
Restorative	Nil
Prosthodontics	Skeletal class II Minimal interarch space
Periodontics	History of treated severe periodontitis
Endodontics	Nil

Treatment objectives

Short term
- Education on oral hygiene.

Long term
- Improve stability, retention and resistance.
- Function and aesthetics.
- Restore occlusal stability.
- Minimise maintenance.
- Cleanliness.
- Increase OVD.

Treatment options
Mandible
Treatment option 1: Removable complete prostheses
- Mandibular removable complete prosthesis with the following features:
  - slight increase of the OVD;
  - increased teeth display;
  - modified peripheral contour to increase stability and retention;
  - use of neutral zone concept to increase stability.

Treatment option 2: Osteotomy and implant-retained overdenture
- Osteotomy.
- Insertion of two implants.
- Implant-retained overdenture.

Treatment option 3: Osteotomy; implant-supported fixed prosthesis
- Osteotomy.
- Insertion of five or six implants between the two mental foramens.
- Restoration of the missing mandibular teeth with provisional fixed implant-supported acrylic prosthesis.
- Implant-supported fixed full-arch prosthesis to be fabricated in porcelain or acrylic on gold alloy; or acrylic on titanium; or porcelain on zirconia.

Maxilla
Treatment option 1: Removable complete prostheses
- Maxillary removable complete prostheses with the following features:
  - slight increase in OVD;
  - increased teeth display;
  - modified peripheral contour to increase stability and retention;
  - use of neutral zone concept to increase stability.

Treatment option 2: Implant-retained overdenture
- Insertion of four or more implants.
- Implant-retained overdenture.

Treatment option 3: Implant-supported fixed prosthesis
- Insertion of four or more implants.
- Restoration of the missing maxillary teeth with provisional fixed implant-supported acrylic prosthesis.
- Implant-supported fixed full-arch prosthesis to be fabricated in porcelain or acrylic on gold alloy; or acrylic on titanium; or porcelain on zirconia.

Treatment plan accepted
Mandible (option 3): Implant-supported fixed prosthesis
- Insertion of four or more implants.
- Restoration of the missing maxillary teeth with provisional fixed implant-supported acrylic prosthesis.

- Implant-supported fixed full-arch prosthesis to be fabricated in porcelain or acrylic on gold alloy; or acrylic on titanium; or porcelain on zirconia.

Maxilla (option 1): Removable complete prostheses
- Maxillary removable complete prostheses with the following features:
  - slight increase of the OVD;
  - increased teeth display;
  - modified peripheral contour to increase stability and retention.

Treatment sequence
Diagnostic phase I
- Chief concerns.
- History.
- Examination.
- Radiographs.
- Diagnosis/problem list.
- Prognosis.
- Treatment options.

Control phase
- Extraction of the teeth.
- Repair of the existing denture.
- Diagnostic set up (Figure 11.1.7)
- Issue new complete diagnostic dentures (Figure 11.1.7)

Treatment planning
- Duplicate of the dentures and construction of radiographic and surgical guides.
- Volumetric analysis (CT scan).
- Treatment plan and sequence.

Surgical and prosthetic phases (3 months after the extractions)
- Osteotomy.
- Insertion of the implants (Figure 11.1.8).
- Immediate loading of implants.
- Conversion of removable mandibular denture into FDP.

Prosthetic phase (at least 3 months after the previous phase)
- Implants and abutments assessment.
- Impressions.
- MMR and articulation.
- Wax-up and set up (Figure 11.1.10).
- Teeth try-in.
- Acrylic frame for CAD/CAM try-in (Figure 11.1.9).
- Zirconia frame try-in.

Prosthetic phase (at least 6 weeks after the previous phase)
- Issue of mandibular zirconia/porcelain fixed prosthesis (Figure 11.1.11).
- Issue of maxillary acrylic removable complete prosthesis (Figures 11.1.12–11.1.14).

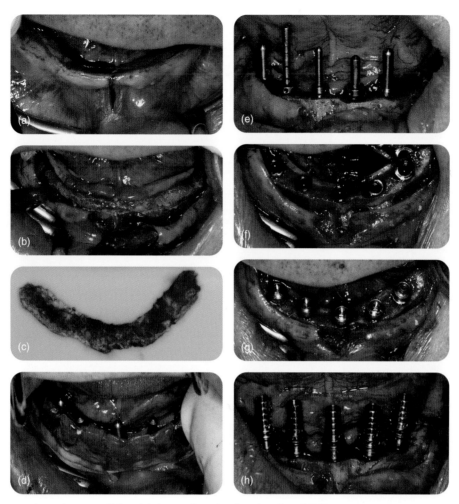

Figure 11.1.8 Treatment phase I – mandible with immediate implant loading. Midline and crestal incision (a). Full thickness flap (b). Fragment of the alveolar crest after osteotomy of the thin ridge (c). Verification of the implant position with the surgical guide and direction indicators (d). Verification the parallelism with direction indicators (e). Insertion of the five implants (f). Multi-unit abutments placed on the implants (g). Titanium temporary abutments mounted on the multi-unit abutments (h).

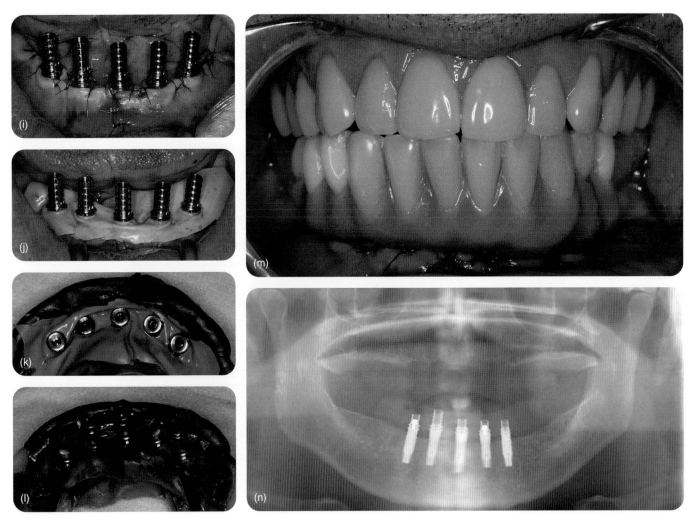

Figure 11.1.8 (*Continued*) The flap is sutured around the multi-unit abutments (i). Sterile rubber dam is placed at the base of the temporary abutments (j). A copy of the removable denture is used to take an impression with the temporary abutments as implant pick-ups (k). The implant replicas are linked together and a model is fabricated using fast setting impression material (l). The denture is then converted into a fixed acrylic prosthesis (m). A panoramic radiograph is taken to verify the fitting of the prosthesis (n).

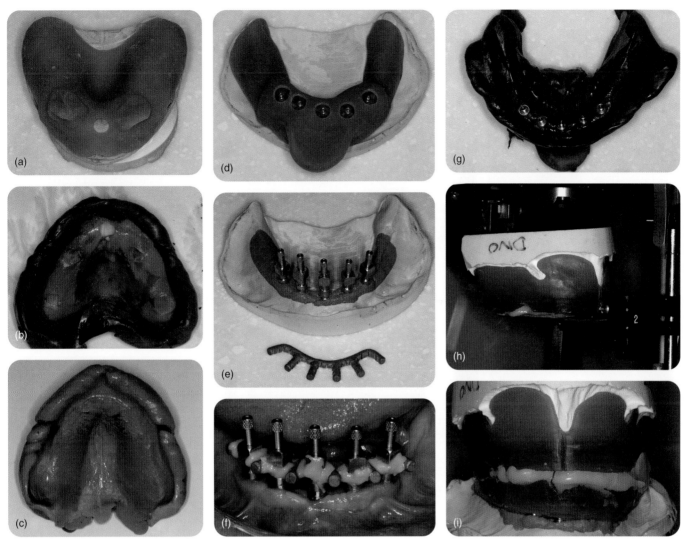

Figure 11.1.9 Treatment phase – maxilla and mandible. Custom tray for maxillary complete removable dental prosthesis (a). Impression of the border detail with thermoplastic material and low-viscosity polyether material (b). Impression of the remaining tissues with high viscosity polyether material injected in the tray (c). A preliminary model of the mandible with the implants (d) is used to fabricate a bar to passively link the impression copings (e) with a light-cured composite (f). Final impression taken with a polyether material (g). Occlusal rims on an articulator (h, i).

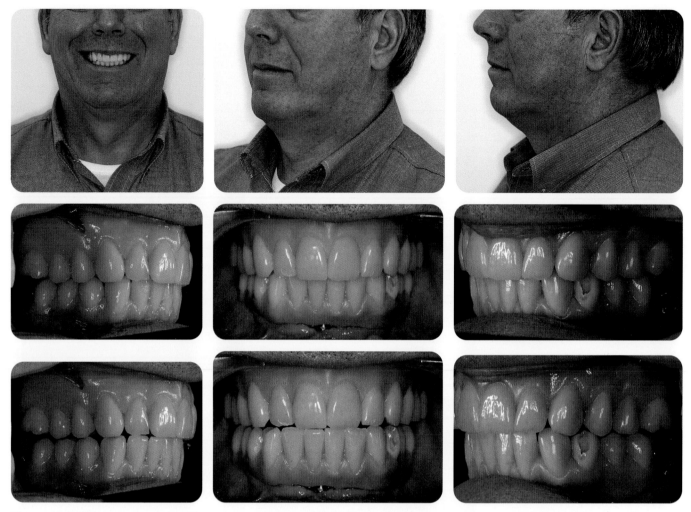

Figure 11.1.10 Treatment phase. The set-up try-in is fitted to verify aesthetics, tissue support and the occlusion.

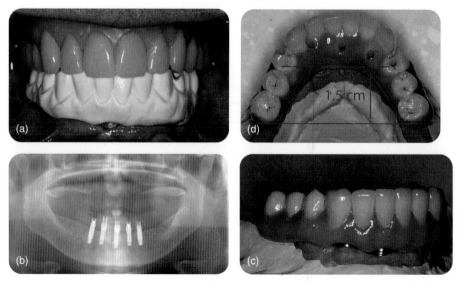

Figure 11.1.11 Treatment phase – final prosthesis. The mandibular set-up is duplicated with acrylic resin used to guide the milling process (a) and fit is verified with a panoramic radiograph (b). The mandibular zirconia-based prosthesis (c), with the distal cantilever limited to 1.5 cm (d).

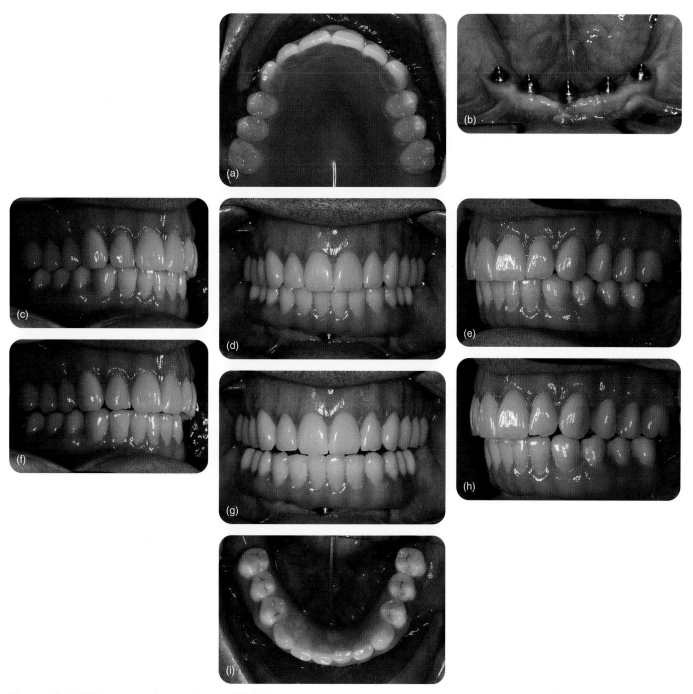

Figure 11.1.12 Treatment phase – issue of definitive prosthesis. Occlusal view of the maxillary complete removable dental prosthesis (a) and zirconia-based mandibular implant-supported fixed dental prosthesis (b). Lateral and frontal views of the prostheses in intercuspal position (c–e). Lateral and frontal views of lateral and protrusive positions (f–h). View of the multi-unit abutments before insertion of the prosthesis (i).

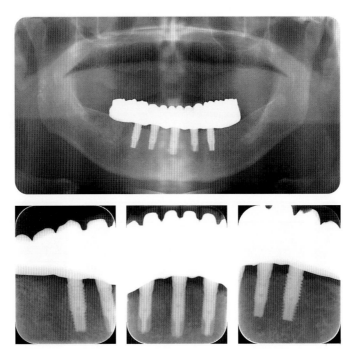

Figure 11.1.13 Panoramic and periapical radiographs with the definitive prostheses.

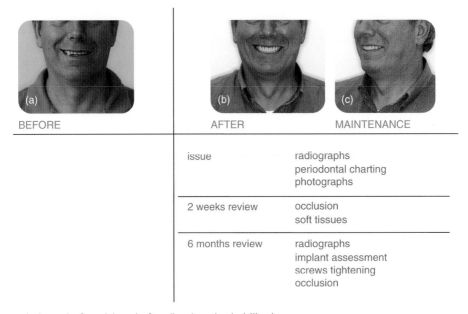

Figure 11.1.14 Extraoral views before (a) and after (b, c) oral rehabilitation.

Discussion
Maxilla
The chief concerns from the patient were the infection in the canine tooth and the poor stability and appearance of the dentures. After extraction of the teeth, the maxilla was restored with a complete removable denture. The patient was satisfied with the stability but would have preferred to have had more tooth display and less lip support. The teeth had been set labially and apically to compensate for the lack of interarch space.

An osteotomy of the anterior mandibular ridge will increase ridge thickness and also increase interarch space. The maxillary teeth will be then reset on the ridge increasing tooth display, reducing lip support and reducing the horizontal discrepancy of the skeletal class II relationship.

In summary, the following treatment options were discussed:

- removable complete prostheses (patient's preference);
- implant-borne overdenture;
- implant-borne FDP.

Mandible
Treatment options required consideration of the patient's profession in public relations and staff training. The following treatment options were discussed:

- removable complete denture;
- implant-supported overdenture;
- implant-supported FDP.

The rationale for the treatment options for the mandibular teeth was based on:

- clinical outcomes of implant-retained overdentures;
- patient satisfaction with implant-retained FDPs; implant-retained overdentures; or conventional prostheses;
- clinical outcomes of implant-supported mandibular FDPs: conventional loading (delayed) protocol;
- clinical outcomes of conventionally loaded (delayed) implant-retained mandibular FDPs;
- clinical outcomes of implant-supported mandibular FDPs: early loading protocol;
- clinical outcomes of implant-supported mandibular FDPs: immediate loading protocol;
- criteria for immediate loading with DIEM protocol;
- material options for the fabrication of implant-supported FDPs;
- risk analysis;
- maintenance and definition of clinical success;
- The AP was not significant. A maximum of 22 mm cantilevered extension was used with the prostheses.

Risk analysis of the preferred treatment options
The risk analysis has been divided in risk analysis for the maxillary prosthesis and risk analysis for the mandibular prosthesis.

The treatment options preferred for this case are:

- upper removable complete prosthesis;
- lower immediate implant insertion, immediate loading zirconia/porcelain fixed full-arch prosthesis.

The maxillary prosthesis
The anatomy of the maxilla is favourable to ensure stability and retention of the prosthesis. In the long term the patient may be disappointed with the outcome, as the stability of the prosthesis is compromised by physiological bone loss. Regular relining and adjustments of the occlusion are required.

The mandibular prosthesis
The risk analysis concerning the restoration of the mandibular arch considers risk factors linked to:

- the patient's medical conditions, parafunctions and habits;
- the surgical procedure;
- the selected prosthetic option.

Risk factors linked to the patient's medical conditions, parafunctions and habits
The medical history does not suggest any contraindications to surgical procedures. Parafunction (nocturnal grinding) has been reported by the patient.

The patient has a history of severe periodontitis. A history of periodontitis is associated with significantly greater risk of implant failure especially when associated to other risk factors such as diabetes, quality of the bone and smoking (Moy et al. 2005).

Risk factors linked to the surgical procedure
Infections (3%), implant loss, poor healing, bleeding, neurosensory disturbance related to damage of the mental or mandibular nerves and increased bone loss have been reported in most of the studies on the clinical outcomes of dental implants and the corresponding literature reviews (Adell et al. 1990, Goodacre et al. 2003, Herrmann et al. 2005). These complications are best prevented by using a sterile protocol during implant insertion and the administration antibiotics and antiseptic mouthwashes. A CT scan and a surgical guide are used to increase the accuracy of the procedure and prevent damage to the adjacent structures.

Risk factors linked to the prosthetic procedure
The use of acrylic or porcelain on gold alloy and hybrid dentures is relatively well documented. Disadvantages in some cases may be the aesthetically unpleasant view

of the metal, the cost of gold, and the possible staining and chipping of the acrylic material (Jemt & Johansson 2006).

The main issues related to the use of a porcelain-veneered to zirconia FDP are:

- lack of long-term clinical studies;
- possibility of porcelain/zirconia chipping fracture;
- screw loosening and fracture;
- cantilever design;
- difficulty in oral hygiene;
- phonetic problems.

Discussion

Full-arch implant-supported prostheses with porcelain fused to zirconia frameworks have been proposed recently in some clinical report articles (Holst et al. 2006, Van Dooren 2007, Wohrle & Cornell 2008). The authors claim that this material/technique offers biocompatibility, accuracy, passive fitting, colour stability, wear resistance and aesthetics. However, chipping of the veneering porcelain has been reported in several clinical studies regarding multi-unit FDPs (Sailer et al. 2007). Unfortunately, there are no long-term studies documenting the clinical outcomes of zirconia/porcelain prostheses used to restore edentulous mandibles. The principles for the design of the zirconia/porcelain prosthesis are based on studies by Guazzato et al. (2004a,b, 2010) regarding thickness, distribution of the core material and veneering porcelain, thermal and surface treatment of the material, fatigue behaviour, accuracy and passivity. According to the in vitro and clinical studies, it is likely that this type of prosthesis will outperform alternative materials.

Implants will be inserted in the interforaminal region of the mandible where the quantity and quality of the bone is optimal and to allow physiological bending movements of the mandible (De Marco & Paine 1974). In order to ensure posterior support, the prosthesis is designed with a distal cantilever. A cantilever design may create an unfavourable lever arm that may be responsible for possible stress and overloading of the implants. The cantilever is related also to the AP spread and an early review by English (1990) on the mechanical consequences of lower full-arch implant-borne prosthesis reported that the AP spread is an important parameter to be considered in the design of the prosthesis. The AP spread is the distance between the centre of the most anterior implant and a line linking the distal edges of the two most distal implants bilaterally. The length of the cantilever should generally be minimised and not greater than a 'factor' (X) multiple to the AP distance. There is some disagreement on what this factor should be (Testori et al. 2003, Misch 2005).

English (1990) indicated that the surgical placement of five implants in the anterior region of the mandible does not guarantee that an FDP with cantilever will be successful long term. A cantilever mandible prosthesis is a class I lever that is efficient (or damaging). To counteract this unfavourable lever it is possible to position the lower anterior teeth more anteriorly than the most anterior implants to create a class II lever where the anterior bending moment competes with the posterior cantilevered section. Excessive cantilever is likely to result in a number of complications. Lindquist et al. (1996) first reported that bone loss was found around the medial implant (most anterior and in tension) rather than in the distal implants.

English pointed out in addition to AP distance, the length of the implants, the occlusal plane to implant length ratio and the strength of the abutments are also important (crown–root ratio). However, no tables or practical indications are available to calculate the influence of these factors. In addition, patient factors such as parafunction (bruxism) and poor hygiene may aggravate the biomechanical factors.

In general, English proposed that a cantilever 1.5 times the AP spread is suitable for a five-implant FDP. This should allow 10–12 mm of cantilever in the mandible. In the maxilla, a shorter cantilever should be considered due to the inferior load capacity.

Lindquist et al. (1996) used an average cantilever extension of 15 mm with a complete FDP opposing and had no failure in 10-year follow-up. Lindquist et al. were of the view that the AP spread was not a very important factor under the conditions tested and the bone loss on the anterior implants was associated with poor oral hygiene and smoking rather than mechanical factors. The AP spread appeared not to be significant.

The criteria of specific protocols (e.g. the DIEM protocol) require an adequate AP spread; however, no indications are given of what an adequate AP spread is. Testori et al. (2003) suggested 1.5 times the AP spread as an ideal and safe extension of the distal cantilevered. Misch (2005) suggested that in the mandible, the distal cantilever calculated as 2.5 times the AP spread is suitable. Neither of the authors supported their conclusions with clinical evidence. Shackleton et al. (1994) elaborated clinical data from previous studies of Adell (1990) to investigate the influence of the length of the distal cantilever on the survival rate of implant-borne mandibular FDPs. The study showed that the survival rate of the prostheses with a cantilevered length of 15 mm or less was significantly better than in prostheses with a cantilever length greater than 15 mm. Of importance is that no implants were lost as a result of longer cantilever and the failures concerned the prosthesis only.

In this case, a conservative approach was used by having no distal cantilever in the provisional prosthesis and by ensuring that the final prosthesis cantilever will not exceed 15 mm.

Rationale for the treatment plan

The rationale for the treatment chosen is summarised as follows:

- The patient wants to use his financial resources to increase the stability of the mandibular denture.
- The patient is willing to try with a maxillary complete removable prosthesis initially and select another option should this be needed.
- The patient strongly prefers an FDP in the mandible.
- The try-in of the mandibular denture with and without a flange does not show any difference in support for the soft tissues and validates from an aesthetic point of view that the use of an FDP is possible.
- An immediate loading protocol will be used, as the criteria for immediate loading are satisfied and the patient prefers this option.
- The patient prefers a final prosthesis of zirconia and porcelain as he favours cleanliness, biocompatibility and lack of metal components. He understands that this option is not supported by 5-year term clinical studies. Should complications arise compromising aesthetics and function, the prosthesis will be replaced at no cost with a hybrid denture.
- The operator has long and proven experience with the procedure and the materials proposed.
- The mandibular prosthesis is placed on multi-unit abutments for two reasons:
  ○ to favour undisturbed attachment of epithelium to the surface of the titanium abutments;
  ○ to create a predictable weak point at the screws holding the prosthesis onto the abutments (loosening of these will be a predictor of instability and poor distribution of the masticatory forces on the prosthesis).

Maintenance and definition of treatment success
- Review at 2 weeks, 1 month, 6 months and 1 year.
- Review every 6 months after the 1st year.
- Radiographs.
- Reinforcement of oral hygiene.
- Examination/occlusion.
- Tightening abutment screws.
- Peri-implant probing.

During the reviews the following parameters will be assessed as reported for implants by Testori et al. (2003):

- no clinically detectable mobility;
- no evidence of peri-implant radiolucency;
- no peri-implant infection;
- no pain;
- no paraesthesia;
- no crestal bone loss exceeding 1.5mm by the end of the first year and exceeding 0.2mm/year in the subsequent years.

Review at 18 months
1. Oral hygiene and plaque control. *Excellent oral hygiene, minimal deposit of plaque and calculus.*

2. Soft tissue health. *No gingival inflammation, no bleeding on probing, and peri-implant tissue is healthy.*
3. Check on home-care programme and advise on frequency of brushing, use of dental floss and mouth rinses. *Patient brushes and flosses regularly twice a day; Superfloss and interproximal toothbrushes are used daily to clean underneath the mandibular FDP; the maxillary complete is soaked overnight in a mild disinfectant solution.*
4. Note and record recurrent dental caries associated with restorations or new carious lesions; note periodontal status – check probing depths and record changes; new PA radiographs to check alveolar bone levels (see below). *The soft tissue is firm and pale; there is no bleeding on probing.*
5. Medical status – change in general health and implications for oral health. *The medical history is unchanged.*
6. Occlusion – check tooth contacts with GHM foil at ICP, RCP, lateral and protrusive excursive contacts – note lateral contact details, especially where there is a fracture of restorative material – record, photograph fracture and contact details with GHM foil and comment on reason for fracture. *The occlusion is stable; the wear of the acrylic teeth opposing the full arch zirconia-based prosthesis is minimal and does not require further attention at this time.*
7. Radiographs – 1-year review. PA views for specific details of the status of crowns on teeth and implants. Check crown margins and alveolar bone levels; measure thread exposure to bone crest around implants and correlate with clinical details as above. *A panoramic radiograph was taken at the 18-month review showing that the bone level had been maintained and no bone loss has occurred.*
8. Discuss oral health related quality of life – comfort, appearance; function – chewing and speech; whether there has been a change in confidence, social interaction and relationships. *The patient ranks comfort, appearance, function as very satisfactory and chewing and speech as satisfactory; the treatment has improved his confidence and social interaction from 2 to 9 on a visual analogue scale (graded from 0 to 10).*
9. Seek any additional comments from the patient about the treatment and whether they would undertake the process again if needed. *The patient was satisfied with the treatment and would undertake the procedure again if required, although he acknowledged that the treatment was significantly invasive and time consuming.*

References
Adell, R., Ericksson, B., Lekholm, U. et al. (1990) A long-term follow-up study of osseointegrated implants in the treatment of totally edentulous jaws. *International Journal of Oral & Maxillofacial Implants*, 5 (4), 347–359.
De Marco, T.J. & Paine, S. (1974) Mandibular dimensional change. *Journal of Prosthetic Dentistry*, 31 (5), 482–485.

English, C.E. (1990) The critical A–P spread. *Implant Society*, 1 (1), 2–3.

Goodacre, C.J., Bernal, G., Rungcharassaeng, K. *et al.* (2003) Clinical complications with implants and implant prostheses. *Journal of Prosthetic Dentistry*, 90 (2), 121–132.

Guazzato, M., Albakry, M., Ringer, S.P. *et al.* (2004a). Strength, fracture toughness and microstructure of a selection of all-ceramic materials. Part II: Zirconia-based dental ceramics. *Dental Materials*, 20 (5), 449–456.

Guazzato, M., Proos, K., Quach, L. *et al.* (2004b). Strength, reliability and mode of fracture of bilayered porcelain/zirconia (Y–TZP) dental ceramics. *Biomaterials*, 25 (20), 5045–5052.

Guazzato, M., Walton, T.R., Franklin, W. *et al.* (2010). Influence of thickness and cooling rate on the development of spontaneous cracks in porcelain fused to zirconia structures. *Australian Dental Journal*, 55 (3), 306–310.

Herrmann, I., Lekholm, U. Holm, S. *et al.* (2005) Evaluation of patient and implant characteristics as potential prognostic factors for oral implant failures. *International Journal of Oral & Maxillofacial Implants*, 20 (2), 220–230.

Holst, S., Bergler, M., Steger, E. *et al.* (2006). The application of zirconium oxide frameworks for implant superstructures. *Quintessence of Dental Technology*, 29, 103–112.

Jemt, T. & Johansson, J. (2006) Implant treatment in the edentulous maxillae: a 15-year follow-up study on 76 consecutive patients provided with fixed prostheses. *Clinical Implant Dentistry & Related Research*, 8 (2), 61–69.

Lindquist, L.W., Carlsson, G.E. & Jemt, T. (1996). A prospective 15-years follow-up study of mandibular fixed prostheses supported by osseointegrated implants. Clinical results and marginal bone loss. *Clinical Oral Implants Research*, 7 (4), 329–336.

Misch, C.E. (2005) *Dental Implant Prosthetics*. Elsevier Mosby, St Louis, Missouri.

Moy, P.K., Medina, D., Shetty, V. *et al.* (2005) Dental Implant failure rates and associated risk factors. *International Journal of Oral & Maxillofacial Implants*, 20 (4), 569–577.

Sailer, I., Feher, A., Filser, F. *et al.* (2007) Five-year clinical results of zirconia frameworks for posterior fixed partial dentures. *International Journal of Prosthodontics*, 20 (4), 383–388.

Shackleton, J.L., Carr, L., Slabert, J.C. *et al.* (1994). Survival of fixed implant-supported prostheses related to cantilever lengths. *Journal of Prosthetic Dentistry*, 71 (1), 23–26.

Testori, T., Del Fabbro, M., Szmukler-Moncler, S. *et al.* (2003) Immediate occlusal loading of Osseotite implants in the completely edentulous mandible. *International Journal of Oral & Maxillofacial Implants*, 18 (4), 544–551.

Van Dooren, E. (2007). Using zirconia in esthetic implant restorations. *Quintessence of Dental Technology*, 30, 119–128.

Wohrle, P.S. & Cornell, D.F. (2008). Contemporary maxillary implant-supported full-arch restorations combining esthetics and passive fit. *Quintessence of Dental Technology*, 31–47.

Case 11.2 Mrs Lehong H

Agnes Lai

Patient: Mrs Lehong H (date of birth 12/04/1954)

Presenting complaint
- Tooth loss and breakdown.
- Does not want dentures – prefers a fixed prosthesis.

Subsidiary complaints
- Current removable dental prosthesis is loose.
- Can only eat soft foods.
- Concern that the abutment teeth are not strong enough.

History of complaints
- First lost mandibular posterior teeth 20 years ago, later maxillary anterior teeth
- Reason for tooth loss was caries and tooth fracture.

Patient's expectations
- No more denture use.
- Replace missing teeth.
- Fixed prosthetic solution.
- A natural appearance.

History
Medical history
- Received a course of Nexium for reflux 6 months ago, otherwise unremarkable.

Social history

Marital status	Single		
Children	Living with father		
Occupation	Laundry cleaning owner		
Recreational drugs	Nil		
Smoking	Nil		
Diet			
	√	Acidic foods	Pomegranate – twice weekly
	√	Water	1.0 L/day
	√	Tea	2 cups/day
	√	Coffee	Alternate days with 1 tsp sugar and milk
	√	Soy milk	1 cup/day
	√	Alcohol	Nil
	√	Hard/brittle foods	Cashews three times a week
Habits/ hobbies	Singing		

Dental history

			Additional information
Date of last examination		With Dr L less than 3 months ago	
Oral hygiene	√	Brushing	Twice daily and if at home, after meals three times/day
	√	Flossing	Twice daily before brushing
		Mouthwash	Nil
Treatment	√	Toothpaste	Sensodyne
	√	Restorations	
	√	Endodontics	
	√	Periodontics	
	√	RDP	
	√	FDP	
	√	Extractions	

Extraoral examination (Figures 11.2.1 & 11.2.2)
Aesthetics

Facial form	Ovoid, mesofacial	
Facial symmetry	Good	
Profile	Convex	
Nasolabial angle	Acute	
Facial folds	Symmetrical	
Midlines	Maxillary centrals	Around 2 mm to left of facial midline
	Maxillary central alignment	Straight
	Maxillary/mandibular centrals	Not coincident – maxillary right of mandible
Lip posture	Symmetry	Good
	Upper lip	Thin
	Lower lip	Thin
Occlusal plane	Undulated	
	Over-eruption	All remaining teeth
Vertical	FWS	3 mm (central bearing pin and swallow, relaxed)
	OVD assessment	Satisfactory
Smile assessment	Symmetry	Higher on the left
	Lip line	Low
	Gingival display	Nil
	Tooth display	70% maxillary; 10% mandibular
	Buccal corridor	Minimal appearance

Phonetics

	Normal	Abnormal
Labial (m)	√	
Labiodental (f/v)	√	
Linguodental (th)	√	
Interdental (s)	√	
Linguopalatal (k/ng)	√	

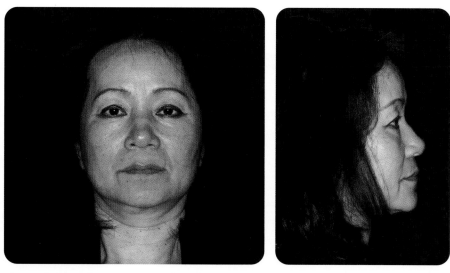

Figure 11.2.1 Extraoral examination. Frontal and profile view.

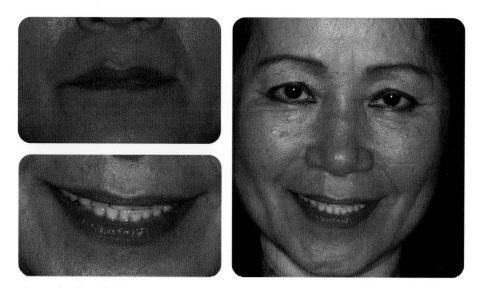

Figure 11.2.2 Extraoral examination. Smile analysis showing low smile line and significant show of anterior mandibular teeth.

Temporomandibular assessment

TMJ	NAD
Muscle tenderness	NAD
Glands and nodes	NAD

Jaw movement	Measurement (mm)	Reference points
Maximal opening	37 (corrected)	Tooth 11
Right laterotrusion	8 (corrected)	
Left laterotrusion	8 (corrected)	
Midline deviation	2 (to the left)	
Maximal protrusion	6	
Opening pathway	Straight	
Overjet	4	
Overbite	2	
Further investigation required	No	

Intraoral examination (Figure 11.2.3)
Soft tissues

Tissue	Healthy	Abnormal	Additional information
Lips	√		
Labial vestibule		√	Sinus tract between 13 and 14
Cheeks	√		
Palate	√		
Oropharynx	√		
Tongue	√		
Floor	√		
Frenal attachments	√		

Ridges	Maxilla	Mandible
Arch shape	U	U
Resorption	Mild	Moderate
Palatal vault	NAD	NAD
Tori	Nil	Nil
Frenal attachments	Normal	Normal
Mucosa	Thick	Thick
Pathology	NAD	NAD

Oral cleanliness

Condition	Yes	No			
Plaque	√		Generalised	Mild	Supragingival
Calculus		√			
Food impaction	√				
Stains	√				
Halitosis		√			

Saliva

Water intake	1 L/day
Quality	Good
Quantity	Good
Pathology	Nil
Medications affecting	Nil

Occlusal assessment

Skeletal classification	Class I			
Dental occlusion	Class 1			
Angle right	Molar class	NAD	Canine	Class I
Angle left	Molar class	NAD	Canine	Class I
Cross-bites	Nil			
Open-bites	Nil			
Curve of Spee	RHS	-ve	LHS	-ve
Curve of Wilson	–			
RP to IP slide	Not present			
FWS	Close/M/swallow test		3 mm	

Tooth guidance

Right laterotrusion

```
 7 6 5 4 3 2 1 |  2 3    6 7
─────────────────────────────
   5 4 3 2 1  1 2 3 4 5    8
```

Left laterotrusion

```
 7 6 5 4 3 2 1 |  2 3    6 7.
─────────────────────────────
   5 4 3 2 1  1 2 3 4 5    8
```

Protrusion

```
 7 6 5 4 3 2 1 |  2 3    6 7
─────────────────────────────
   5 4 3 2 1  1 2 3 4 5    8
```

Tooth surface loss

General

```
 7 6 5 4 3 2 1 |  2 3    6 7
─────────────────────────────
   5 4 3 2 1  1 2 3 4 5    8
```

Attrition

```
 7 6 5 4 3 2 1 |  2 3    6 7
─────────────────────────────
   5 4 3 2 1  1 2 3 4 5    8
```

Erosion

```
 7 6 5 4 3 2 1 |  2 3    6 7 8
──────────────────────────────
   5 4 3 2 1  1 2 3 4 5    8
```

Abrasion

```
 7 6 5 4 3 2 1 |  2 3    6 7
─────────────────────────────
   5 4 3 2 1  1 2 3 4 5    8
```

Bruxofacets

```
 7 6 5 4 3 2 1 |  2 3    6 7 8
──────────────────────────────
   5 4 3 2 1  1 2 3 4 5    8
```

Periodontium

Diagnosis	Localised mild chronic periodontitis: 16, 14, 43, 38	
Gingiva	Biotype	Thick
	Colour	Pink
	Contour	Receded
	Consistency	
Papillae	Colour	Pink
	Contour	Receded
Symmetry		Acceptable

Periodontal examination (14/08/2008) (Figures 11.2.4 & 11.2.5)

	03	04	05
CPITN	2	1	2
	1	3	3
	06	08	07

Facial upper

Tooth no.	17	16	15	14	13	12	11	22	23	26	27
Recession	222	321	11-	-1-	1--		-1-		-1-	23-	
Pocket	323	232	223	323	222	232	111	111	223	222	222
Bleeding		√√√		-√	-√	√√√	√-√	-√	—		-√-	—
Suppuration											
Buccal furcation											
Distal furcation											
Mobility							II		I		
Restoration											
Vitality	-	-	-	-	-		+		-	-	-

Palatal upper

Tooth no.	17	16	15	14	13	12	11	22	23	26	27
Recession			11-				11-		-11		-11
Pocket	333	334	333	322	323	332	323	222	333	333	333
Bleeding	√√√	√√√	√√√	√-√	√-√	√√√	√√√	√√√	√√√	√√√	√-√
Suppuration											
Mesial furcation											

Lingual lower

Tooth no.	45	44	43	42	41	31	32	33	34	35	38
Recession				-1-	-1-	-2-	-1-	-1-	-2-	22-	
Pocket	113	323	533	222	222	222	222	222	222	322	533
Bleeding		√√√	√√√	√-	-√			-√-	√√√		√√√
Suppuration											
Furcation											
Mobility											
Restoration											
Vitality	+	+	+	+	+	+	+	+	+	+	+

Facial lower

Tooth no.	45	44	43	42	41	31	32	33	34	35	38
Recession	—	-1-	-1-	-2-	—	—	—	-1-	-1-	-1-	—
Pocket	223	323	323	323	322	323	323	323	323	322	522
Bleeding	-√	-√	—	√√-	√-	—	—	—	—	√√-	√√√
Suppuration											
Furcation											

Mobility component	Grade I = ≤1 mm; II = >1 mm; III = >1 mm including vertical
Furcation	Class I = ≤3 mm; II = >3 mm; (horizontal probing, e.g. 3H, 4H, 5H); III = through and through
Recession	Distance (mm) from CEJ to FGM. If not clear CEJ, from restorative margin
BOP	√ or red highlight
Suppuration	√ or yellow highlight

Dental charting

Tooth	Clinical findings	Comments
18	Absent	Nil
17	Amalgam restoration	Nil
16	Over-hang and overcontour PFM crown	Secondary caries present, over-erupted
15	PFM crown	Over-erupted, gingival recession
14	PFM crown	Gingival recession
13	Large composite resin with leakage	Associated with sinus tract with GP
12	Root remnant	Secondary caries
11	PFM	Nil
21	Absent	Nil
22	Root remnant	Secondary caries present
23	Large composite resin with leakage	Nil
24	Absent	Nil
25	Absent	Nil
26	Temporary crown	Overhang present splinted to 27
27	Temporary crown fracture distal aspect	Abutment to existing P/-
28	Absent	Nil
38	Mesial tilt with large composite	Pseudopocket in mesial
37	Absent	Nil
36	Absent	Patient wants replacement
35	PFM	Margins are underhung but cleansable
34	Composite resin	Require redo
33	Mild wear	Nil
32	Mild wear	Nil
31	Mild wear	Nil
41	Mild wear	Nil
42	Mild wear	Nil
43	Mild wear	Nil
44	Composite resin	Require redo
45	Lost MODB restoration	Wear in dentine
46	Absent	Patient wants replacement
47	Absent	Nil
48	Absent	Nil

Previous dentures

Teeth replaced

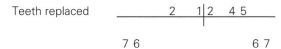

	Maxilla	Mandible
Age/number	4–5 over 20 years	2 over 8 years
Type	2 years	5 years
Kennedy classification	Class IV mod 2	Class I mod I
Appearance	Poor	Poor
LFH	Reasonable	Nil
Stability	Fair	Poor
Support	Fair	Poor
Retention	Fair	Fair
Hygiene	Fair	Fair
Patient opinion	Negative	Negative

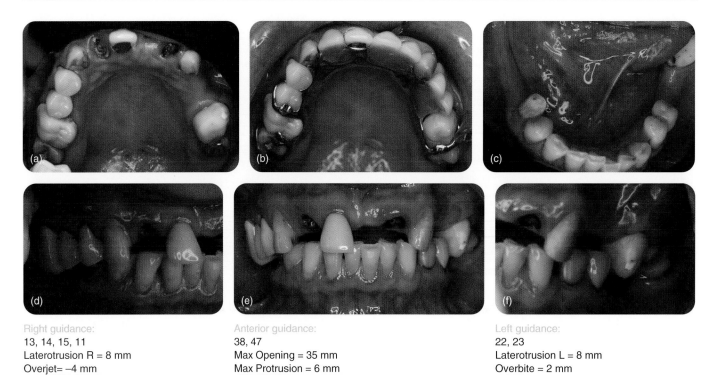

Right guidance:
13, 14, 15, 11
Laterotrusion R = 8 mm
Overjet= −4 mm

Anterior guidance:
38, 47
Max Opening = 35 mm
Max Protrusion = 6 mm

Left guidance:
22, 23
Laterotrusion L = 8 mm
Overbite = 2 mm

Figure 11.2.3 Intraoral examination. (a–c) Maxillary occlusal views of the maxilla and mandible and indicate the presenting status of teeth and with the maxillary prosthesis. (d–f) Anterior (middle) and lateral view of intercuspal position – note uneven occlusal plane with reduced inter-arch space on the right and extrusion of tooth 26 on the left.

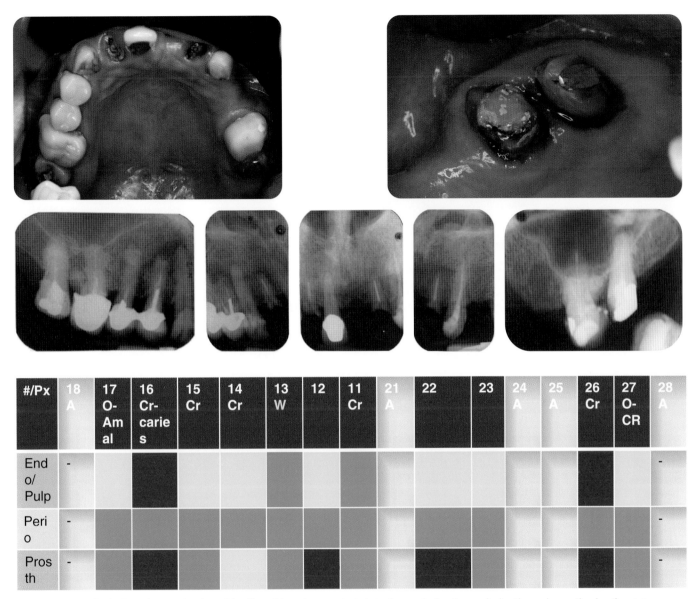

#/Px	18 A	17 O-Am al	16 Cr-carie s	15 Cr	14 Cr	13 W	12	11 Cr	21 A	22	23	24 A	25 A	26 Cr	27 O-CR	28 A
Endo/Pulp	-															-
Perio	-															-
Prosth	-															-

Figure 11.2.4 Periodontal examination. Maxilla with colour-coded data for endodontic, periodontic and prosthodontic status (green, no treatment; yellow, treatment needed; red, hopeless situation).

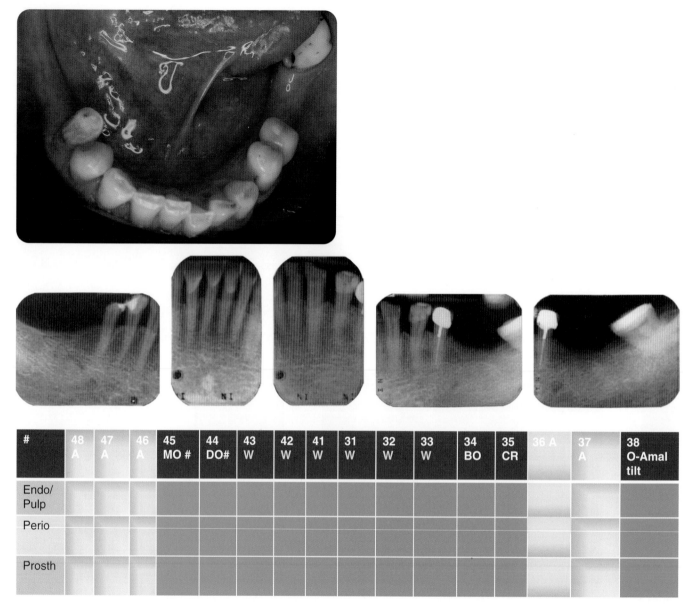

#	48 A	47 A	46 A	45 MO #	44 DO#	43 W	42 W	41 W	31 W	32 W	33 W	34 BO	35 CR	36 A	37 A	38 O-Amal tilt
Endo/Pulp																
Perio																
Prosth																

Figure 11.2.5 Periodontal examination. Mandible with colour-coded data for endodontic, periodontic and prosthodontic status; the green-coloured boxes confirm that no intervention is needed.

Radiographs (Figure 11.2.6)
Periapical films (23/09/2008)

Tooth no.	Findings	Tooth no.	Findings
18	Absent	38	Mesial angular bone loss, mesial tilt
17	Endodontically treated, inadequate obturation Questionable core material	37	Absent
16	Endodontically treated, inadequate obturation, Secondary caries, overhang with PFM	36	Absent
15	Endodontically treated, inadequate obturation, PFM	35	Endodontically treated with short post and PFM
14	Endodontically treated, inadequate obturation, post and crown	34	Composite resin restoration B and occlusion
13	Large composite restoration with PAL	33	Mild wear
12	Root remnant, endodontically treated, secondary caries	32	Mild wear
11	PFM, widened PDL space	31	Mild wear
21	Absent	41	Mild wear
22	Root remnant, endodontically treated, secondary caries	42	Mild wear
23	Endodontically treated with large composite	43	Mild wear
24	Absent	44	DO composite restoration
25	Absent	45	Lost MODB composite – exposed dentine with wear
26	Caries in mesial aspect and core Temporary crown with over hang	46	Absent
27	Amalgam core, inadequate endodontic treatment PAL	47	Absent
28	Absent	48	Absent

Orthopantomogram (23/09/2008)

General bone loss	Mild in areas
Sinuses	Clear
Retained roots	12, 22
Pathology	14 and 13 associated with sinus tract, 27 PAL
Caries	16, 12, 22, 26
Restorations	17, 16, 15, 14, 13, 11, 23, 26, 27, 38, 35, 34, 44, 45

Study casts and diagnostic wax-up

>Articulation	Position	RP
	Face bow	Yes
Diagnostic wax-up	OVD change	0 mm
	Occlusal plane	Flat
	Occlusal adjustment	Additive to mandibular premolars

Special tests

Test	Performed
Percussion	√
Palpation	√
Vitality	√
Saliva	√

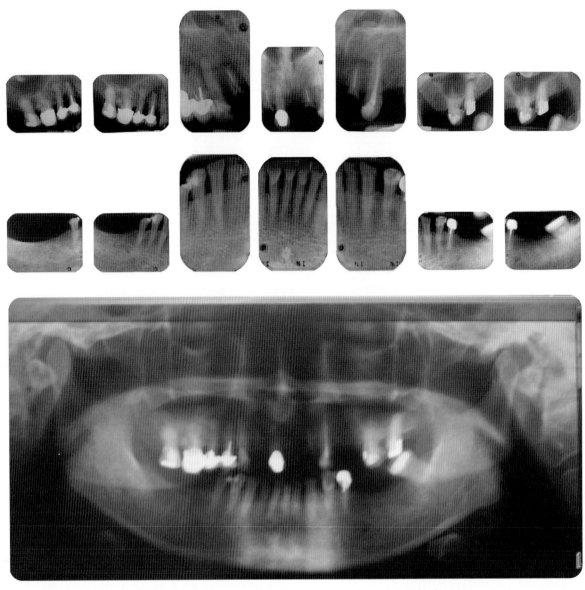

Figure 11.2.6 Radiographs. Periapical and orthopantomogram indicating tooth and alveolar bone status.

Provisional diagnosis

- Localised mild chronic periodontitis: 14, 16, 38, 43.
- 12 and 22 root remnants with secondary caries.
- Inadequate endodontic treatment of teeth 17, 16, 15, 26, 27.
- Periapical lesions on 13, 14 and 27.
- Secondary caries on 16 and 26.
- Kennedy class II mod I in mandible.
- Kennedy class III in maxilla.
- Class I anterior and L-molar, Class II R-molar.
- Lost restoration 45.

Problem list
Patient perceived

- Tooth loss.
- Would like to have an FDP.
- Aesthetics – midline correction.

Dentist perceived

- Aesthetics – low lip line.
- Biological – disease control.
- Motivation – highly motivated and co-operative.
- Time – attending a wedding party in August and would like to have a temporary or fixed restoration by then.
- Financial – able to contribute to costs.

Treatment goals
Short term

- Improve aesthetics and retentive solution for maxillary anterior teeth:
  - redo temporary crowns on abutment.
- Oral hygiene instructions and education.
- Removal of teeth with poor prognosis.
- Restore and conserve teeth with good prognosis:
  - immediate P/- removable;
  - restore 34, 44, 45.

Long term

- Maintainable prosthesis that provides reasonable longevity, catering for patient's lifestyle, eating pattern, general health and oral hygiene ability.
- Increase patient knowledge and awareness of oral health requirements and regular dental visits, as well as ongoing maintenance.
- Deliver an aesthetic outcome in accordance with patient's expectations.
- FDP.
- Maintenance (6-monthly prophylaxis and yearly review of rehabilitation).

Treatment options
Maxilla (patient only wants fixed definitive options)

Option 1. Sequential planning
- Retreatment of endodontics: 17, 15, 14, 13, 22, 23, 27.
- Crown lengthening 22.
- Implant bridge 24–26.
- Single tooth implant 21, 12, 16.
- Single crowns 17, 15, 14, 13, 11, 22, 23, 27.

Advantages
- Single tooth implants with adjacent natural dentition have demonstrated a predictable 5-year outcome: a meta-analysis reported survival rate of 96.8% at 5 years (Jung *et al.* 2008); failure rate at 10 years may be expected to be 10%, due to biological problems, late failure such as overloading of implants or peri-implantitis (Brägger *et al.* 2005).
- Endodontic retreatment by a specialist may have a success rate of up to 70%, with the success rate for first-time treatment of 98% at 5 years (Alley *et al.* 2004). With maintenance of periodontal health around these teeth, the expected survival rate is comparable to vital teeth (Torabinejad *et al.* 2007).
- Will allow retaining of the natural dentition. High physiological and functional responses can be maintained including jaw tap reflex, bite-force, etc. (Lundqvist 1993).
- Further treatment possible – additional implant at 13 position – six-implant full-arch prosthesis.

Disadvantages
- Extensive treatment involving high cost for endodontic retreatment, and prosthodontic work involving implants, full-arch FDPs have a high initial treatment cost, even in a hospital setting.
- When natural teeth fail over the next 10 years, progressive changes of the prosthesis are possible.

Option 2. Removal of teeth 16–26 and providing a six-implant full-arch prosthesis (fixed or removable to be determined)
Advantages
- Predictable outcome at a lower cost. A predictable outcome has been reported in a 15-year study on 6–8 implant-supported FDPs with implant survival rate of 90.9%, prostheses survival of 90.6% and mean marginal bone loss around implants of 0.5 mm at 5 years (Jemt & Johansson 2006). Review in 2009 indicated that in four well-designed studies, the 2–10 year implant survival in conventionally loaded maxillary fixed prostheses is 95–97% and prostheses survival is 96–100% (Gallucci *et al.* 2009).
- Patient previously demonstrated high caries risks that resulted in loss of teeth.
- Is easier to develop a satisfactory aesthetic.
- Maintenance cost outcome is lower.

Disadvantages
- More radical treatment involving loss of teeth.
- Need for a removable provisional appliance for 4–6 months.
- Implant therapy is not without complications; including surgical, prostheses, biological, mechanical and aesthetic complications and implant loss (10% in maxillary

fixed complete prosthesis) (Goodacre *et al.* 2003). It is important to note that the maxilla, having a softer bony structure, has a higher complication risk compared with the mandible.

Mandible
- Laboratory work will be completed in-house.
- 36 and 46 implants with CMCs:
  ○ patient's wish for further occluding units;
  ○ survival data as given above.

Treatment discussion
Fixed treatment options were discussed. Patient selected option 2 due to cost and understands that depending on fixture placement outcomes, a number of materials may be used for the definitive prosthesis. According to the scan, implants in tooth positions 13, 11, and 23 may require angulation corrections with customised abutments and would be most appropriately restored with CMCs. Although scans and planning are carried out to the highest detail, variations of the anatomy in relation to bone quality and volume are to be expected. The patient understands and accepts these considerations and the consequences including cost, material choice and time.

The patient also understands that currently she has good function with remaining 35–45 and 38, and 36 and 46 are also not part of the aesthetic zone. However, the patient has a strong wish to replace these two teeth. A staged approach was agreed where maxillary treatment was commenced first, and patient may choose to include 36 and 46 implants at a future time.

Treatment sequence
Urgent phase
- Fabricated temporary crowns in 26 and 27.

Control phase (Figure 11.2.7)
- OHI and prophylaxis.
- Removal of teeth: 16, 15, 14, 13, 12, 11, 22, 23, 26.
- Composite resin on 45.
- Provisional phase.
- Immediate complete denture.
- Further additional diagnostics:
  ○ further diagnostic considerations for definitive tooth set-up;
  ○ flange or no flange assessment;
  ○ patient has adapted well to increased OVD for phonetics and function;
  ○ i-CAT – implant assessment in maxilla and mandible.
- Treatment discussion.

Definitive phase (Figure 11.2.8)
- Implant surgery in maxilla (submerged or non-submerged implants: to be decided at time of surgery).
- No dentures for 2 weeks.
- Soft reline of denture weekly for following 6 weeks.

- If non-submerged technique employed – will require two-stage surgery.
- 2 months post-implant placement – provisional acrylic appliance fixed to implants (Figure 11.2.9).
- Final diagnostic fixed prosthesis to be carried out with provisional appliance after 3–4 weeks.
- Definitive prosthesis fabrication and insertion – maxillary implant bridge and 35 and 45 crowns.
- Timeframe: 4–6 months.
- Mandibular implants in 36 and 46 position are optional and can be commenced at any stage:
  ○ implant surgery with healing abutments;
  ○ after 8 weeks – impressions taken;
  ○ definitive crowns fabricated (Figures 11.2.10 & 11.2.11).

Maintenance phase
- 6-monthly prophylaxis (Figures 11.2.12 & 11.2.13).
- Yearly check of rehabilitation (Figures 11.2.14 & 11.2.15).

Procedural complication
During placement of maxillary implants, the thin labial wall of 23 fractured. The surgeon considered that implants could still be placed and procedure was carried out as a two-stage protocol. Unfortunately, during the tissue healing phase, fenestration occurred and the site had not fully epithelialised. As implant over the 4–6 months of osseointegration demonstrated increased resonance frequency analysis values at second-stage surgery and the PA of the area showed maintained bone level (although compromised initial bone height due to surgical and site factors), maxillary implants were loaded at 5 months post-insertion and the definitive bridge was issued 2 months later.

Unfortunately, at the definitive prosthesis issue, 23 implants osseointegration was disrupted by the abutment torque of 30 Ncm. The prosthesis was issued with a further 1-month and 5-month follow-up, which equates to a 7-month follow-up since initial loading.

The peri-implant soft tissue remains healthy with no tenderness to palpation and there is no bleeding on probing. However, there is possible marginal bone loss that may be seen since initial loading on the mesial aspect with an already compromised level to begin with, while the distal aspect seems to have increased bone to implant contact and the bone density surrounding this implant has demonstrated a steady increase with time. As the periapical radiographs have not been taken in a standardised manner, it is impossible to draw definitive conclusions radiographically. Clinically, the patient has demonstrated excellent hygiene and has been advised of the guarded prognosis of this implant (its failure should be expected sooner than other implants). In such a scenario, early detection may enable planning for implant removal, healing, grafting and placement of another implant in the same site with guided surgery.

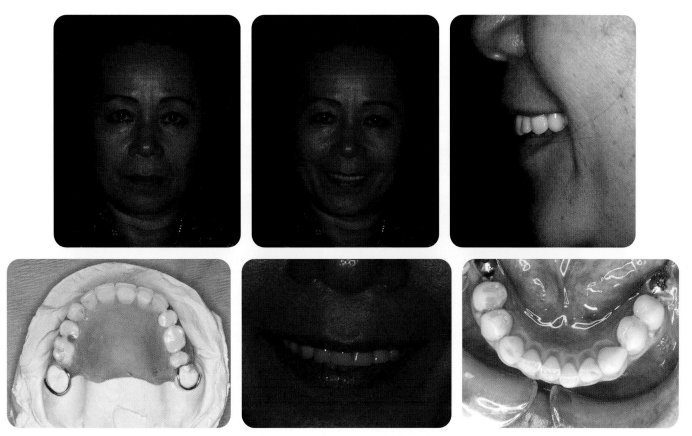

Figure 11.2.7 Control phase showing facial view with maxillary temporary acrylic partial prosthesis and composite addition to selected mandibular teeth to restore occlusal vertical dimension and improve aesthetics.

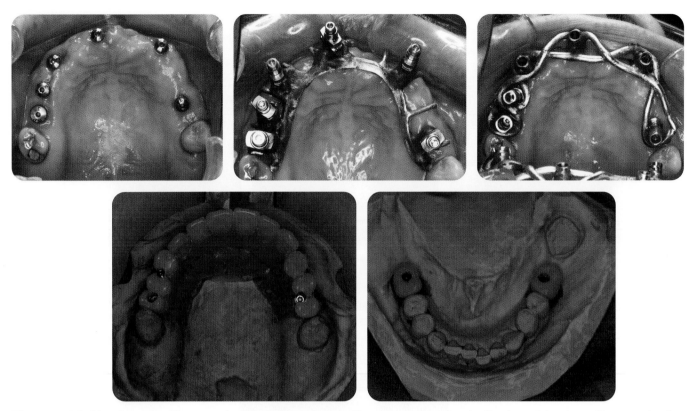

Figure 11.2.8 After 8 weeks. The upper images indicate the maxillary impressions for the fixed provisional maxillary prosthesis; the lower images show the occlusal views of the maxillary and mandibular prostheses.

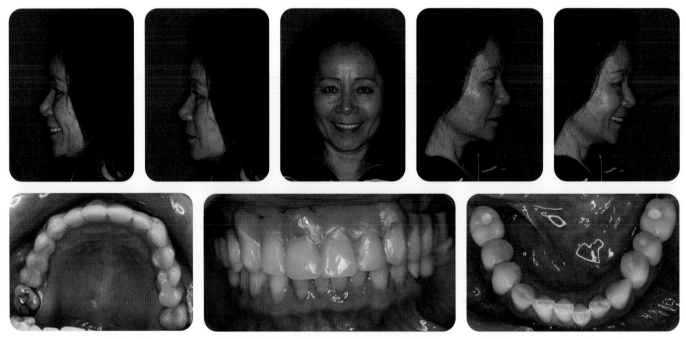

Figure 11.2.9 Provisional phase to provide long-term stabilisation for each dental arch at the determined occlusal vertical dimension. Note that implant-supported crowns are in place for teeth 36 and 46.

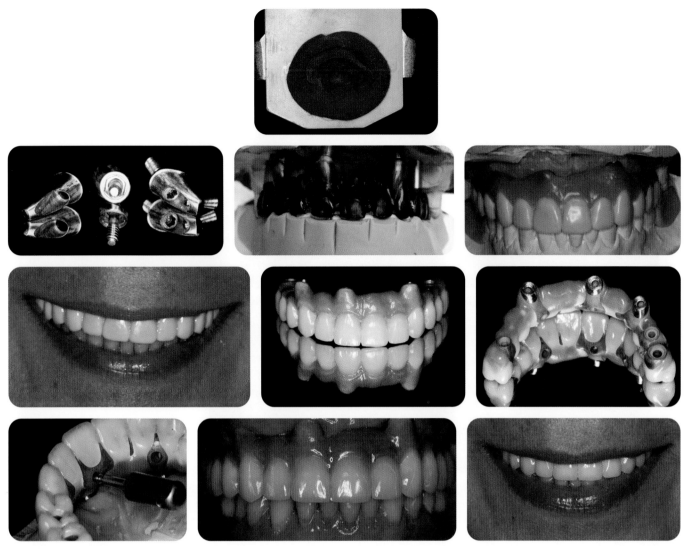

Figure 11.2.10 Patient agreement with the provisional tooth arrangement and satisfactory aesthetics allowed the customised occlusal table to be prepared. The definitive wax-up of the maxillary substructure was then finalised according to the provisional tooth arrangement. The final gold substructure was verified with the wax trial insertion and aesthetic details were revised at chairside. The definitive porcelain–gold prosthesis was finalised and acrylic resin was processed to support the dental arch. Note the cross-pinning to link the anterior dental components with the gold substructure.

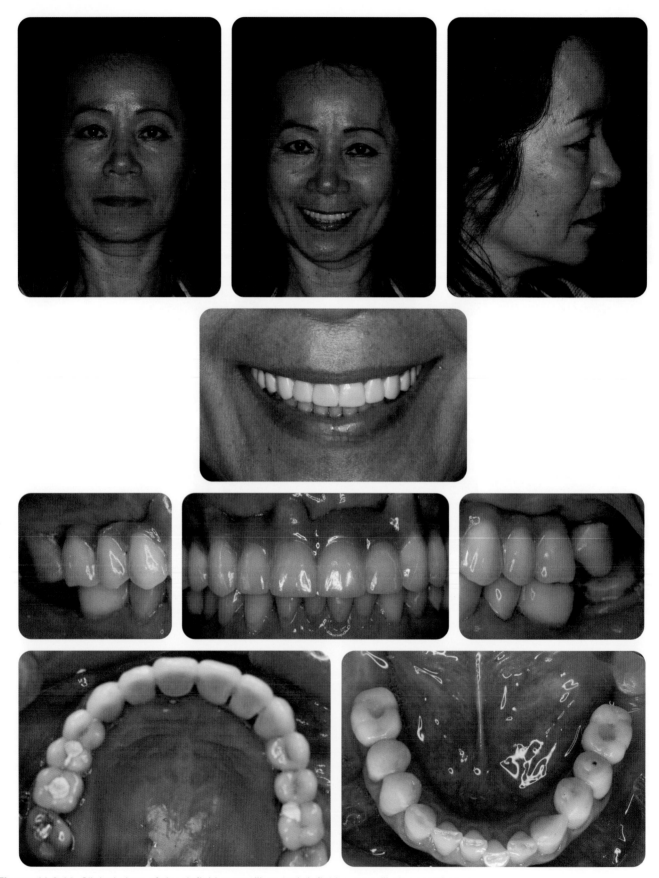

Figure 11.2.11 Clinical view of the definitive maxillary and definitive mandibular prostheses.

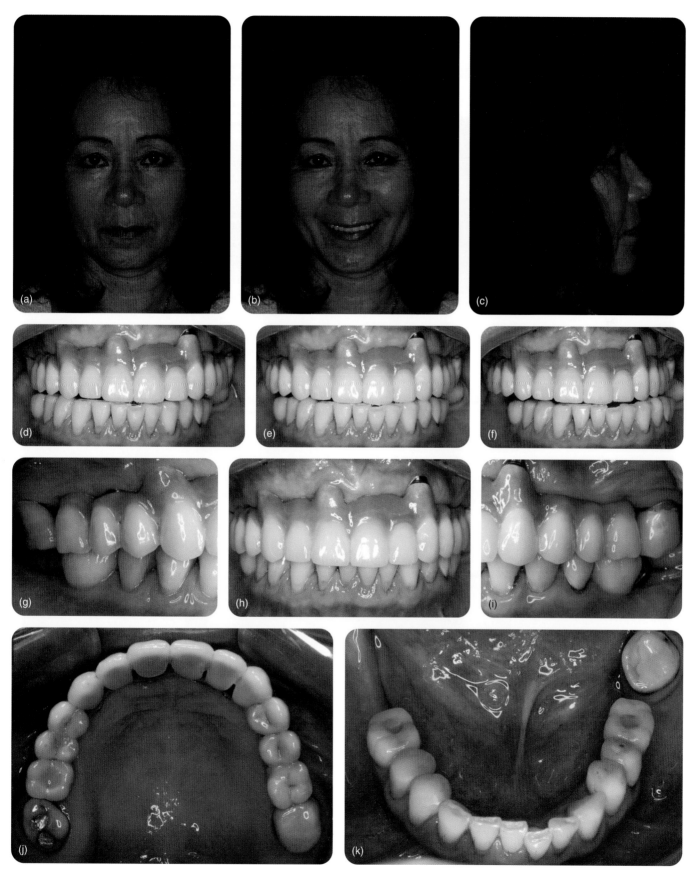

Figure 11.2.12 These images are at 5-month follow-up. (a–c) Extraoral presentation at rest, with smile and profile views. (d–f) Images demonstrate excursive movements preserved as designed. (g–i) Frontal and buccal views with intercuspation. (j, k) Maxillary and mandibular occlusal views.

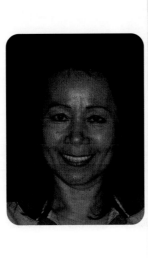

Satisfaction on her new teeth	Issue	5 months
Eating or enjoyment of food	Good	Very good
Appearance	Good	Good
Speech	Good	Good
General health	Good	Very good
Ability to relax or sleep	Good	Very good
Social life	Good	Good
Romantic relationship	Good	Good
Smiling or laughing	Very good	Good
Confidence	Very good	Very good
Carefree manner (lack of worry)	Good	Good
Mood	Very good	Good
Work or ability to do your usual job	Good	Very good
Finances	None	Very good
Personality	Good	Very good
Comfort	Good	Good
Breath odour	Good	Very good

Figure 11.2.13 Review at 6 months. Patient was pleased with the result at issue and at 6 months (see table). Further improvements in comfort and function were noted at 12 months – see review notes.

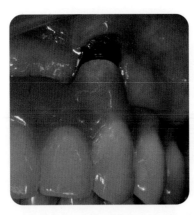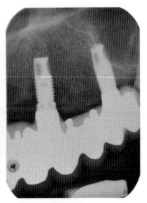

Figure 11.2.14 Review at 12 months. There was evidence of soft tissue inflammation at the 23 site with gingival recession which correlated with the PA radiograph.

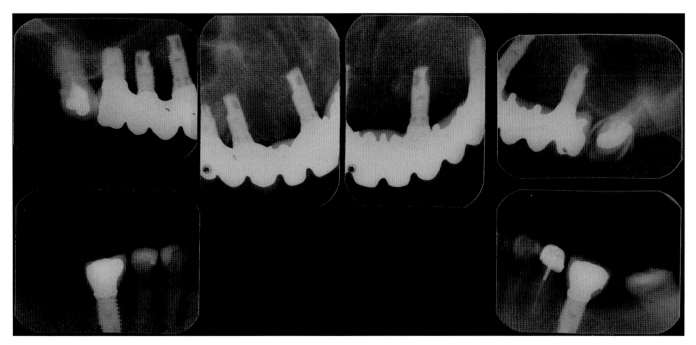

Figure 11.2.15 Review PA views at 12 months indicated no change in bone levels with the exception of the bone around the 23 implant.

Review at 1 year

1. Oral health status. Oral hygiene and plaque control; soft tissue health – note gingival inflammation, colour change – check on home-care programme and advise on frequency of brushing, use of dental floss and mouth rinses. Note and record recurrent dental caries associated with restorations or new carious lesions; note periodontal status – check probing depths and record changes; new PA radiographs to check alveolar bone levels (see 3 below).

   Oral hygiene was well maintained and there was no secondary caries in the mandibular teeth.

   Implant at 23 position showed signs of chronic peri-implantitis, which required surgical intervention due to progressive bone loss and peri-implantitis.

   Eighteen months later the patient developed a swelling around 23 implant site. Periodontal surgery was required to debride the area, which was grafted with bone ceramics. Several months later, although the gingivae appeared healthy and firm, buccal recession had occurred with exposure of three implant threads and radiographically vertical bone loss remained. The patient was also aware of occasional buccal tenderness of the 23 site with palpation.

   Probing depths around 23 was 5 mm mesially and distally with bleeding on probing.

   This is an interesting outcome that correlates with the procedural complication (see above) at the time of implant placement. At that time the decision was made to proceed with delayed loading of 12 months and careful monitoring of the site.

   A full-arch occlusal splint was issued to be used at night to ensure that the loading at implant at 23 position was not excessive. At review examination of the splint wear marks were apparent confirming sleep bruxism.

2. Medical status. Change in general health and implications for oral health.

   No change – generally healthy and a feeling of well-being (see 5 below).

3. Occlusion. Check tooth contacts with GHM foil at ICP, RCP, lateral and protrusive excursive contacts – note lateral contact details preserved.

   There was no fracture or prosthetic complication noted. Occlusal contacts were bilateral and balanced at ICP and RCP. Protrusion was guided anteriorly and laterotrusion was guided by ipsilateral anterior teeth.

4. Radiographs. 1-year review PA views for specific details of the status of crowns on teeth and implants. Check crown margins and alveolar bone levels; measure thread exposure to bone crest around implants and correlate with clinical details as in 1 above. At 2 years an OPG may add global information.

   Radiographs showed good integration of the implants at 16, 15 and 26. Mild bone loss was noted around implant 13; however, this bone level remained unchanged following the healing period. Radiograph of 23 showed slight further bone loss as discussed in 1 above.

Radiographs of the mandibular dentition showed unchanged bone levels of the dentition and implants.

5. Discuss oral health related quality of life – comfort, appearance, function – chewing and speech; whether there has been a change in confidence, social interaction and relationships.

On immediate insertion, the patient reported that her rehabilitation provided marked improvement and increased satisfaction of eating and enjoyment of food.

As well as improved appearance, speech and general health, and the ability to relax and sleep, the patient reported that her social life had improved and there was improved work confidence.

Her improved satisfaction was reflected in more smiling and laughing, self-confidence and mood.

6. Seek any additional comments from the patient about the treatment and whether they would undertake the process again if needed.

The patient was afraid of the surgical procedures involved and disliked the removable provisionalisation period waiting for osseointegration. However, she reported that the benefits of the definitive treatment was worthwhile and positively transformed all aspects of her life.

Despite the need for further intervention with implant 23, and its relatively uncertain prognosis, the patient understood and accepted the limitation given the anatomical situation, aesthetic requirement and surgical requirements.

In addition a 'different' sensation was felt in the cheeks after implant placement, which was initially uncomfortable; however, after months of no change in the sensation, the patient has become accustomed to it and it does not affect her daily activities or quality of life.

The patient would choose to undertake the process again if needed.

References

Alley, B.S., Kitchens, G.G., Alley, L.W. *et al.* (2004) A comparison of survival of teeth following endodontic treatment performed by general dentists or by specialists. *Oral Surgery, Oral Medicine, Oral Pathology, Oral Radiology and Endodontology*, 98 (1), 115–118.

Brägger, U., Karoussis, I., Person, R. *et al.* (2005) Technical and biological complications/failures with single crowns and fixed partial dentures on implants: a 10 year prospective cohort study. *Clinical Oral Implants Research*, 16 (3), 326–334.

Gallucci, G.O., Morton, D., Weber, H.P. *et al.* (2009) Loading protocols for dental implants in edentulous patients. *International Journal of Oral & Maxillofacial Implants*, 24 (Suppl.), 132–146.

Goodacre, C.J., Bernal, G., Runcharassaeng, K. *et al.* (2003) Clinical complications with implants and implant prostheses. *Journal of Prosthetic Dentistry*, 90 (2), 121–132.

Jemt, T. & Johansson, J. (2006) Implant treatment in the edentulous maxillae: a 15-year follow-up study on 76 consecutive patients provided with fixed prostheses. *Clinical Implant Dentistry & Related Research*, 8 (2), 61–69.

Jung, R.E., Pjetursson, B.E., Glauser, R. *et al.* (2008) A systematic review of the 5-year survival and complication rates of implant-supported single crowns. *Clinical Oral Implants Research*, 19 (2), 119–130.

Lundqvist, S. (1993) Speech and other oral functions. Clinical and experimental studies with special reference to maxillary rehabilitation on osseointegrated implants. *Swedish Dental Journal – Supplement*, 91, 1–39.

Torabinejad, M., Anderson, P., Bader, J. *et al.* (2007) Outcomes of root canal treatment and restoration, implant-supported single crowns, fixed partial dentures, and extraction without replacement: a systematic review. *Journal of Prosthetic Dentistry*, 98 (4) 285–311.

Case 11.3 Ms Cynthia B

Michael Lewis

Patient: Ms Cynthia B (date of birth 09/12/1942)

Presenting complaints

Chief complaint	'I can't eat, I can't smile . . . I can't enjoy my life.'
Subsidiary complaints	'I bite my lips and tongue . . . it affects my sleep.'
	Ms B complained of left jaw pain: 'It clicks and everything . . . to touch it hurts.'
	'The look is terrible, I don't go out.'
History of complaints	History of orofacial pain and restorative treatment with prosthodontic postgraduates at the Centre for Oral Health from 1987 to 1993. Ms B reports smashing her teeth in a car crash in 1998
Patient's expectations	'I just want to be able to eat . . . I can't chew.'
	'Function and looks are equally important.'

History
Medical history

Medical Practitioner	Dr L		
Respiratory	Chronic bronchitis	Asthmatic	
Cardiovascular	History rheumatic and scarlet fever	Hypertension	
	Endocarditis – cardiologist has recommended antibiotic prophylaxis		
Gastrointestinal	NAD		
Neurological	History of depression and social isolation after loss of daughter and mother in 1998		
Endocrine	Patient reports dilation of one kidney		
Musculoskeletal	Rheumatoid arthritis in hands, ankles and spine	Fractured jaw in motor vehicle accident many years ago	Three spinal surgeries – last one 15 years ago
Genitourinary	NAD		
Haematological	NAD		
	Bleeding	Prior history of warfarin use	
	Immune	NAD	
Other	Allergies	Valium, Fortral	
	Smoking	20–40 cigarettes/day	
	Infectious diseases	Hepatitis C	
	Pregnancy	N/A	
	Hospitalisation	Back operation 15 years ago	
	Medications	Sinequan (doxepin) 25 mg/day	
		Karveside (ibersartan HCl) 300 mg/day	
		Cardizem (diltiazem) 360 mg/day	
		Panadiene forte prn	
		Ventolin prn	

Social history

Marital status	Widowed		
Children	2 (daughter deceased/one 30-year-old son)		
Occupation	Pensioner. Retired animator, actress and model		
Smoking	Type	'Stradbroke' brand; 8 mg	
	Frequency	20–40 cigarettes/day	
	Period	20 years	
Recreational drugs	Nil		
Diet		Soft drinks	Nil
		Sports drinks	Nil
		Lemons	Nil
		Acidic foods	Nil
	√	Sweet foods	2 tsp sugar in tea/coffee. Nil sweets
	√	Water	>2 L/day
	√	Tea	2 cups coffee or tea/day
	√	Coffee	As for tea
		Alcohol	Nil
		Hard/brittle foods	Nil
		Ice crunching	Nil
Habits/hobbies	√	Musical instrument	Nil
		Exercise	Nil now – used to be an athlete
	√	Oral habits	Gum chewing

Dental history

		Additional information	
Date of last examination	10/05/2007		
Oral hygiene	√	Brushing	Twice daily
		Flossing	Nil
		Mouthwash	Nil
	√	Toothpaste	Sensodyne or Colgate
Treatment	√	Restorations	Build up teeth 13, 12, 21, 22, 33, 32, 41, 42, 43
	√	Endodontics	13, 12, 22 RCT
		Periodontics	Nil
		Orthodontics	Nil
	√	RDP	P/P transitional dentures
	√	FDP	Single crowns on teeth 14, 13, 12, 21, 22, 26
			Implant-supported single crowns in 15, 11, 23, 24 sites
			Complete mandibular implant-supported FDP
	√	TMD	Self-care management for chronic pain
	√	OMFS	Extraction teeth 11, 33, 32, 41, 42, 43
			Implant placement in 15, 11, 23, 24 sites; four implants placed in the 34, 32, 42, 44 sites

Extraoral examination (Figures 11.3.1 & 11.3.2)
Aesthetics

Facial symmetry	Symmetrical	
Profile	Straight	
Nasolabial angle	110°	
Facial folds	Marked folds at the corners of the mouth	
Midlines	Face/maxillary centrals	Maxillary dental midline is 1 mm to the right of the facial midline
	Maxillary central alignment	Perpendicular to interpupillary line
	Maxillary/mandibular centrals	Mandibular dental midline is 1 mm to the left of maxillary dental midline
Lip posture	Symmetry	Symmetrical
	Upper lip	Moderate thickness
	Lower lip	Moderate thickness
	Competence	Yes
	Tooth display	50% mandibular incisors
Occlusal plane	Parallel to ala tragus line	Yes
	Parallel to interpupillary line	No (anticlockwise cant)
	Over-eruption	Maxillary posterior teeth
Vertical	FWS	10 mm
	OVD assessment	Decreased
Smile assessment	Symmetry	Yes
	Lip line	Low
	Gingival display	Minimal
	Tooth display	50–70% maxillary anterior teeth. 50% mandibular anterior teeth.
	Buccal corridor	Moderate

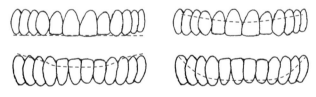

At rest   Broad smile

Phonetics

	Normal	Abnormal
Labial (m)	√	
Labiodental (f/v)		√
Linguodental (th)	√	
Interdental (s)		√
Linguopalatal (k/ng)	√	

Temporomandibular assessment

TMJ			Additional information
Click	LHS	Hard	Hard click on protrusion and LHS excursion
Crepitus			NAD
Tenderness	LHS		Moderate extraoral/mild intrameatal tenderness to 0.5 kg palpation pressure

Muscle tenderness	Right	Left
Temporalis	Nil	Mild in anterior/posterior/tendon
Masseter	Mild in superior/body	Mild in superior/inferior Moderate in body
Posterior mandible	Nil	Nil
Anterior mandible	Nil	Nil
Glands	NAD	
Nodes	NAD	

Jaw movement	Measurement (mm)	Reference points
Maximal opening	52	21–41 incisal edges
Right laterotrusion	52	Midlines
Left laterotrusion	12	Midlines
Midline deviation	1	21–41 incisal edges
Maximal protrusion	10	21–41 incisal edges
Opening pathway	Corrected 'S' deviation to LHS	Frontal view
Overjet	0	21–41 incisal edges
Overbite	5	21–41 incisal edges
Further investigation required	Yes	Assessment in orofacial pain clinic

Intraoral examination (Figure 11.3.3)
Soft tissues

Soft tissue	Healthy	Abnormal	Additional information
Lips		√	Bilateral moderate angular cheilitis
Labial vestibule	√		NAD
Cheeks	√		NAD
Palate		√	Palatal graft from previous biopsy
Oropharynx	√		NAD
Tongue		√	Ulcer on left ventral surface 2 mm in diameter
Floor	√		NAD
Frenal attachments	√		NAD

Ridges	Maxilla	Mandible
Arch shape	U	Tapered
Resorption	Mild	Moderate
Palatal vault	Moderate	
Tori	Nil	
Frenal attachments	Labial	Labial and buccal
Mucosa	Firm	Firm
Pathology	Palatal graft	NAD

Oral cleanliness

Condition	Yes	No	Additional information		
Plaque		√	Nil	Nil	Nil
Calculus		√	Nil	Nil	Nil
Food impaction	√		Self report		
Stains	√		Arrested decay 11, 21, 22, 33, 42		
Halitosis		√	Nil		

Saliva

Water intake	More than 2 L a day
Quality	Moderate – resting saliva frothy/bubbly in consistency with a resting salivary pH of 6.0–6.6; stimulated salivary pH 6.8–7.8, with 10–12 buffering capacity
Quantity	Moderate – hydration <30 s from rest; 3.5–5.0 ml stimulated saliva
Pathology	Nil
Medications affecting	Hypertension medication
Further investigation required	Yes Referred to oral medicine speciality

Periodontium

CPITN

1	1	1
–	1	–

Gingiva	Biotype	Moderate
	Colour	Coral pink
	Contour	Receded
	Consistency	Firm
Papillae	Colour	Coral pink
	Contour	Flattened

Periodontal charting (Figures 11.3.4 & 11.3.5)

Maxillary buccal

Tooth no.	18	17	16	15	14	13	12	11	21	22	23	24	25	26	27	28
Pocket			323		213	211	212	222	222	222				222	222	
Bleeding			---		---	---	---	---	---	---				---	---	
Suppuration			-		-	-	-	-	-	-				-	-	
Recession			542		332	212	200	000	313	203				332	232	
Buccal furcation			I												I	
Distal furcation			-		-									-	-	
Mobility			I		I	I	I	I	I	I				I	I	

Maxillary palatal (Figure 11.3.4)

Tooth no.	18	17	16	15	14	13	12	11	21	22	23	24	25	26	27	28
Pocket			212		111	212	221	211	212	222				312	222	
Bleeding			---		---	---	---	---	---	---				---	---	
Suppuration			-												-	
Recession			132		322	211	111	111	313	223				051	274	
Mesial furcation			-		-									-	-	

Mandibular lingual

Tooth no.	48	47	46	45	44	43	42	41	31	32	33	34	35	36	37	38
Pocket						211	112	111		111	111					
Bleeding						---	---	---		---	---					
Suppuration						-	-	-		-	-					
Recession						442	233	343		232	333					
Furcation																

Mandibular buccal

Tooth no.	48	47	46	45	44	43	42	41	31	32	33	34	35	36	37	38
Pocket						111	111	111		111	211					
Bleeding						---	---	---		---	---					
Suppuration						-	-	-		-	-					
Recession						101	022	123		210	222					
Furcation																
Mobility						I	I	II		I	I					

Occlusion

Skeletal classification	Class I			
Dental occlusion	Class III (edge-to-edge due to worn dentition)			
Angle right	Molar	N/A	Canine	Class N/A
Angle left	Molar	N/A	Canine	Class III
Anterior overbite	−5 mm			
Anterior overjet	0 mm			
Cross-bites	Anterior cross-bite			
Open-bites	Nil			
Curve of Spee	RHS -		LHS -	
Curve of Wilson	+			
RP to IP slide	Nil			
FWS	IO/EO measurement		10 mm	

Tooth guidance

Right laterotrusion

8 7 6 5 4 3 2 1 | **1** 2 3 4 5 6 7 8

8 7 6 5 4 3 2 1 1 **2** 3 4 5 6 7 8

Left laterotrusion

8 7 6 5 4 **3** 2 1 | 1 2 3 4 5 6 7 8

8 7 6 5 4 **3** 2 1 1 2 3 4 5 6 7 8

Protrusion

8 7 6 5 4 3 2 1 | **1 2** 3 4 5 6 7 8

8 7 6 5 4 **3 2** 1 **1** 2 3 4 5 6 7 8

Tooth surface loss

Caries

8 7 6 5 4 3 2 **1** **1** 2 3 4 5 **6** 7 8

8 7 6 5 4 3 2 1 1 2 3 4 5 6 7 8

Attrition

8 7 6 5 **4 3 2 1** **1 2** 3 4 5 **6** 7 8

8 7 6 5 4 **3 2 1** 1 **2 3** 4 5 6 7 8

Erosion

8 7 **6** 5 4 **3 2** 1 | **1 2** 3 4 5 6 7 8

8 7 6 5 4 **3 2 1** 1 **2 3** 4 5 6 7 8

Abrasion

8 7 6 5 4 3 2 1 | 1 2 3 4 5 6 7 8

8 7 6 5 4 3 **2 1** 1 2 3 4 5 6 7 8

Abfraction

8 7 6 5 4 3 2 1 | 1 2 3 4 5 6 7 8

8 7 6 5 4 3 2 1 1 2 3 4 5 6 7 8

Dental charting

Tooth no.	Clinical findings	Comments
18		
17		
16	MOD amalgam	Good prognosis – vital, PPD <3 mm, mobility I, 1 mm supragingival tooth structure
15		
14	RCT, post and core, CMC	Fair prognosis – stable RCT/post and core/CMC. Short post and RCT 2 mm short of apex
13	BDP carious lesion	Fair prognosis – vital, PPD <3 mm, mobility I, equigingival distal carious lesion
12	Retained root	Fair prognosis – vital, PPD <3 mm, mobility I, 1 mm supragingival tooth structure
11	RCT retained root	Poor prognosis – RCT, nil supragingival tooth structure
21	DPI carious lesion	Good prognosis – vital, PPD <3 mm, mobility I
22	MIDP erosion/M caries	Good prognosis – vital, PPD <3 mm, mobility I
23		
24		
25		
26	CMC with 15 cantilever pontic. Caries around the mesial margin	Good prognosis – vital, PPD <3 mm, mobility I
27	MODP amalgam	Fair prognosis – vital, PPD<3 mm, Grade I furcational involvement, mobility I
28		
38		
37		
36		
35		
34		
33	Incisal erosion and attrition	Good prognosis – vital, PPD <3 mm, mobility I
32	MIDBP erosion and attrition	Questionable prognosis – vital, PPD <3 mm, mobility I, substantial loss of tooth structure and moderate recession
31		
41	MIDBP erosion and attrition	Good prognosis – vital, PPD <3 mm, mobility I
42	MIDBP erosion and attrition	Poor prognosis – non-vital, PPD <3 mm, mobility I, substantial loss of tooth structure and moderate recession
43	I CR/MIDBP erosion and attrition	Questionable prognosis – vital, PPD <3 mm, mobility I, substantial loss of tooth structure and moderate recession
44		
45		
46		
47		
48		

Special tests

Test	Performed	Additional information
Percussion	√	Tested positive to percussion: 17, 14, 12, 11, 21, 22, 42
Palpation	√	Nil
Vitality	√	Tested positive to CO_2: 17, 13, 12, 21, 22, 27, 33, 32, 41, 43

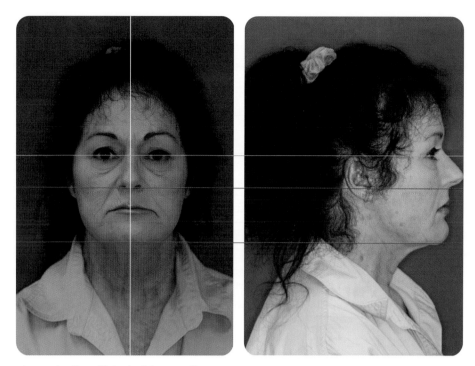

Figure 11.3.1 Extraoral examination. Note facial proportions.

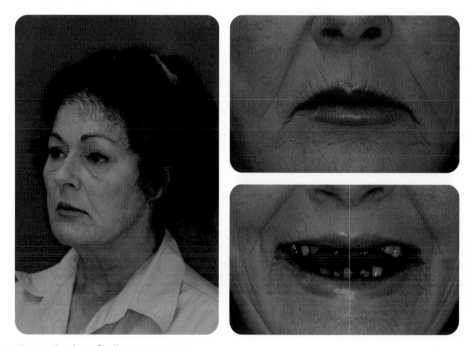

Figure 11.3.2 Extraoral examination. Smile assessment.

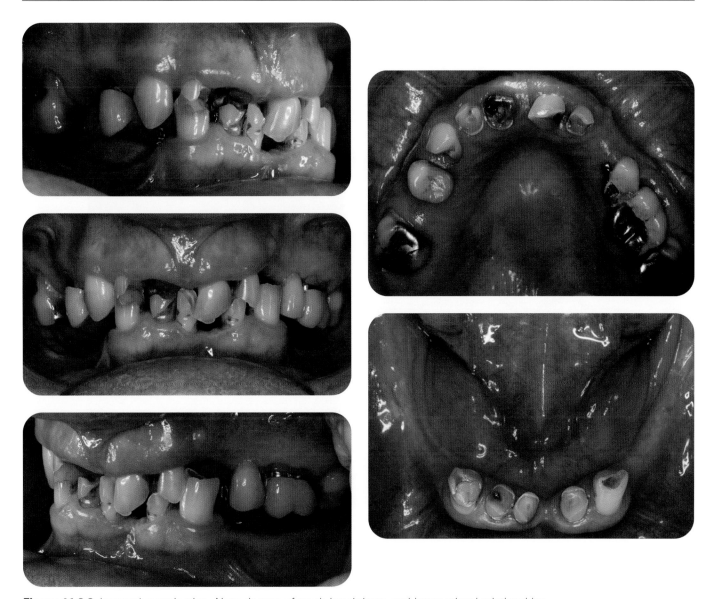

Figure 11.3.3 Intraoral examination. Note degree of tooth breakdown and interocclusal relationships.

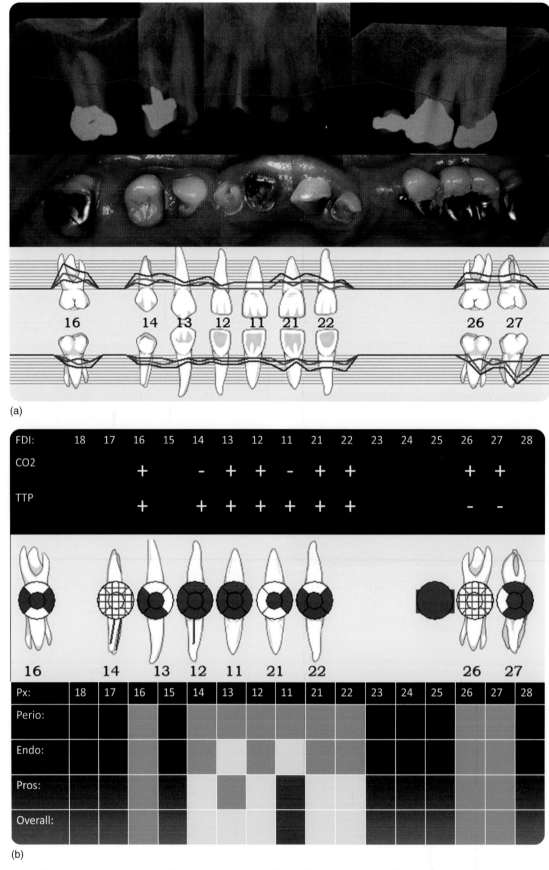

(a)

(b)

Figure 11.3.4 (a) Periodontal assessment of the maxillary dentition. (b) Restorative and endodontic assessment of maxillary dentition.

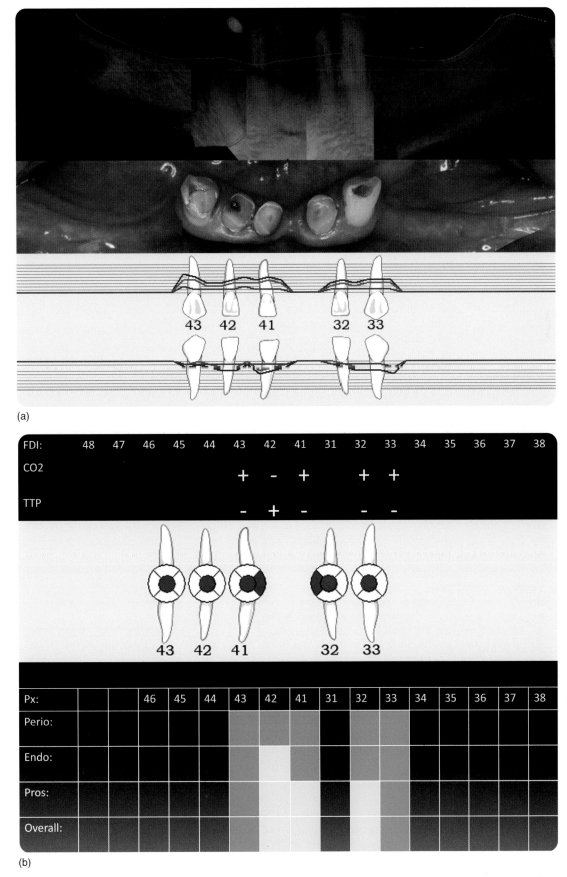

(a)

(b)

Figure 11.3.5 (a) Periodontal and radiographic assessment of mandibular dentition. (b) Restorative and endodontic assessment of mandibular dentition.

Radiographs
Periapical films (17/01/2008) (Figures 11.3.4 & 11.3.5)

Tooth no.	Information	Tooth no.	Information
18	Tooth absent. NAD	38	Tooth absent. NAD
17	Tooth absent. NAD	37	Tooth absent. NAD
16	Heavily restored tooth. Horizontal bone loss to the Buccal furcation. Nil periapical pathology	36	Tooth absent. NAD
15	Tooth absent. NAD	35	Tooth absent. NAD
14	Previous RCT/post/crown. RCT is 2–3 mm short of ideal apical seal. Mild horizontal bone resorption. Nil periapical pathology	34	Tooth absent. NAD
13	Deep distal tooth loss not extending to the pulp. Mild periodontal bone loss. Nil periapical pathology	33	Mild incisal tooth loss not extending to the pulp. Mild periodontal bone loss. Nil periapical pathology
12	Heavy incisal tooth loss not extending to the pulp. Mild periodontal bone loss. Nil periapical pathology	32	Moderate incisal tooth loss not extending to the pulp. Moderate periodontal bone loss. Nil periapical pathology
11	Previously root-treated tooth with equigingival tooth loss. Root therapy exposed to the oral environment. Mild periodontal bone loss. Nil periapical pathology	31	Tooth absent. NAD
21	Disto-incisal tooth loss not involving the pulp. Mild periodontal bone loss. Nil periapical pathology	41	Heavy incisal tooth loss not extending to the pulp. Moderate periodontal bone loss. Nil periapical pathology
22	Heavy incisal tooth loss not extending to the pulp. Mild periodontal bone loss. Nil periapical pathology	42	Moderate incisal tooth loss not extending to the pulp. Moderate periodontal bone loss. Nil periapical pathology
23	Tooth absent. NAD	43	Mild incisal tooth loss not extending to the pulp. Incisal restoration present. Mild periodontal bone loss. Nil periapical pathology
24	Tooth absent. NAD	44	Tooth absent. NAD
25	Tooth absent. NAD	45	Tooth absent. NAD
26	Bridge abutment with CMC and mesial cantilever pontic attached. Crown margins extend to the furcation. Horizontal bone loss to the buccal furcation. Nil periapical pathology	46	Tooth absent. NAD
27	Heavily restored tooth with pin placed. Moderate horizontal bone loss to the buccal furcation, extending to the apical third on the distal. Nil periapical pathology	47	Tooth absent. NAD
28	Tooth absent. NAD	48	Tooth absent. NAD

Orthopantomogram (23/09/2008) (Figure 11.3.6)

Features	Radiographic data
TMJ	NAD
Bone loss	Minimal bone loss in maxilla/ moderate bone loss in mandible
Sinuses	NAD
Mandibular foramen and canal	Visible. NAD
Mental foramen	Visible. NAD
Retained roots	21
Pathology	NAD

Other radiographs

Radiograph	Date	Radiographic data
OPG	17/08/1987	Teeth 27, 26, 14, 13, 12, 11, 21, 23, 26, 27, 38, 34, 33, 32, 31, 41, 42, 43, 44 present Radiopacity present at the apex of tooth 38 Posterior dentition moderately restored Post-core crown on tooth 14
FMS	28/11/1988	No changes to previous findings Mild horizontal bone loss localised to maxillary posterior teeth
OPG	04/03/1992	Endodontic therapy completed for teeth 16, 13, 38, 34 FDP on teeth 24 and 26
FMS	30/2/1993	Tooth 16 has been extracted Endodontic therapy completed for tooth 11
OPG	19/10/1993	Nil change from previous

Study casts (Figure 11.3.7)

Articulation	Position	RCP
	Face bow	Yes
Diagnostic wax-up	OVD change	+6 mm
	Occlusal adjustment	26/27
	Crown lengthening	13, 12, 21

Problem list

Problem list	Details
Medical condition	Rheumatic fever – requires antibiotic prophylaxis Chronic bronchitis – smokes 20–40 cigarettes a day Hepatitis C
Aesthetics	Poor dental aesthetics Dentofacial midline discrepancy Low smile line
Speech	Some problems pronouncing words since her teeth broke Distortions of 'f', 'v' and 's' sounds
TMD	Left subluxation on opening Left disc displacement with reduction on lateral movements Bilateral myofascial pain and arthralgia
Soft tissue	Moderate angular cheilitis
Oral hygiene	Good
Saliva	Moderate salivary quality and quantity
Periodontal	Lower anterior recession Class I furcational involvement associated with teeth 16 and 27
Edentulism	Patient missing several teeth in aesthetic areas Patient has no posterior occlusal support
Occlusion	Interarch and intra-arch occlusal collapse Lack of favourable tooth guidance
Tooth surface loss	Moderate to severe tooth-surface loss localised to the maxillary and mandibular anterior teeth
Restorative	11 decayed to the equigingival level
Prosthetic	Excessive decrease in OVD Patient has a poor history with three previous partial dentures
Endodontic	11 RCT exposed to the oral cavity 14 RCT and short post

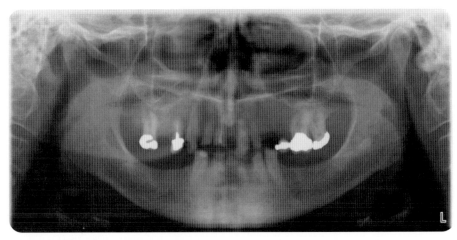

Figure 11.3.6 Preoperative radiograph – orthopantomogram.

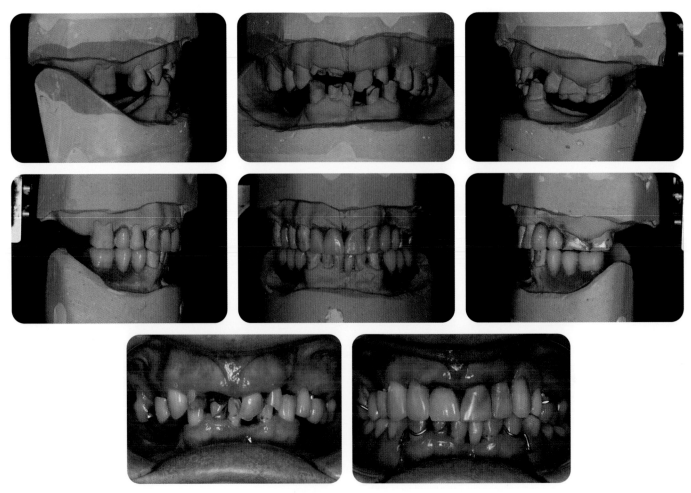

Figure 11.3.7 Diagnostic wax-up and initial determination of a stable occlusal vertical dimension.

Treatment options
Maxilla
Treatment option 1 (treatment time short, 2 months)
- Systemic and hygiene phase (see definitive treatment plan for details).
- Extract tooth 11.
- Replace crown on tooth 26.
- Build up teeth 13, 12, 21, 22 in composite resin.
- P/- RPD replacing teeth 15, 11, 23, 24.

Treatment option 2 (treatment time moderate, 4 months)
- Systemic and hygiene phase (see definitive treatment plan for details).
- Extract tooth 11.
- Elective endodontic therapy on teeth 13, 12, 22.
- Cast post core restorations on teeth 13, 12, 22.
- Crowns on teeth 13, 12, 21, 22, 26.
- Milled P/- denture replacing teeth 15, 11, 23, 24.

Treatment option 3 (treatment time moderate, 3–4 months)
- Systemic and hygiene phase (see definitive treatment plan for details).
- Extract tooth 11.
- Elective endodontic therapy on teeth 13, 12, 22.
- Cast post core restorations on teeth 13, 12, 22.
- Telescopic crowns on teeth 13, 12, 21, 22, 26.
- Telescopic crown-retained denture replacing teeth 15, 11, 23, 24.

Treatment option 4 (treatment time long, 6–9 months)
- Systemic and hygiene phase (see definitive treatment plan for details).
- Extract tooth 11.
- Elective endodontic therapy on teeth 13, 12, 22.
- Cast post core restorations on teeth 13, 12, 22.
- Crowns on teeth 13, 12, 21, 22, 26.
- Implant-borne single crowns in the 11, 23, 24 sites.
- FDP on teeth 16, 14.

Treatment option 5 (treatment time long, 6–9 months)
- Systemic and hygiene phase (see definitive treatment plan for details).
- Extract tooth 11.
- Elective endodontic therapy on teeth 13, 12, 22.
- Cast post core restorations on teeth 13, 12, 22.
- Crowns on teeth #15, 13, 12, 21, 22, 26.
- Implant-borne single crowns in the 15, 11, 23, 24 sites.

Mandible
Treatment option 1 (treatment time short, 1–2 months)
- Systemic and hygiene phase (see definitive treatment plan for details).
- Build up teeth 33, 21, 41, 42, 43 in composite resin.
- -/P RPD replacing teeth 36, 35, 34, 31, 44, 45, 46.

Treatment option 2 (treatment time moderate, 3–4 months)
- Systemic and hygiene phase (see definitive treatment plan for details).
- Build up teeth 33, 21, 41, 42, 43 in composite resin.
- Telescopic crowns on teeth 33, 43.
- Telescopic crown-retained RPD replacing teeth 36, 35, 34, 31, 44, 45, 46.

Treatment option 3
- Systemic and hygiene phase (see definitive treatment plan for details).
- Extract teeth 32, 41, 42.
- FDP on teeth 33, 43.
- FDP on implants in sites 36, 34, 44, 46.

Treatment option 4
- Systemic and hygiene phase (see treatment plan for details).
- Extract teeth 33, 32, 41, 42 and 43.
- Complete mandibular implant-supported FDP on four interforaminal implants.

Treatment plan

Treatment phase	Detail	Time between phases
Systemic phase	Refer to Oral Medicine – establish need for antibiotic prophylaxis Refer patient to Quitline Refer to Clinical Psychologist Referral to the Orofacial Pain Clinic	Concomitant
Hygiene phase	Preventative strategy: • oral hygiene instruction • remineralisative protocols (nightly tooth mousse) Extract 11 retained root	Concomitant
Pre-prosthetic pretreatment: phase I	Endodontic therapy teeth 13, 12, 22 Build up teeth 13, 12, 21, 22, 33, 32, 41, 42, 43 in composite resin at an increased OVD of +6 mm P/P acrylic transitional dentures	0
Pre-prosthetic pretreatment: phase II	Cast post and core in teeth 13, 12, 22 Refer to Periodontics for implant placement: • place implants in the 15, 11, 23, 24 sites • extract teeth 11, 33, 32, 41, 42, 43 and place four interforaminal implants	2 months
Prosthetic phase	Single crowns on teeth 14, 13, 12, 21, 22, 26 Implant-borne single crowns in 15, 11, 23, 24 sites Complete mandibular FDP on implants (milled titanium superstructure/ acrylic veneered)	3/12 post insertion 0–3/12 post insertion
Maintenance	Occlusal splint Recall 6/12	

			I	C	C	C	I	C	C	I	I	–	C		
18	**17**	**16**	**15**	**14**	**13**	**12**	**11**	**21**	**22**	**23**	**24**	**25**	**26**	**27**	**28**
48	**47**	**46**	**45**	**44**	**43**	**42**	**41**	**31**	**32**	**33**	**34**	**35**	**36**	**37**	**38**
Complete mandibular implant-borne FDP															
				I	P	I	P	P	I	P	I	P			

Treatment sequence

Appointment no.	Duration	Appointment objectives
1	120	Approve treatment plan Obtain any missing information for complete treatment plan Obtain informed consent Control phase Make appointments for stabilisation phase
2	240	Build up 12, 21, 22 in CR Extract 11 Cut off 25 pontic Enameloplasty 16, 26, 27 Issue P/- immediate/reline as required
3	240	Build up 33, 32, 41, 42, 43 in CR Issue -/P acrylic dentures

Appointment no.	Duration	Appointment objectives
4	90	Secondary issue of transitional dentures
5	60	Fit surgical guides. Refer for a cone-beam CT scan
6	60	Definitive treatment plan
7	120	Take new diagnostic models for construction of an immediate -/F
8	120	Extract mandibular teeth and issue immediate complete denture
9	90	Review extraction and Viscogel reline 1/52 post-extraction
10	120	Review extraction and Viscogel reline 1/52 post-extraction Duplicate maxillary RDP
11	60	Issue maxillary radiographic guide and sent for cone-beam scan
12	60	Joint consult with implant surgeon
13	All day	Implant surgery and immediate provisionalisation of FDP in mandible (Figure 11.3.8)
14	60	Review FDP in mandible
15	180	Implant surgery for fixtures in 15, 11, 23, 24 sites (Figure 11.3.9)
16	60	Postoperative review
17	240	Heat out 14, 13, 12, 22 Rough preparation 14, 13, 12, 11 Post and core preparation Prepare temporary crowns
18	180	Try-in post and cores Cement Remake provisional crowns (Figure 11.3.10)
19	120	Remove 14 crown and reprepare Impression and provisional crown
20	180	Definitive preparation 13, 12, Impression and provisional crown
21	120	Definitive preparation 21, 22 Impression and provisional crown
22	180	Remove 26 CMC Definitive preparation 26 Impression and provisional crown
23	240	Take maxillary pick-up impression of crowns/implant-retained single crown (Figure 11.3.11) Take face bow
24	120	Take mandibular pick-up impression using splinted copings (Figure 11.3.12) Take MMR
25	240	Cement 14, 13, 12, 21, 22, 36 single crowns Insert 15, 11, 23, 24 implant-retained single crowns Adjust occlusion
26	120	Issue mandibular prosthesis Adjust occlusion
27	120	Impressions for maxillary stabilisation splint
28	120	Issue maxillary stabilisation splint
29	60	Secondary issue stabilisation splint
30	60	Review V1/12 (Figure 11.3.13)

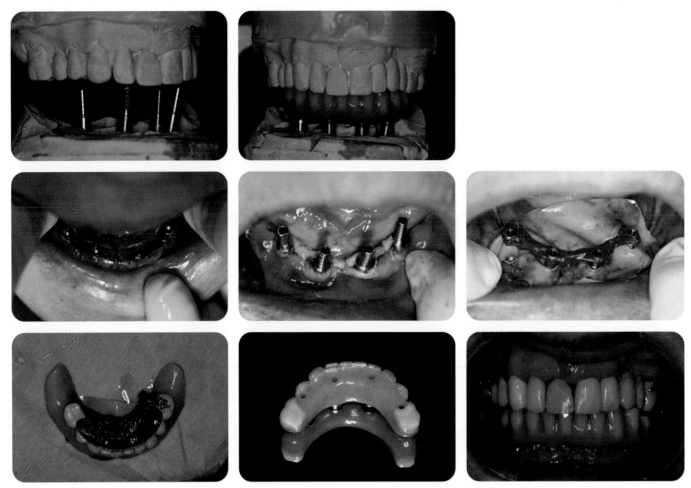

Figure 11.3.8 NobelGuide planned implant positions and mandibular implant surgery guided by the diagnostic wax-up.

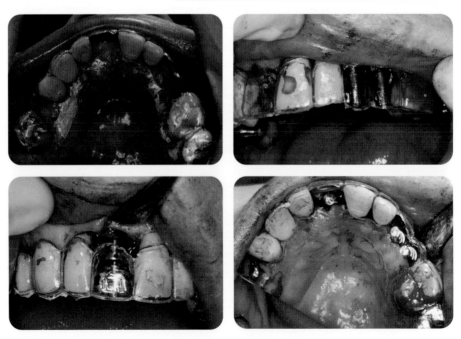

Figure 11.3.9 NobelGuide planned implant positions and maxillary implant surgery and immediate loading.

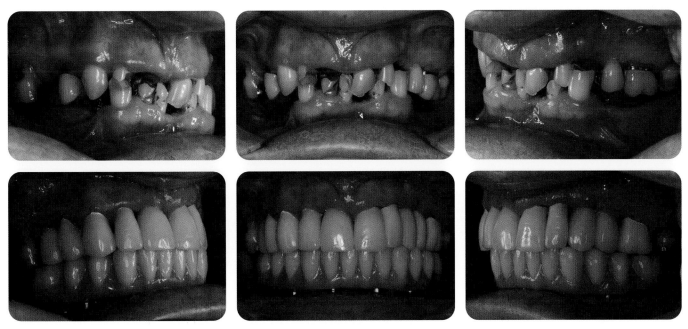

Figure 11.3.10 Provisional implant crowns and fixed dental prosthesis.

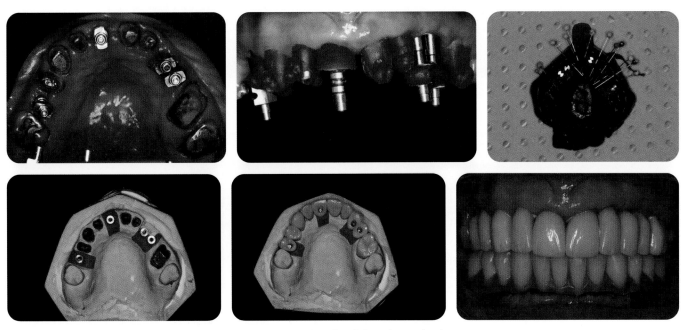

Figure 11.3.11 Construction of maxillary crowns and implant fixed dental prosthesis.

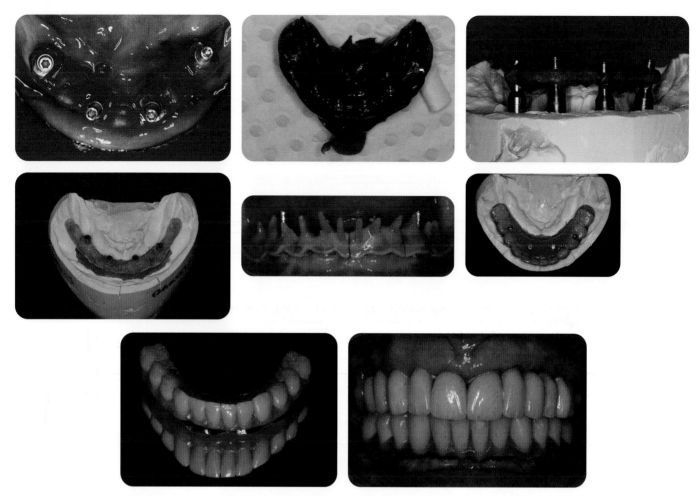

Figure 11.3.12 Construction of the mandibular implant-borne fixed dental prosthesis.

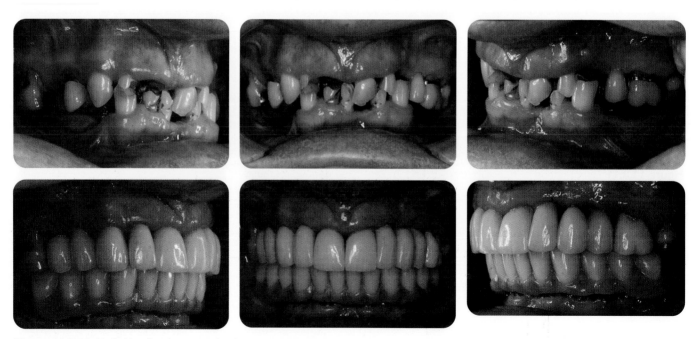

Figure 11.3.13 Definitive implant prosthesis.

Treatment discussion

Ms B presented with a chief complaint of 'I can't eat, I can't smile . . . I can't enjoy my life'. She stated in the initial consultation that function and aesthetics are equally important in her future rehabilitation. She advised that she has had three previous lower dentures and could not wear any of them.

Ms B presented with an extensive medical and dental history. She has suffered rheumatic fever/scarlet fever, for which her cardiologist requests antibiotic prophylaxis prior to dental treatment. For the past 20 years she has been a heavy smoker (20–40 cigarettes/day), suffers from chronic musculoskeletal problems and contracted hepatitis C from a blood transfusion. Ms B has been a patient of the Oral Restorative Sciences Department of the Dental Hospital for the past 20 years. She received oral rehabilitation and treatment for orofacial pain in the late 1980s, oral medicine consultations and endodontic treatment. Her attendance at the Dental Hospital ceased in the mid-1990s, coinciding with the death of her daughter and mother. Ms B reports emotional trauma and social isolation coinciding with these events.

Extraoral examination reveals a symmetrical face with a marked reduction in OVD. Dental examination revealed a severely broken down dentition, with complete inter- and intra-arch collapse. Ms B reports that her restorations failed due to the physical trauma of a car accident. She has excellent oral hygiene, a stable periodontium and minor caries in a few teeth. All teeth except 11 and 41 have a good prognosis with treatment as single-unit restorations; all mandibular posterior teeth are missing and occlusal contact is on anterior teeth only. Her teeth are fractured such that her occlusion interdigitates tightly and there is no ability for excursive movement. At present, the patient does not have a minimum number of posterior occluding units to ensure occlusal stability (Witter et al. 1999, 2001).

Several options are available to replace missing teeth, at a variation of cost and complexity of treatment. Tooth replacement options included fixed and removable solutions. Ms B. requested a fixed solution only to replace missing teeth – the treatment option of FDPs supported by teeth and/or implants. In a systematic review of survival of implant-supported single crowns (Jung et al. 2008) the 5-year survival data were 94.5%. In a large prospective case series (Walton et al. 2002, 2003) of up to 15 year follow-up of tooth-supported FDPs, 85% of FDPs were surviving at 15 years. However, it must be noted that tooth-borne FDPs are associated with increased failure if abutment teeth have minimal tooth structure, previous RCT and support long-span prostheses. As the existing posterior FDPs in the maxilla are stable, a single-tooth implant is to be placed in the 14 site.

In the mandible, two options are available: to maintain the mandibular anterior teeth and place posterior FDPs on implants in quadrants three and four and a six-unit FDP on teeth 33 and 43; or extract the remaining mandibular dentition and place a mandibular complete FDP on four implants. The systematic review by Pjetursson et al. (2007) reported that the 5- and 10-year survival data for FDP on implants was 95.2% and 86.7%, respectively. Ekelund et al. (2003) conducted a 20-year prospective case series study on the longevity of mandibular complete FDPs on implants, with reported 97.5% success. Lindquist et al. (1996) conducted a case series report on 47 complete mandibular implant-borne FDPs. They reported a cumulative survival rate of 100% for all prosthesis. In a retrospective, cross-sectional study, Walton et al. (1986) found that the canine-to-canine bridge had the highest level of service of all tooth-borne bridges with a lifespan average of 10.4 years. Cone-beam CT scans indicate that both solutions are possible. In light of good long-term data, the patient selected the mandibular complete FDP on implants.

The restorations on teeth 13, 12, 21 and 22 will require replacement due to caries and attrition. Several approaches are available to restore lost tooth structure, including a direct and indirect approach. A direct approach will allow the use of composite resin, while an indirect approach will allow use of all-ceramic or ceramo-metal materials. Limited evidence is available on the long-term clinical service of large composite resin reconstruction of anterior teeth. Poyser et al. (2007) conducted a case series on 168 composite resin build-ups at an increased OVD. Over a 2.5-year follow-up period, 6% required replacement. Hemmings et al. (2000) conducted a randomised control trial to test the clinical service of microfill and microhybrid composite resin restorations used to restore anterior teeth at an increased OVD. 89.4% of restorations were still successful after 30 months, with substantially better results when a microhybrid composite resin was used. In a systematic review by Pjetursson et al. (2007), 5-year survival rates for ceramo-metal restorations and all-ceramic restorations were 95.6% and 93.3%, respectively. When Procera copings were used, results were comparable. In a large prospective case series (Walton 1999) of up to 10-year follow-up of tooth-supported CMCs, 94% were surviving at 10 years, with a 3% repair and failure rate, respectively. Owing to financial constraints and in light of excellent clinical service offered by the previous direct restorations, it was agreed to replace the composite resin restorations with the same material.

Restoring dental appearance and function is of utmost importance to the patient in getting on with her life after traumatic events. She acknowledges that an alternative solution would entail a large cost. It is essential that the rehabilitation selected ensures ongoing maintenance can be provided as required. The definitive treatment plan for the maxilla involved restoring 13, 12, 21 and 22 with indirect restorations and implant-borne single crowns in the 15, 11, 23 and 24 sites. The definitive reconstruction incorporated canine guidance to prevent loading of the posterior implants on excursive movements. Preventative strategies for failure included remineralisative measures, oral hygiene instruction and nightly occlusal splint wear to protect against nocturnal parafunction.

The patient requires maintenance at 6-monthly recalls for the first year, then annually, at which the crown margins and occlusal contacts would be carefully inspected at the implant sites. Plaque disclosing and oral hygiene would be carried out at 6-monthly recall appointments. It is expected that the reconstruction would have longevity in excess of 10 years, based on the literature which cites 90% survival at 10 years for all prospective treatments.

Review at 1 year (Figure 11.3.14)

1. Oral health status – oral hygiene and plaque control – check on home-care programme and advise on frequency of brushing, use of dental floss and mouth rinses; note recurrent dental caries associated with restorations or new carious lesions; note periodontal status – check probing depths and record changes; new PA radiographs to check alveolar bone levels.

   Intraoral examination of soft and hard tissues revealed generalised moderate tooth-brush trauma on the buccal gingiva. Oral hygiene was excellent with absence of soft and hard deposits.

   The patient reports adequate oral hygiene practices: brushing twice a day with an electric toothbrush and flossing after every meal. Periodontal probing depths were 3mm or less, with absence of bleeding on probing. No recession was noted and tooth mobility remains unchanged.

   No new carious lesions were noted, and restorative margins remained intact. Neither the prostheses nor the teeth had developed a change in mobility.

2. Medical status – change in general health and implications for oral health.

   Recent blood serology shows that the patient is not hepatitis C positive. In addendum to the patient's existing conditions she is suffering with chronic back pain and may have a fourth spinal operation in the near future.

3. Occlusion – check tooth contacts with GHM foil at ICP, RCP, lateral and protrusive excursive contacts.

   Neither the prosthesis nor the crowns showed any signs of material fracture. Occlusal analysis revealed a heavier load on the left than the right. The left hand side cantilever was in full occlusion. The maxillary dentition showed no signs of wear; however, the mandibular prosthesis showed moderate to severe wear of acrylic teeth.

4. Radiographs – 1-year review PA views for specific details of the status of crowns on teeth and implants. Check crown margins and alveolar bone levels; measure thread exposure to bone crest around implants and correlate with clinical details as in 1 above; at 2 years an OPG may add global information.

   Periapical radiographs demonstrated consistent bone levels around the teeth as well as the implants. No change in the apical periodontal ligament was recorded. Implant prosthesis did not demonstrate an opening between the implant–prosthetic junction.

5. Discuss oral health related quality of life – comfort, appearance, function – chewing and speech; whether there has been a change in confidence, social interaction and relationships.

   The patient reported improvement in comfort, appearance and function since initial examination. The patient considered that her teeth look 'fantastic'; however wished that her teeth were whiter. The patient remarked 'The shape of my face is much better than it was' and 'I can smile now and I'm not afraid to go out or do anything'.

6. Seek any additional comments from the patient about the treatment and whether they would undertake the process again if needed.

   When asked if she would have the treatment again, the patient replied 'Of course!'. The only note the patient advised of was the acrylic veneer on the mandibular FDP, which collects stain and feels rougher than the ceramic teeth.

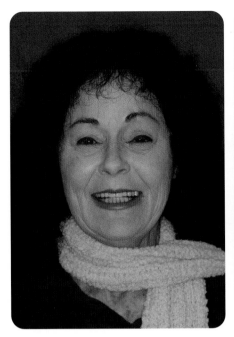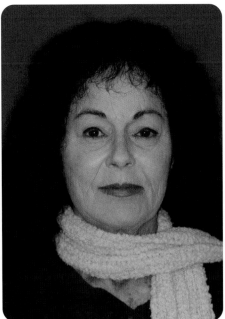

Figure 11.3.14 Extraoral view of completed treatment.

References

Ekelund, J.A., Lindquist, L.W., Carlsson, G.E. *et al.* (2003) Implant treatment in the edentulous mandible: a prospective study on Branemark system implants over more than 20 years. *International Journal of Prosthodontics*, 16 (6), 602–608.

Hemmings, K.W., Darbar, U.R. & Vaughan, S. (2000) Tooth wear treated with direct composite restorations at an increased vertical dimension: results at 30 months. *Journal of Prosthetic Dentistry*, 83 (3), 287–293.

Jung, R.E. Pjetursson, B.E., Glauser R. *et al.* (2008) A systematic review of the 5-year survival and complication rates of implant-supported single crowns. *Clinical Oral Implants Research*, 19 (2), 119–130.

Lindquist, L.W., Carlsson, G.E. & Jemt, T. (1996) A prospective 15-year follow-up study of mandibular fixed prostheses supported by osseointegrated implants. Clinical results and marginal bone loss. *Clinical Oral Implants Research*, 7 (4), 329–336.

Pjetursson, B.E., Bragger, U., Lang, N.P. *et al.* (2007) Comparison of survival and complication rates of tooth-supported fixed dental prostheses (FDPs) and implant-supported FDPs and single crowns (SCs). *Clinical Oral Implants Research*, 18 (Suppl. 3), 97–113.

Poyser, N.J., Briggs, P.F., Chana, H.S. *et al.* (2007) The evaluation of direct composite restorations for the worn mandibular anterior dentition – clinical performance and patient satisfaction. *Journal of Oral Rehabilitation*, 34 (5), 361–376.

Walton, J.N., Gardner, F.M. & Agar, J.R. (1986) A survey of crown and fixed partial denture failures: length of service and reasons for replacement. *Journal of Prosthetic Dentistry*, 56 (4), 416–421.

Walton, T.R. (1999) A 10-year longitudinal study of fixed prosthodontics: clinical characteristics and outcome of single-unit metal-ceramic crowns. *International Journal of Prosthodontics*, 12 (6), 519–526.

Walton, T.R. (2002) An up to 15-year longitudinal study of 515 metal-ceramic FPDs: Part 1. Outcome. *International Journal of Prosthodontics*, 15 (5), 439–445.

Walton, T.R. (2003) An up to 15–year longitudinal study of 515 metal-ceramic FPDs: Part 2. Modes of failure and influence of various clinical characteristics. *International Journal of Prosthodontics*, 16 (2), 177–182.

Witter, D.J., van Palenstein Helderman, W.H., Creugers, N.H. *et al.* (1999) The shortened dental arch concept and its implications for oral health care. *Community Dentistry and Oral Epidemiology*, 27 (4), 249–258.

Witter DJ, Creugers NH, Kreulen CM, *et al.* (2001) Occlusal stability in shortened dental arches. *Journal of Dental Research*, 80 (2), 432–436.

Case 11.4 Ms Pamela C

Alan Yap

Patient: Ms Pamela C (date of birth 18/11/1946)

Presenting complaints

Chief complaint	'I will be losing teeth'
Subsidiary complaints	'My top teeth look big and ugly', in particular the 'shape' and 'gum line' of maxillary anteriors
History of complaints	Periodontal disease treated around 15 and 30 years ago. Maxillary anterior crowns constructed 12–15 years ago for aesthetic reasons (recession)
Patient's expectations	Replacement of terminal teeth with fixed prostheses. 'I do not mind wearing a removable denture but only temporarily'

History
Medical history

Medical Practitioner	Dr TD	
Respiratory	Nil	
Cardiovascular	Nil	
Endocarditis	Nil	
Gastrointestinal	Nil	
Neurological	Nil	
Endocrine	Nil	
Musculoskeletal	Osteoporosis	Fosamax (1 tablet/fortnight, started August 2004)
Genitourinary	Nil	
Haematological	Nil	
	Bleeding	Nil
	Immune	Nil
Other	Allergies	Nil
	Smoking	Nil
	Infectious diseases	Nil
	Pregnancy	Nil
	Hospitalisation	Nil
	Medications	Fosamax (1 tablet/fortnight, started August 2004) Folate supplements Vitamin D injection once/year

Social history

Marital status	Married		
Children	Two (aged 36 and 34 years)		
Occupation	Self-employed jeweller		
Smoking	Type	Nil	
	Frequency	Nil	
	Period	Nil	
Recreational drugs	Nil		
Diet		Soft drinks	Nil
		Sports drinks	Nil
		Lemons	Nil
		Acidic foods	Nil
	√	Sweet foods	Lollies (jellies, marshmallows) twice daily
	√	Water	>1 L/day
	√	Tea	Chinese and green occasionally
		Coffee	Nil
		Alcohol	Nil
		Hard/brittle foods	None – lifestyle choice, mainly vegetarian
		Ice crunching	Nil
Habits/hobbies		Musical instrument	Nil
	√	Exercise	Walking
		Oral habits	Nil

Dental history

			Additional information
Date of last examination	30/06/2005		
Oral hygiene	√	Brushing	Twice daily, manual toothbrush
	√	Flossing	Once daily
		Mouthwash	Nil
	√	Toothpaste	Sensodyne
Treatment	√	Restorations	Multiple
	√	Endodontics	11, 21
	√	Periodontics	Currently treated, periosurgery October 2005, 15 and 30 years ago
		Orthodontics	Nil
		RDP	Nil
	√	FDP	Multiple crowns 12–15 years ago
		TMD	Nil
	√	OMFS	Multiple extractions

Extraoral examination (Figures 11.4.1 & 11.4.2)
Aesthetics

Facial symmetry	Symmetrical	Nil
Profile	Straight	Nil
Nasolabial angle	130°	Nil
Facial folds	Normal	Nil
Midlines	Face/maxillary centrals	Coincident
	Maxillary central alignment	Right cant
	Maxillary/mandible centrals	Coincident
Lip posture	Symmetry	Yes
	Upper lip	Moderate
	Lower lip	Moderate
	Competence	Yes
Occlusal plane	Parallel to ala tragus line	Yes
	Parallel to interpupillary line	Yes
	Over-eruption	12, 32, 31, 41, 42
Vertical	FWS	3 mm
	OVD assessment	Optimal
Smile assessment (Figure 11.4.2)	Symmetry	Yes
	Lip line	High
	Gingival display	Moderate to high
	Tooth display	100%
	Buccal corridor	Wide

Phonetics

	Normal	Abnormal
Labial (m)	√	
Labiodental (f/v)	√	
Linguodental (th)	√	
Interdental (s)	√	
Linguopalatal (k/ng)	√	

Temporomandibular assessment

TMJ		Additional information
Click	Nil	
Crepitus	Nil	
Tenderness	Nil	

Muscle tenderness	Right	Left
Temporalis	Anterior/mid/posterior	Anterior/mid/posterior
Masseter	Superior/body/inferior	Superior/body/inferior
Posterior mandible	Nil	Nil
Anterior mandible	Nil	Nil
Glands	Nil	
Nodes	Nil	

Jaw movement	Measurement (mm)	Reference points
Maximal opening	38	11 and 41
Right laterotrusion	9	11 and 41
Left laterotrusion	10	11 and 41
Midline deviation	0	11 and 41
Maximal protrusion	7	11 and 41
Opening pathway	Straight	11 and 41
Overjet	4	11 and 41
Overbite	6	11 and 41
Further investigation required	No	

Intraoral examination (Figures 11.4.3, 11.4.4 & 11.4.5)
Soft tissues

Tissue	Healthy	Abnormal	Additional information
Lips	√		Nil
Labial vestibule	√		Nil
Cheeks	√		Nil
Palate	√		Nil
Oropharynx	√		Nil
Tongue	√		Nil
Floor	√		Nil
Frenal attachments	√		Nil

Ridges	Maxilla	Mandible
Arch shape	Parabolic	Parabolic
Resorption	N/A	N/A
Palatal vault	Moderate	Nil
Tori	Nil	Nil
Frenal attachments	Moderate	Moderate
Mucosa	N/A	N/A
Pathology	Nil	Nil

Oral cleanliness

Condition	Yes	No			
Plaque	√		Local (molars)	Mild	Supragingival
Calculus		√			
Food Impaction		√			
Stains	√		Mild generalised root stains (tannin)		
Halitosis		√			

Saliva

Water intake	>1 L/day
Quality	Good (clear, low viscosity)
Quantity	Good (<30 s lower lip)
Pathology	Nil
Medications affecting	Nil
Further investigation required	No

Periodontium

CPITN

4	4	4
4	4	4

Gingiva	Biotype	Thin
	Colour	Pink
	Contour	Blunted upper ants, scalloped lower ants
	Consistency	Firm anteriorly, spongy/oedematous 14, 15
Papillae	Colour	Pink
	Contour	Generally receded and flat

Periodontal charting (13/04/2005) 4–5 mm, 6–7 mm, 8–9 mm

Maxillary buccal

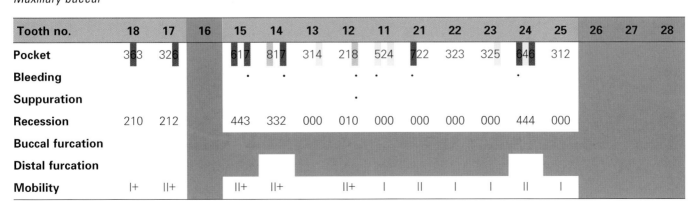

Tooth no.	18	17	16	15	14	13	12	11	21	22	23	24	25	26	27	28
Pocket	363	326		617	817	314	218	524	722	323	325	646	312			
Bleeding					•	•		•	•			•				
Suppuration							•									
Recession	210	212		443	332	000	010	000	000	000	000	444	000			
Buccal furcation																
Distal furcation																
Mobility	I+	II+		II+	II+		II+	I	II	I	I	II	I			

Maxillary palatal

Tooth no.	18	17	16	15	14	13	12	11	21	22	23	24	25	26	27	28
Pocket	335	525		756	857	512	329	524	742	312	225	726	322			
Bleeding		• •		• • •	• •	•	•	•	• •			• •				
Suppuration													• •			
Recession	000	022		444	443	000	122	000	000	000	002	233	011			
Mesial furcation																

Mandibular lingual

Tooth no.	48	47	46	45	44	43	42	41	31	32	33	34	35	36	37	38
Pocket		326	525	623	322	222	212	613	312	217	412	324	324	637	733	
Bleeding			•		•			• •		• •				•	•	
Suppuration																
Recession		000	000	300	000	000	000	030	010	020	020	000	000	000	000	
Furcation														I		

Mandibular buccal

Tooth no.	48	47	46	45	44	43	42	41	31	32	33	34	35	36	37	38
Pocket		324	725	612	113	113	213	732	312	127	423	422	212	535	323	
Bleeding			•	•				•		•		•		•	•	
Suppuration			•					•								
Recession		000	334	030	000	000	022	020	040	000	000	020	020	433	200	
Furcation			I											I		
Mobility			I+	I			I+	I	I	I=				I	I	

Occlusion

Skeletal classification	~Class I			
Dental occlusion	Class I			
Angle right	Molar	Half class III	Canine	Class I
Angle left	N/A		Canine	Class I
Anterior overbite	6 mm (11, 41)			
Anterior overjet	4 mm (11, 41)			
Cross-bites	Nil			
Open-bites	Nil			
Curve of Spee	RHS	+ve	LHS	+ve
Curve of Wilson	+ve			
RP to IP slide	1 mm			
FWS	M test		3 mm	

Tooth guidance

Right laterotrusion

```
8 7 6 5 4 3 2 1 | 1 2 3 4 5 6 7 8
8 7 6 5 4 3 2 1   1 2 3 4 5 6 7 8
```

Left laterotrusion

```
8 7 6 5 4 3 2 1 | 1 2 3 4 5 6 7 8
8 7 6 5 4 3 2 1   1 2 3 4 5 6 7 8
```

Protrusion

```
8 7 6 5 4 3 2 1 | 1 2 3 4 5 6 7 8
8 7 6 5 4 3 2 1   1 2 3 4 5 6 7 8
```

Tooth surface loss

Caries

```
8 7 6 5 4 3 2 1 | 1 2 3 4 5 6 7 8
8 7 6 5 4 3 2 1   1 2 3 4 5 6 7 8
```

Attrition

```
8 7 6 5 4 3 2 1 | 1 2 3 4 5 6 7 8
8 7 6 5 4 3 2 1   1 2 3 4 5 6 7 8
```

Erosion

```
8 7 6 5 4 3 2 1 | 1 2 3 4 5 6 7 8
8 7 6 5 4 3 2 1   1 2 3 4 5 6 7 8
```

Abrasion

```
8 7 6 5 4 3 2 1 | 1 2 3 4 5 6 7 8
8 7 6 5 4 3 2 1   1 2 3 4 5 6 7 8
```

Abfraction

```
8 7 6 5 4 3 2 1 | 1 2 3 4 5 6 7 8
8 7 6 5 4 3 2 1   1 2 3 4 5 6 7 8
```

Dental charting

Tooth no.	Clinical findings	Comments
18		
17	MOD amalgam, DP GIC	
16		
15	MOD amalgam	
14	MOD amalgam with P cusp cap	
13	Nil	
12	CMC	
11	CMC, root filled	
21	CMC, root filled	
22	CMC	
23	D amalgam	
24	DO amalgam	
25	CMC	
26		
27		
28		
38		
37	MO amalgam	
36	MOD amalgam with DB cusp cap	Requires onlay or full coverage restoration
35	MOD amalgam	Requires onlay or full coverage restoration
34	Nil	
33	Nil	
32	Nil	
31	Nil	
41	Nil	
42	Nil	
43	Nil	
44	DO amalgam	
45	MOD amalgam	Requires onlay or full coverage restoration
46	MOD amalgam with MB and DB cusp cap	Distal root caries, buccal abrasion lesion
47	MO amalgam	
48		

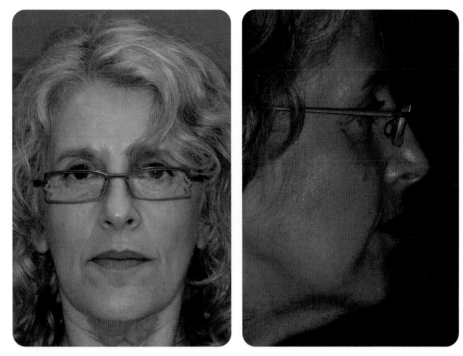

Figure 11.4.1 Extraoral examination.

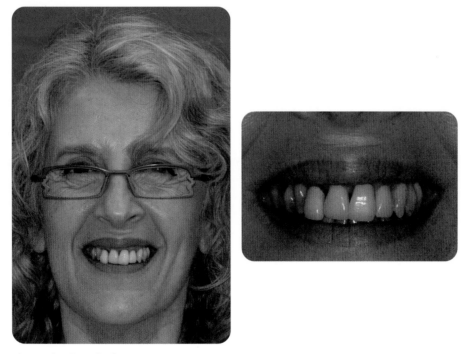

Figure 11.4.2 Extraoral examination. Smile assessment.

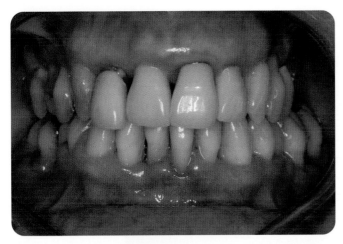

Figure 11.4.3 Intraoral examination. Frontal view of dental arches at intercuspal position.

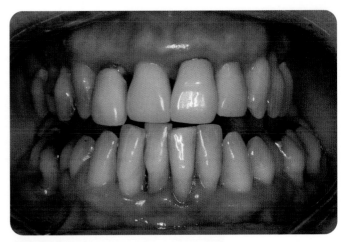

Figure 11.4.4 Intraoral examination. Frontal view of dental arches in protrusive contact.

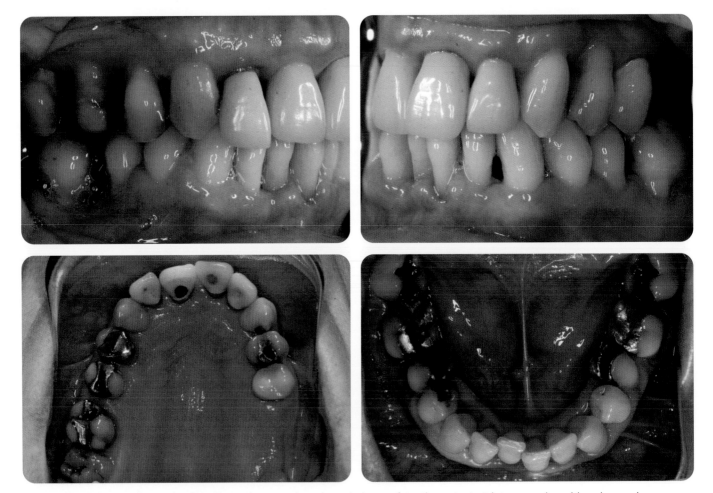

Figure 11.4.5 Intraoral examination. Upper images show lateral views of tooth contact at intercuspal position. Lower images show full arch occlusal views indicating tooth alignments and restorations.

Radiographs
Orthopantomogram (27/02/2006) (Figure 11.4.6)

Features	Radiographic data
TMJ	NAD
Bone loss	Moderate–advanced sextant 1, 2, 3, 4, 6
Sinuses	NAD
Mandible foramen and canal	Unclear
Mental foramen	Unclear
Retained roots	Nil
Pathology	24, 46 PA radiolucency

Periapical films

Tooth no.	Information	Tooth no.	Information
18	Not visible	38	Missing
17	Deep D proximal box, advanced horizontal BL	37	Advanced horizontal BL
16	Missing	36	Moderate horizontal BL
15	Advanced horizontal BL, PA radiolucency	35	Mild horizontal BL
14	Advanced horizontal BL	34	Mild horizontal BL
13	Moderate horizontal BL	33	Moderate horizontal BL
12	Advanced vertical BL	32	Advanced horizontal BL, adj roots close proximal
11	Advanced horizontal BL	31	Moderate BL, adj roots close proximal
21	Advanced vertical BL	41	Moderate BL, adj roots close proximal
22	Moderate horizontal BL	42	Moderate BL
23	Moderate horizontal BL	43	Mild BL
24	Advanced vertical BL, PA radiolucency	44	Radiopacity (possible hypercementation)
25	Mild horizontal BL	45	Advanced horizontal BL
26	Missing	46	Advanced horizontal BL, M and D root caries
27	Missing	47	Moderate horizontal BL
28	Missing	48	Missing

Study casts

Articulation	Position	ICP
	Face bow	Yes
Diagnostic wax-up	OVD change	Not required
	Occlusal adjustment	Not required
	Crown lengthening	Not required

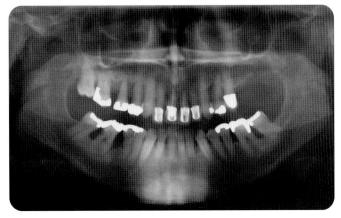

Figure 11.4.6 Radiographs. Orthopantomogram demonstrates severe generalised periodontal bone loss (see above in Periapical films data – in the maxilla and furcation involvement of teeth 36, 46).

Problem list

Problem list	Details
Medical condition	Osteoporosis (bisphosphonate – Fosamax)
Aesthetics	Misalignment: 12, 11, 21, 22
	Recession and exposed CMC margins: 12, 11, 21, 22
	Interproximal 'black triangles': maxillary anteriors
	Over-eruption: 12
	Colour mismatch: 12, 11, 21, 22
	High smile line
Speech	Nil
TMD	Nil
Soft tissue	Nil
Oral hygiene	Nil
Saliva	Nil
Periodontal	Periodontitis: generalised moderate to severe chronic periodontitis, terminal maxillary dentition
Edentulism	Kennedy class II
Occlusion	Over-eruption 12, 32, 31, 41, 42
	Mild loss of left posterior support
	Right molar half class III
Tooth surface loss	Caries: 46 M and D root
	Attrition (mild)
	Abrasion (toothbrush): 46B and 14P
Restorative	Weakened cusps: 15, 16, 36, 35, 45
Prosthetic	Nil
Endodontic	24, 46 PA radiolucency

Treatment options

Option 1: Removable complete denture
- Maxillary removable full denture.
- Replace restorations in 36, 35, 45:
  - type: onlay/full coverage restoration;

material: gold/porcelain/amalgam/composite resin.

Advantages	Disadvantages
Lowest financial cost	Psychological effect of removable prosthesis
Simplified treatment	Decreased masticatory efficacy
Low maintenance cost	Lower comfort with palatal coverage and denture mobility
Aesthetics	Continued bone loss

Option 2: Removable overdenture
- Maxillary bar-retained overdenture on four implants:
  - implant placement: immediate/early/delayed;
  - loading: immediate/early/delayed;
  - material:
    - teeth: acrylic/porcelain;
    - framework: gold/titanium/chrome.

- Replace restorations in 36, 35, 45:
  - type: onlay/full coverage restoration;
  - material: gold/porcelain/amalgam/composite resin.

Advantages	Disadvantages
Access for oral hygiene	Psychological effect of removable prosthesis
Masticatory efficacy (retention and stability)	Lower comfort (partial palatal coverage for denture support)
Aesthetics	Moderate maintenance cost
Speech (peripheral seal)	

Option 3: Complete fixed prosthesis
- Complete maxillary implant-supported screw-retained FDP on six implants:
  - implant placement: immediate/early/delayed;
  - loading: immediate/early/delayed;
  - material:
    - teeth: acrylic/porcelain;
    - framework: gold/titanium/chrome.
- Replace restorations in 36, 35, 45:
  - type: onlay/full coverage restoration;
  - material: gold/porcelain/amalgam/composite resin.

Advantages	Disadvantages
Psychological effect of FDP	Higher financial cost
Masticatory efficacy (retention, stability and support)	Moderate maintenance cost
Comfort	Poor access for oral hygiene
Higher flexibility for implant position and hence lower chance of requiring bone graft	Possible speech difficulty (air escape at peripheries)
Cross-arch stabilisation	Aesthetics (above FDP)

Option 4: Fixed three-unit prosthesis
- Maxillary implant-supported three-unit FDP × 4 (16–14, 13–11, 21–23, 24–26) on eight implants:
  - sequence: staged/full clearance;
  - implant placement: immediate/early/delayed;
  - loading: immediate/early/delayed;
  - material:
    - teeth: porcelain;
    - framework: gold/titanium.
- Replace restorations in 36, 35, 45:
  - type: onlay/full coverage restoration;
  - material: gold/porcelain/amalgam/composite resin;

Advantages	Disadvantages
Psychological effect of fixed prosthesis Masticatory efficacy (retention, stability and support) Comfort Psychological effect of staged approach Aesthetics of porcelain teeth	Highest financial cost Higher risk of implant failure with staged approach Crown and implant position must coincide and hence higher chance of requiring bone graft Poor access for oral hygiene Wear of opposing dentition Highest maintenance cost Possible speech difficulty (air escape at peripheries) Aesthetics (above and between FDPs) Length of treatment

Treatment plan
Option 4: Fixed three-unit prosthesis
- Maxillary implant-supported three-unit FDP × 4 (16–14, 13–11, 21–23, 24–26) on eight implants:
  - sequence: staged/full clearance;
  - implant placement: delayed;
  - loading: delayed;
  - material:
    - teeth: porcelain;
    - framework: gold alloy.

Treatment sequence
- Healing phase.
- Osseointegration.
- Prosthetic phase.

Date	Procedure
13/03/2006	Consultation
03/2006	Endodontic treatment of 46
03/2006	Secondary impressions, shade, MMR for P/- immediately
04/2006	Supportive periodontal therapy
04/2006	Extraction of 16, 15, 14, 24, 25 (Figure 11.4.7) Immediate issue of P/- replacing 16, 15, 14, 24, 25, 26, 27 clasping 16, 13, 23
04/2006	Denture review
05/2006	Secondary impressions, MMR for F/- immediately
05/2006	Wax try-in for F/-

Date	Procedure
05/2006	Extraction of 18, 13, 12, 11, 21, 22, 23 Immediate issue of F/- (Figure 11.4.8)
06/2006	Reline F/-
06/2006	Denture review and radiographic guide (Figures 11.4.9 & 11.4.10)
06/2006	CT scan (Figure 11.4.11)
07/2006	Supportive periodontal therapy
07/2006	Surgical guide preparation (Figure 11.4.12)
07/2006	Implant surgery, single stage (Figure 11.4.13)
08/2006	Review
10/2006	Supportive periodontal therapy
11/2006	Implant-level impression (Figure 11.4.14)
11/2006	Provisional implant bridge (Figures 11.4.15–11.4.17)
11/2006	Verification record (Figure 11.4.18)
12/2006	Casting try-in (Figure 11.4.19)
01/2007	Supportive periodontal therapy
01/2007	MMR, shade selection
02/2007	Definitive bridge (Figures 11.4.20 & 11.4.21) Review and maintenance (Figures 11.4.22 & 11.4.23)

The proposed treatment sequence is dependent upon the success of each step. Throughout treatment, complications may be encountered requiring modification of the sequence and an extension of treatment time. The patient will be advised of all modifications progressively if required.

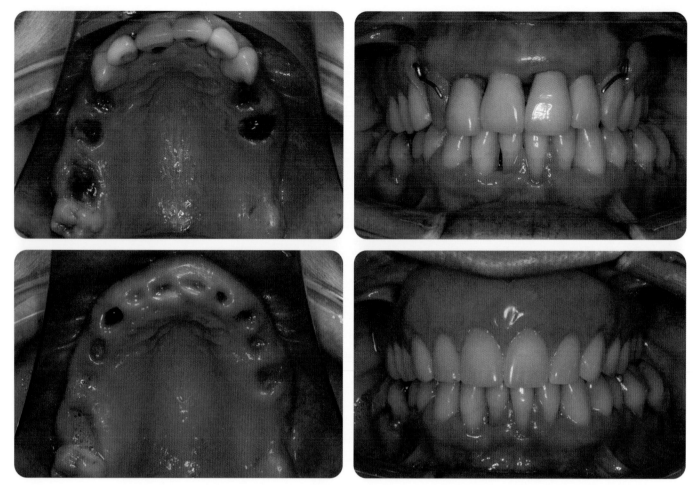

Figure 11.4.7 A staged approach to management with extraction of 16, 15, 14, 24, 25 and an immediate transitional partial maxillary removable dental prosthesis; followed by extraction of the remaining maxillary anterior teeth and the fitting of an immediate complete maxillary removable prosthesis.

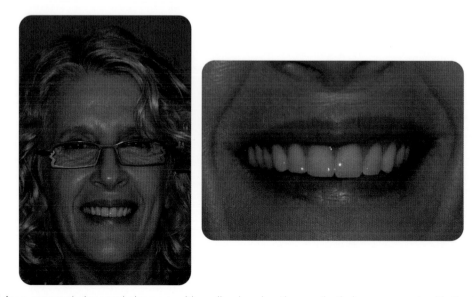

Figure 11.4.8 Full face extraoral view and close up with smile showing the aesthetic improvement with the immediate complete maxillary removable dental prosthesis *in situ*.

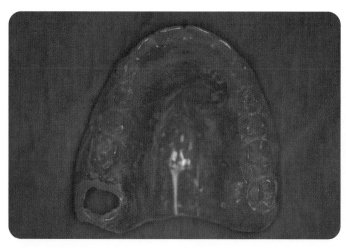
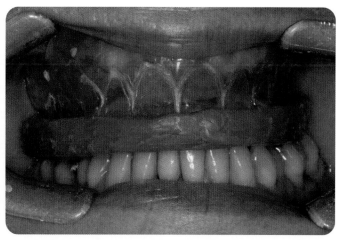

Figure 11.4.9 Maxillary clear acrylic resin radiographic guide with gutta percha markers. Clinical view of the guide in position with interocclusal wax record for positional location of the guide.

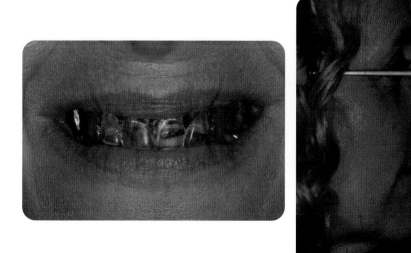

Figure 11.4.10 Smile assessment including buccal position of posterior teeth (to show buccal corridor space) and lip position of maxillary anterior teeth; and profile view of lip support.

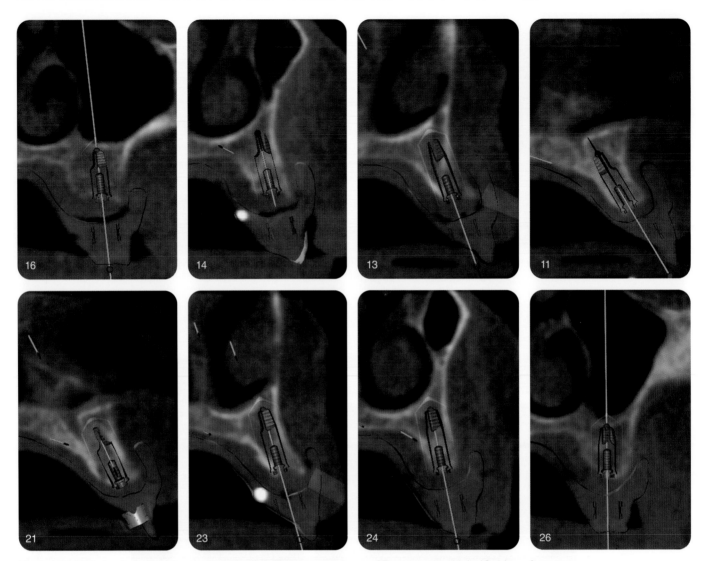

Figure 11.4.11 Implant planning to optimise location on cone-beam CT scan using NobelGuide software.

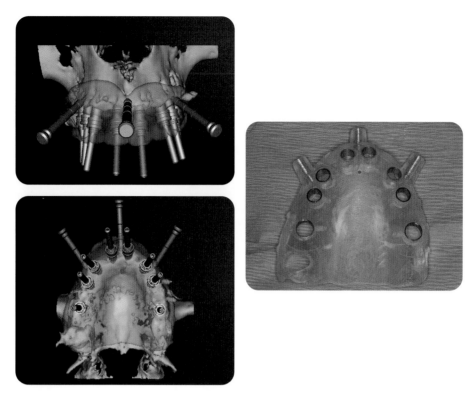

Figure 11.4.12 Left images show the surgical guide completed in NobelGuide software; the right image shows the fabricated complete maxillary surgical guide.

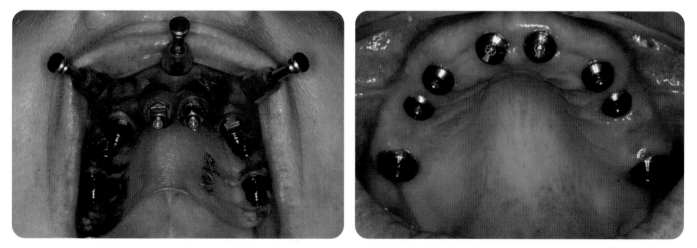

Figure 11.4.13 Guided implant placement (x8) and immediate postoperative view with healing abutments (x8) in place.

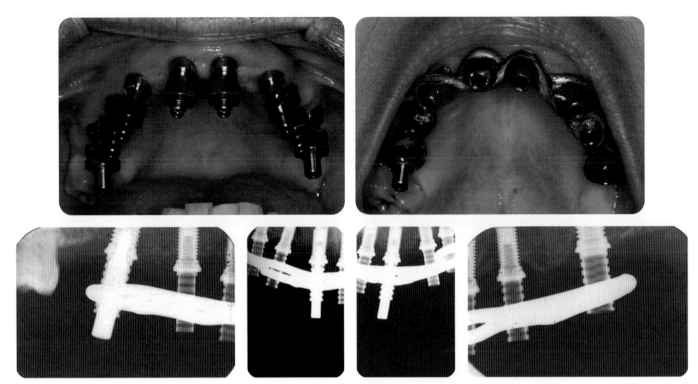

Figure 11.4.14 Implant-level impression copings in place. Right upper image shows the verification jig constructed on the master cast using temporary abutments luted with Duralay resin to a cast cobalt chrome framework. Periapical radiographs using a paralleling technique to check the fit. Note the use of only two guide pins. In addition, with one guide pin placed in the most distal abutment, the guide pin 'end-feel' (to determine whether there is an absolute passive fit of the casting) was checked at all abutments.

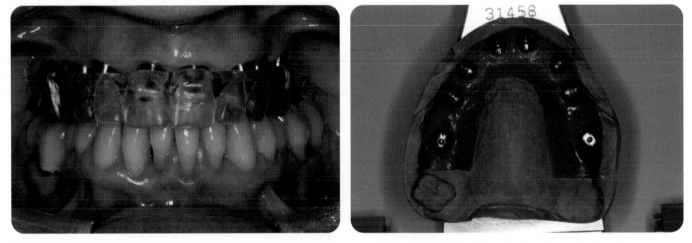

Figure 11.4.15 Left image shows the maxillomandibular relation record taken against healing abutments and using the radiographic guide without a buccal flange. Right image shows the maxillary cast with healing abutments in place.

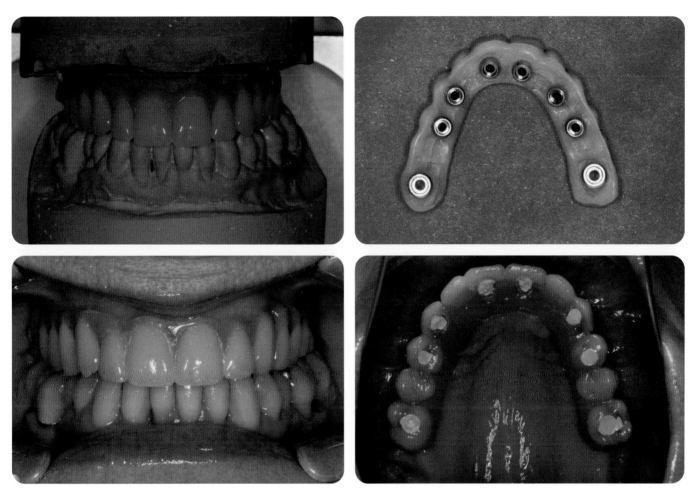

Figure 11.4.16 Provisional acrylic resin implant-supported bridge (upper images). Note clinical views (lower images) of provisional prosthesis in place and the occlusal view (right lower) indicating optimum screw-access locations following planning with NobelGuide software.

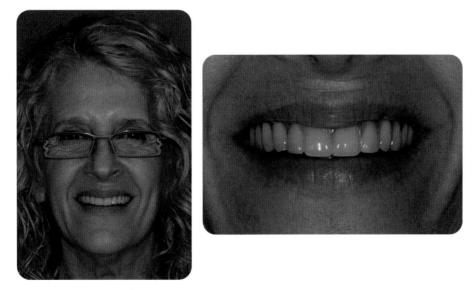

Figure 11.4.17 Provisional implant bridge. Smile assessment.

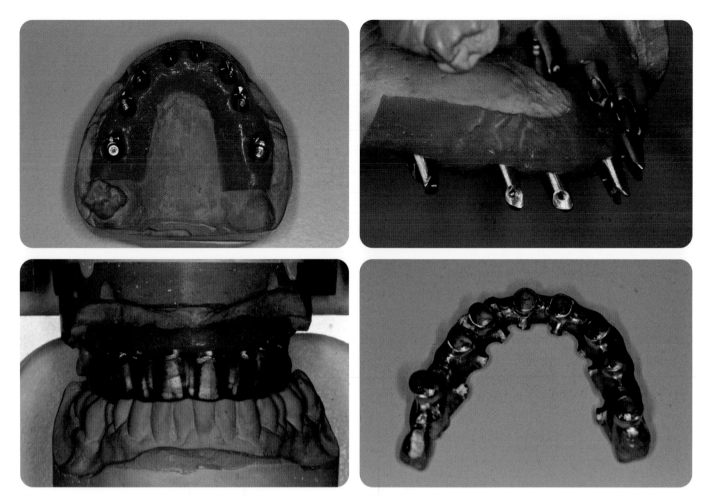

Figure 11.4.18 Custom abutments with transverse screws (cross-pins). Cast gold–alloy framework finely sectioned, luted with acrylic resin and verified by intraoral placement. Maxillo-mandibular relationship retaken on cast framework and used to verify the articulation of the master casts.

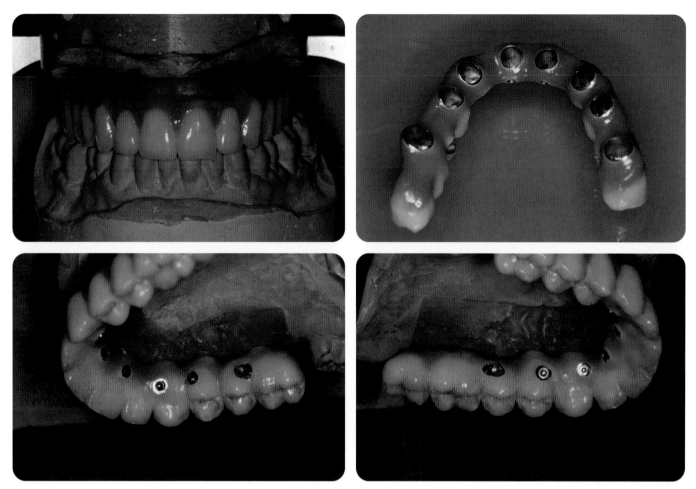

Figure 11.4.19 Definitive bridge on master cast. Note the transverse screw access on the palatal.

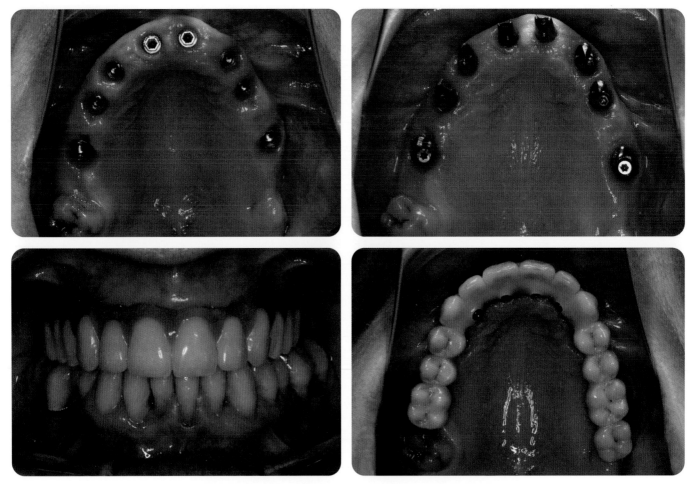

Figure 11.4.20 Definitive bridge screwed in position in the mouth. No adjustments were required.

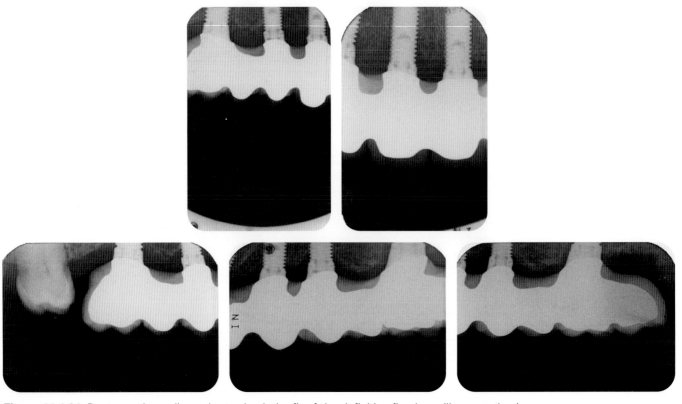

Figure 11.4.21 Postoperative radiographs to check the fit of the definitive fixed maxillary prosthesis.

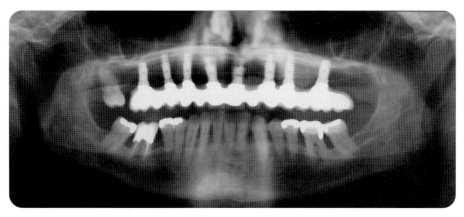

Figure 11.4.22 Postoperative radiograph orthopantomogram of completed oral rehabilitation.

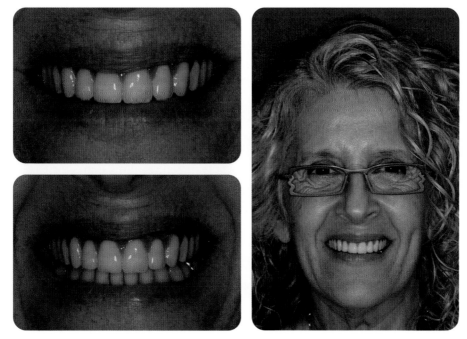

Figure 11.4.23 Review of facial characteristics with smile (upper left image) and 'grimace' (lower left image) with full face smile (right image).

Treatment discussion

Osteoporosis and bisphosphonates

Osteoporosis affects over 8 million females and 2 million males in America. Many patients are concerned that osteoporosis will preclude them from considering dental implant treatment because of a lack of bone density and lack of confidence with respect to risk. As dental implants become more in demand, the prognosis for and potential complications of implant therapy in patients with osteoporosis are a matter of intense interest. Although osteoporosis has been considered a risk factor, particularly for postmenopausal women, no clinical studies on this matter have been published. Future studies of the effect of bisphosphonates on the jaw bone mineral content, bone mineral density and alveolar bone loss in relation to implant treatment, with or without bone grafting, are required.

Currently, such patients are advised that treatment is indeed possible, but prolonged healing periods and careful conservative prosthetic management are desirable (Henry 2002).

Periodontal disease and implants

Periodontal pockets around teeth and implants with equal depths are strikingly similar in their microbial composition (Papaioannou et al. 1996). The microbiota on remaining teeth has been found to be the major influence on peri-implant microbiota (Lee et al. 1999). This confirms the hypothesis that pockets around teeth act as a reservoir. Several studies have confirmed the transmission of microorganisms from teeth to implants, some occurring in as little as 14 days (Koka et al. 1993).

These observations highlight the importance of periodontal health around the natural dentition before as well as after implant installation. Elimination of these periodontal pathogens from the patient's oral cavity before administering dental implant treatment may inhibit colonisation by these pathogens and reduce the risk of peri-implantitis (Sumida et al. 2002).

Success rates

The success rates of implants and their prosthesis have been well published in the literature. In the edentulous maxilla, the success rate of the prostheses is greater than 95% at 10 years and greater than 92% at 15 years (Adell et al. 1990).

Material and wear

There are two main types of fixed bridges available: a resin-gold bridge or a porcelain–gold bridge. The latter type is more suitable for the reconstruction of a jaw with minimal bone loss and the former can be used when more substantial bone loss has occurred and when cost is prohibitive. Porcelain wears down enamel and dentine considerably more than resin (Jagger & Harrison 1995). Furthermore, enamel has been shown to wear down porcelain more rapidly than resin (Jagger & Harrison 1995).

Segmented full-arch prosthesis versus splinted full-arch prosthesis

The rationale for having four separate three-unit bridges was to improve retrievability, reduce repair costs and reduce replacement costs. At the time of provisionalisation, the patient decided that she would not accept the aesthetics of margins between the three-unit bridges and opted for a splinted full-arch prosthesis despite its disadvantages. Furthermore, the patient disliked the aesthetics of the occlusal-access abutment screw holes on the provisional prosthesis so transverse screws were used in the definitive prosthesis.

Proprioception

Following initial periodontal therapy tooth 17 was given a good prognosis; thus 17 was retained to provide greater proprioception in the maxilla as a means of protecting the maxillary prosthesis.

Flapless guided surgery

CAD–CAM surgical guides was relatively new technology at the time of treatment. The NobelGuide planning software and surgical guide were used to optimise prosthetically driven implant placement and reduce the morbidity associated with implant surgery. The patient experienced no post-surgery swelling, bruising or pain. Mrs C was the first patient in the Centre for Oral Health to be treated using NobelGuide technology.

Review at 4 years

Complications

- Minor single complication at 38 months involving bleeding of the mucosa after using Oral B Super Floss. The maxillary bridge was subsequently detached from the implant abutments to assess the implants and soft tissue. All probing depths around implants were within normal limits and without bleeding in probing. The soft tissue beneath the bridge was healthy and was found to have been traumatised from flossing in the maxillary right premolar region.

Oral hygiene

- Excellent.
- Continued daily use of Oral B Super Floss and brushing twice daily, in conjunction with Waterpik Water Jet.

Soft tissue health

- Good.

CPITN	0		
	0	0	0

Occlusion
- ICP: contacts on all teeth except central and lateral incisors.
- RCP: coincident with ICP.

Guidance

Right laterotrusion

8 7 6 5 4 3 2 1 | 1 2 3 4 5 6 7 8

8 7 6 5 4 3 2 1   1 2 3 4 5 6 7 8

Left laterotrusion

8 7 6 5 4 3 2 1 | 1 2 3 4 5 6 7 8

8 7 6 5 4 3 2 1   1 2 3 4 5 6 7 8

Protrusion

8 7 6 5 4 3 2 1 | 1 2 3 4 5 6 7 8

8 7 6 5 4 3 2 1   1 2 3 4 5 6 7 8

Oral health related quality of life
- Comfort: completely satisfied.
- Aesthetics: completely satisfied.
- Function:
  - mastication: completely satisfied;
  - speech: completely satisfied.

- Social interaction:
  - increased confidence levels.
- Would you undertake the process again if needed? – 'Yes, definitely. It has changed my life.'

References

Adell, R., Eriksson, B., Lekholm, U. *et al.* (1990) Long-term follow-up study of osseointegrated implants in the treatment of totally edentulous jaws. *International Journal of Oral & Maxillofacial Implants*, 5 (4), 347–359.

Henry, P.J. (2002) A review of guidelines for implant rehabilitation of the edentulous maxilla. *Journal of Prosthetic Dentistry*, 87 (3), 281–288.

Jagger, D.C. & Harrison, A. (1995) An in vitro investigation into the wear effects of selected restorative materials on dentine. *Journal of Oral Rehabilitation*, 22 (5), 349–354.

Koka, S., Razzoog, M.E., Bloem, T.J. *et al.* (1993) Microbial colonization of dental implants in partially edentulous subjects. *Journal of Prosthetic Dentistry*, 70 (2), 141–144.

Lee, K.H., Tanner, A.C., Maiden, M.F. *et al.* (1999) Pre- and post-implantation microbiota of the tongue, teeth, and newly placed implants. *Journal of Clinical Periodontology*, 26 (12), 822–832.

Papaioannou, W., Quirynen, M. & van Steenberghe, D. (1996) The influence of periodontitis on the subgingival flora around implants in partially edentulous patients. *Clinical Oral Implants Research*, 7 (4), 405–409.

Sumida, S., Ishihara, K., Kishi, M. *et al.* (2002) Transmission of periodontal disease-associated bacteria from teeth to osseointegrated implant regions. *International Journal of Oral & Maxillofacial Implants*, 17 (5), 696–702.

12

Complete Edentulism

Introduction by Iven Klineberg

The state of complete edentulism was common and the widespread use of complete dentures persisted in developed countries until preventive dentistry promoted oral health care at the time of the introduction of fluoride applications, fluoride toothpastes and fluoride at 1 part per million in reticulated water supplies for regular intake through drinking water. The introduction of fluoride was variable but from the late 1950s and early 1960s the momentum began.

The use of complete dentures was a common expectation until that time and was linked with an era of limited oral health knowledge and expectation and was accepted as a clinician-driven treatment decision. Some patients were able to manage adequately while others experienced difficulty initially or over time.

In reflecting on this period of dental and oral health, complete dental extractions can now be recognised as a condition of total dental deafferentation (Klineberg & Murray 1999a,b) with physiological and psychological complications for function (mastication, swallowing, speech) and nutrition, facial aesthetics, social interaction, psychosocial well-being and oral health related quality of life. The emotional effects of tooth loss and complete denture use have been comprehensively investigated by the Davis and Fiske group with cross-cultural studies of English and Chinese cohorts (Fiske et al. 1998, Davis et al. 2000) and a Polish study (Likeman et al. 2002), which yielded consistent data notwithstanding sample size variation. The common and profoundly significant outcome was the varying degree of difficulty in accepting the edentulous state with loss of confidence, reduced self-image with greater inhibition in daily activities, and difficulty in accepting the inevitable changes in facial appearance with premature ageing. The collective effect was a dramatic negative impact on general quality of life, emphasising the importance of the mouth and face on general well-being. In addition, the association of poor nutrition with complete denture use was reported by two thirds of the participants studied, with negative impact on general health (Scott et al. 2001).

Implant application had a transformational effect on edentulism and particularly on mandibular complete RDP stability with significant improvement in physiological function and psychological well-being and enhanced oral health related quality of life. This development was led by the McGill Consensus (Feine & Carlsson 2003) and championed by the Feine group (Emami et al. 2009). Other studies consistently supported the outcomes (Allen et al. 2006, Ma & Payne 2010, Thomason 2010), as well as improved nutritional status reported by Sánchez-Ayola et al. (2010), and improved maxillary RDP function with implant anchorage (Slot et al. 2010).

References

Allen, P.F., Thomason, J.M., Jepson, N.J. et al. (2006) A randomized controlled trial of implant-retained mandibular overdentures. Journal of Dental Research, 85 (6), 547–551.

Davis, D.M., Fiske, J., Scott, B. et al. (2000) The emotional effects of tooth loss: a preliminary quantitative study. British Dental Journal, 188 (9), 503–506.

Emami, E., Heydeke, G., Rompré, P.H. et al. (2009) Impact of implant support for mandibular dentures on satisfaction, oral and general health-related quality of life: a meta-analysis of randomized-controlled trials. Clinical Oral Implants Research, 20 (6), 533–544.

Feine, J.S. & Carlsson, G.E. (eds) (2003) Implant Overdentures: The Standard of Care for edentulous Patients. Quintessence, Chicago.

Fiske, J., Davis, D.M., Frances, C. et al. (1998) The emotional effects of tooth loss in edentulous people. British Dental Journal, 184 (2), 90–93.

Klineberg, I. & Murray, G. (1999a) Dental deafferentation – a paradox in proprioception. In: Osseoperception and Musculo-Skeletal Function (ed. P.- I. Branemark), pp.34–48. Tranemo Typo-Tryck AB, Gothenburg.

Oral Rehabilitation: A Case-Based Approach, First Edition. Edited by Iven Klineberg, Diana Kingston.
© 2012 Blackwell Publishing Ltd. Published 2012 by Blackwell Publishing Ltd.

Klineberg, I. & Murray, G. (1999b) Osseoperception: sensory function and proprioception. *Advances in Dental Research*, 13, 120–129.

Likeman, P., Friske, J. & Davis, J. (2002) Use of internet as a research method in a study of the emotional effects of tooth loss in Poland. *European Journal of Prosthodontics & Restorative Dentistry*, 10 (1), 33–35.

Ma, S. & Payne, A.G. (2010) Marginal bone loss with mandibular two-implant overdentures using different loading protocols: a systematic literature review. *International Journal of Prosthodontics*, 23 (2), 117–126.

Sánchez-Ayola, A., Lagravère, M.O., Gonçalves, T.M. *et al.* (2010) Nutritional effects of implant therapy in edentulous patients – a systematic review. *Implant Dentistry*, 19 (3), 196–207.

Scott, B.J., Leung, K.C., McMillan, A.S. *et al.* (2001) A transcultural perspective on the emotional effect of tooth loss in complete denture wearers. *International Journal of Prosthodontics*, 14 (5), 461–465.

Slot, W., Raghoebar, G.M., Vissink, A. *et al.* (2010) A systematic review of implant-supported maxillary overdentures after a mean observation period of at least 1 year. *Journal of Clinical Periodontology*, 37 (1), 98–110.

Thomason, J.M. (2010) The use of mandibular implant-retained overdentures improve patient satisfaction and quality of life. *Journal of Evidence-based Dental Practice*, 10 (1), 61–63.

Case 12.1 Mr Arthur T

Tuan Dao

Patient: Mr Arthur T (date of birth 10/01/1940)

Presenting complaints

Chief complaint	'My top denture is loose and I do not have a well-fitting bottom denture'
Subsidiary complaints	'I would like to eat nuts as they are my favourite food and I am unable to do so with my current dentures'
History of complaints	
Patient's expectations	The patient would prefer a functional outcome in regard to his fully edentulous state

History
Medical history

Medical Practitioner		
Respiratory	Nil	
Cardiovascular	Hypercholesterolemia Hypertension	
Gastrointestinal	Gastric reflux	
Neurological	Nil	
Endocrine	Diabetes mellitus type 2	
Developmental	Nil	
Musculoskeletal	Nil	
Genitourinary	Nil	
Haematological	Nil	
Other	Allergies	
	Smoking	Previous smoker for 30 years but has ceased smoking for the past 12 months
	Infectious diseases	Nil
	Pregnancy	N/A
	Hospitalisation	Nil
	Medications	Diabex 1000 mg/day
		Lipitor 40 mg/day
		Ascartin one capsule/day
		Ikorel 20 mg/day
		Losec 20 mg/day

Social history

Marital status	Married	
Children	2	
Occupation	Retired truck driver	
Smoking	Type	Cigarettes
	Frequency	25/day
	Period:	For 30 years but has ceased smoking for 12 months
Recreational drugs	Nil	
Diet	Soft drinks	Nil
	Sports drinks	Nil
	Lemons	Nil
	Acidic foods	Nil
	Sweet foods	Nil
	Water	2 cups/day
	Tea	1 cup/day
	Coffee	Nil
	Alcohol	Nil
	Hard/brittle foods	Nil
	Ice crunching	Nil
Habits/hobbies	Musical instrument	Nil
	Exercise	Minimal
	Oral habits	Nil

Dental history

		Additional information
Date of last examination		
Oral hygiene	Brushing	Nil
	Flossing	N/A
	Mouthwash	Nil
	Toothpaste	Nil
Treatment	Restorations	Nil
	Endodontics	Nil
	Periodontics	Nil
	Orthodontics	Nil
	RDP	Current one is 6 years old
	FDP	Nil
	TMD	Nil
	OMFS	Multiple extractions performed over past 20 years

Extraoral examination (Figure 12.1.1)

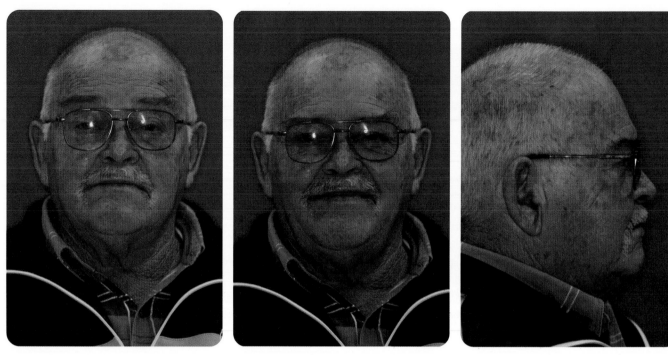

Figure 12.1.1 Extraoral examination. Note reduced occlusal vertical dimension at tooth contact (right frontal view). Profile shows jaw posture and adequate lower facial height.

Aesthetics

Facial symmetry	Present	
Profile	Straight – convex	
Nasolabial angle	Obtuse	
Facial folds	Present	
Midlines	Face/maxillary centrals	Coincident
	Maxillary central alignment	Aligned
	Maxillary/mandible centrals	N/A
Lip posture	Symmetry	Asymmetrical
	Upper lip	Adequate
	Lower lip	Adequate
	Competence	Present
	Tooth display	Minimal
Occlusal plane	Parallel to ala tragus line	Yes
	Parallel to interpupillary line	Yes
	Over-eruption	N/A
Vertical	FWS	2 mm
	OVD assessment	Over-closed by 2 mm
Smile assessment	Symmetry	Present
	Lip line	Low
	Gingival display	Nil
	Tooth display	Minimal
	Buccal corridor	Present

Phonetics

	Normal	Abnormal
Labial (m)	√	
Labiodental (f/v)	√	
Linguodental (th)	√	
Interdental (s)	√	
Linguopalatal (k/ng)	√	

Temporomandibular assessment

TMJ	Additional information
Click	Nil
Crepitus	Nil
Tenderness	Nil

Muscle tenderness	Right	Left
Temporalis	Nil	Nil
Masseter	Nil	Nil
Posterior mandible	Nil	Nil
Anterior mandible	Nil	Nil
Glands	Nil	
Nodes	Nil	
Further investigation required	No	

Intraoral examination (Figures 12.1.2 & 12.1.3)
Soft tissues

Tissue	Healthy	Abnormal	Additional information
Lips	√		Nil
Labial vestibule	√		Nil
Cheeks	√		Nil
Palate	√		Nil
Oropharynx	√		Nil
Tongue	√		Nil
Floor	√		Nil
Frenal attachments	√		Nil

Ridges	Maxilla	Mandible
Arch shape	Regular U-shape	Regular U-shape
Resorption	Average	Minimal
Palatal vault	Average	–
Tori	Nil	Nil
Frenal attachments	High	High
Mucosa	Healthy	Healthy
Pathology	Nil	Nil

Oral cleanliness

Condition	Yes	No
Plaque		√
Calculus		√
Food impaction		√
Stains		√
Halitosis		√

Saliva

Water intake	2 cups water/day
Quality	
Quantity	Adequate
Pathology	Nil
Medications affecting	Antihypertensive

Further investigation required   No

Previous dentures

Teeth replaced   <u>8 7 6 5 4 3 2 1 | 1 2 3 4 5 6 7 8</u>

8 7 6 5 4 3 2 1   1 2 3 4 5 6 7 8

	Maxilla	Mandible
Age/number	6 years old	N/A
Type	Complete denture	N/A
Kennedy classification	N/A	N/A
Appearance	Unaesthetic	N/A
LFH	N/A	N/A
Stability	Poor	N/A
Support	Poor	N/A
Retention	Poor	N/A
Hygiene	Poor	N/A
Patient opinion	Unfavourable	N/A

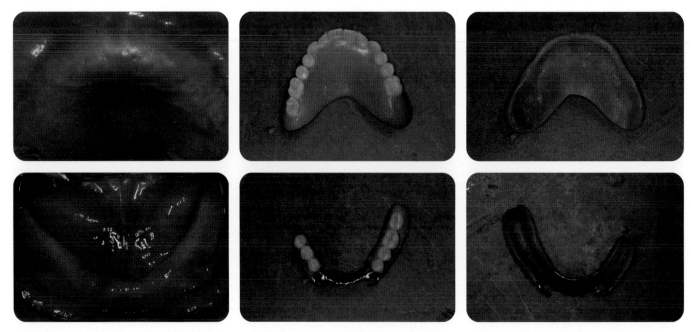

Figure 12.1.2 Remaining bone height is adequate with minimal resorption of maxillary ridge. Previous complete maxillary removable dental prosthesis has reduced palatal extension resulting in loss of post dam seal and denture retention.

Treatment options

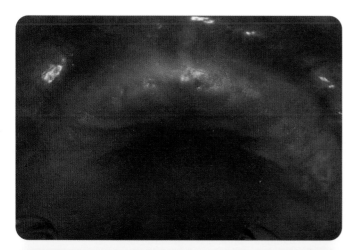

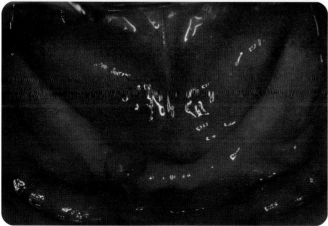

Maxilla and mandible

- Option 1:

  - Complete removable dental prostheses

- Option 2:

  - Implant retained and soft tissue supported removable dental prostheses

- Option 3:

  - Implant retained and supported fixed dental prostheses

Figure 12.1.3 Option 1 was agreed to be the most appropriate.

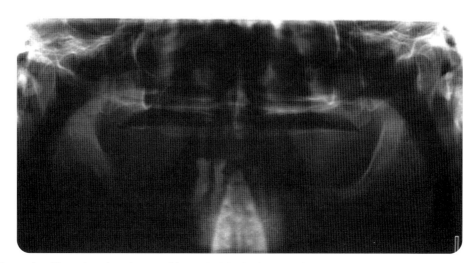

Figure 12.1.4 Radiographs. Note the abundance of bone height in the anterior mandible; there is also adequate maxillary bone.

Special tests

	Performed	Additional information
Percussion		N/A
Palpation		N/A
Vitality		N/A
Cusp loading		N/A
Transillumination		N/A
Selective anaesthesia		N/A
Other		N/A

Radiographs (Figure 12.1.4)
Orthopantomogram

Features	Radiographic data
TMJ	Clear and delineated
Bone loss	Minimal
Sinuses	Clear and present
Mandibular foramen and canal	Identified and no abnormalities detected
Mental foramen	Identified
Retained roots	Nil
Pathology	Nil

Study casts

Articulation	Position	
Diagnostic wax-up	Face bow	
	OVD change	2 mm
	Occlusal adjustment	Nil
	Crown lengthening	Nil

Problem list

Problem list	Details
Medical condition	Hypertension
	Diabetes mellitus type 2
	Hypercholesterolaemia
Aesthetics	No mandibular denture
Speech	Nil
TMD	Nil
Soft tissue	Nil
Oral hygiene	Nil
Saliva	Nil
Periodontal	Nil
Edentulism	Completely edentate
Occlusion	Nil
Tooth surface loss	Nil
Restorative	Nil
Prosthetic	Nil
Endodontic	Nil

Treatment options
Maxilla
Treatment option 1 (5 weeks)
- Conventional complete maxillary.

Treatment option 2 (4.5 months)
- Implant retained and soft tissue supported maxillary overdenture.

Treatment option 3 (9 months)
- Implant retained and supported FDPs in the maxillary; 6 to 8 fixtures to be placed in the maxillary

Mandible
Treatment option 1 (5 weeks)
- Conventional complete mandibular denture

Treatment option 2 (4.5 months)
- Implant retained and soft tissue supported complete mandibular denture.

Treatment option 3 (9 months)
- Implant retained and supported FDP supported by 5–6 dental implants.

Treatment plan

- Maxilla: treatment option 3.
- Mandible: treatment option 2.

Treatment phase	Detail	Timeline
Hygiene phase	Denture hygiene	3 weeks
Pre-prosthetic pretreatment phase I		
Pre-prosthetic pretreatment phase II	A final complete set of maxillary and mandibular dentures made	5 weeks
Prosthetic phase	Following implant surgery, a healing period of 3 months occurred prior to attaching denture attachments to implants	25 weeks
Maintenance	Review 12, 24 months, continuing	

Treatment sequence

Appointment	Procedure	Time (minutes)
1	Primary impressions (Figure 12.1.5)	60
2	Secondary impressions (Figure 12.1.5)	60
3	Maxillomandibular records and shade	60
4	F/F try-in (Figure 12.1.7)	60
5	Issue of dentures (Figure 12.1.8)	60
6	Review (Figure 12.1.9)	30
7	Review	30
8	2 months later, radiographic guide fabricated and iCat scan (Figure 12.1.10)	30
9	Consult for implant surgery with Periodontist	60
10	Implant surgery	150
11	OPG to confirm mandibular implant placement (Figure 12.1.11)	30
12	Review of dentures following surgery	30
13	Matrix attachments luted to mandibular denture (Figure 12.1.12)	90
14	Review at 1 year	30
15	Review at 2 years (Figure 12.1.13)	30

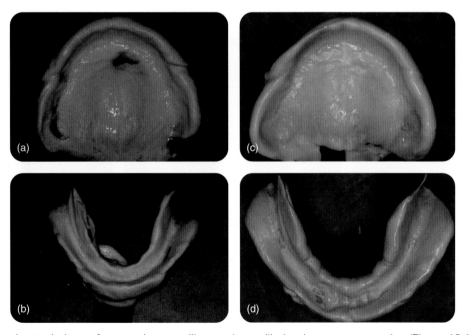

Figure 12.1.5 Impression techniques for complete maxillary and mandibular denture construction (Figure 12.1.6). (a,b) Spaced secondary impression trays have been disclosed with light body alginate to determine border extensions. (c,d) Zinc oxide and Eugenol paste have been applied to the borders for tissue moulding. Light body polyvinyl siloxane is then used as a wash technique to record the fine tissue detail. This approach yields slight compression of the traditional mucostatic impression.

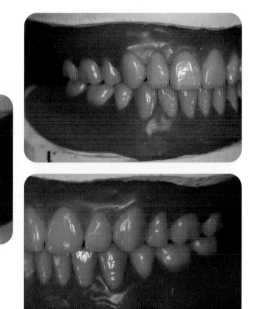

Figure 12.1.6 Complete denture construction. Note that the maxillary teeth have been aligned to provide a more natural appearance, with the teeth being aligned with varying degrees of overlap to provide the appearance of anterior crowding and three anterior tooth shades were used to again reflect a more natural appearance.

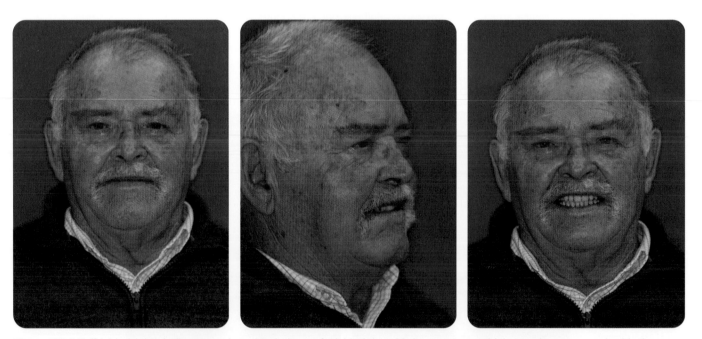

Figure 12.1.7 Trial insertion indicates an increase in lower facial height with jaw posture which may be compared with the previous extraoral views in Figure 12.1.1.

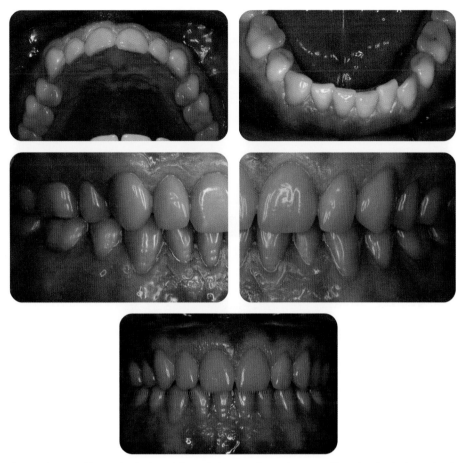

Figure 12.1.8 Issue of prostheses. Note gingival staining of the acrylic resin as well as the inclusion of palatal rugae.

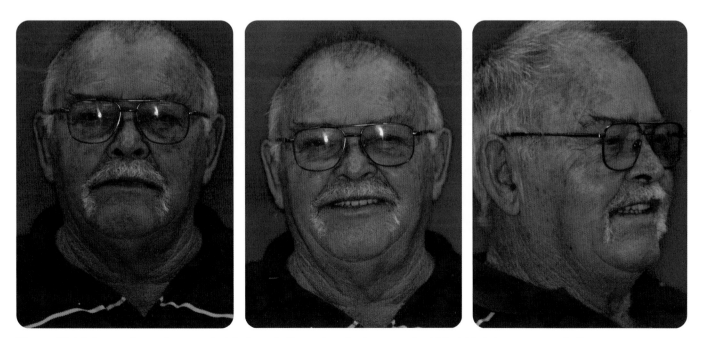

Figure 12.1.9 Issue of prostheses – facial views indicate that the lower and mid facial heights are now similar.

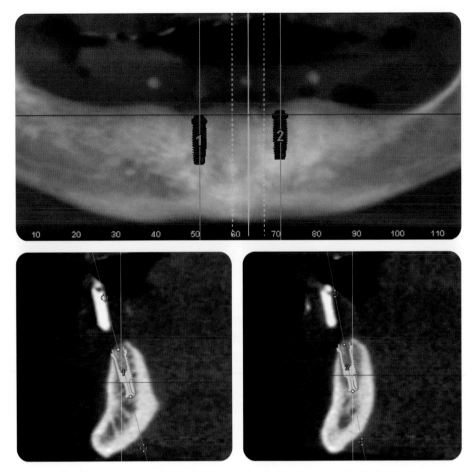

Figure 12.1.10 Surgical planning – of significance is the abundance of anterior mandibular bone.

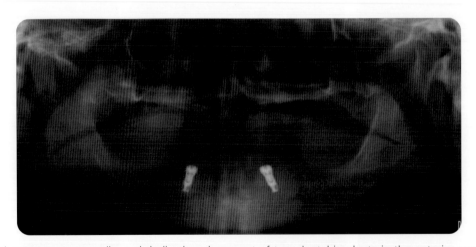

Figure 12.1.11 Orthopantomogram radiograph indicating placement of two dental implants in the anterior mandible.

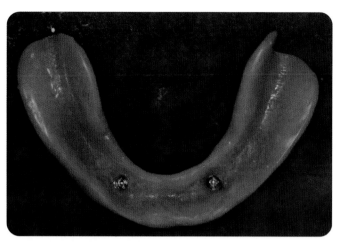

Figure 12.1.12 Reline of the tissue surface of the mandibular prosthesis to include the internal units (matrices) for the overdenture denture attachments.

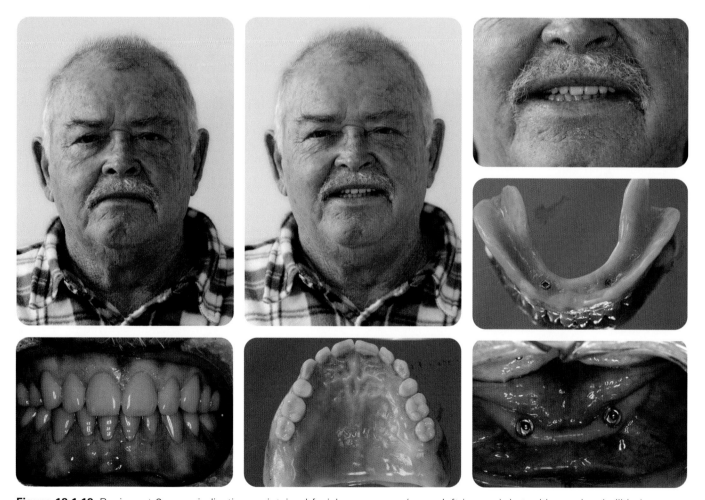

Figure 12.1.13 Review at 2 years indicating maintained facial appearance (upper left images), but with angular cheilitis (upper right image) as a reflection of general health. Prostheses *in situ* indicating appropriate tooth arrangement and contact relationships (lower left images). The mandibular prosthesis tissue surface indicates the matrix attachments and the intraoral view confirms soft tissue health.

Treatment discussion

The McGill Consensus Statement is that 'the 2-implant overdenture should become the first choice treatment for the edentulous mandible' (Feine et al. 2002).

Awad et al. (2003a) conducted a randomised clinical trial comparing general satisfaction of patients treated with conventional dentures and those with mandibular implant overdentures. There were 54 patients in the treatment group and 48 patients in the control group. A visual analogue scale was used to determine patients' general satisfaction. The authors concluded that 'a mandibular implant overdenture opposed by a maxillary conventional complete denture is a more effective treatment . . . than conventional dentures on both arches'.

In a follow-up study comparing oral health impact profile, Awad et al. (2003b) showed that the implant overdenture group had a significantly better oral health related quality of life than the conventional denture group. This is reflective in the oral health impact profile recorded pretreatment (Figure 12.1.10) and at 1-year review.

Kapur et al. (1999) conducted a randomised clinical trial comparing the efficacy of mandibular implant overdentures with conventional dentures in diabetic patients. There were two groups: a control group of 37 patients and a treatment group of 52 patients. A questionnaire was taken at baseline, 6 and 24 months following completion. Improvements were higher in the implant overdenture group. There was a significant improvement in eating enjoyment as well as general satisfaction in the treatment group. A significant difference was detected for speech in favour of the implant overdenture group.

Fitzpatrick (2006) conducted a systematic review of the literature in relation to the standard of care for the edentulous mandible and concluded that 'There is no evidence for a single universally superior treatment modality for the edentulous mandible'.

DeLuca et al. (2006) investigated the effects of smoking on osseointegrated dental implants. Patients who at the time of surgery were smokers had a higher rate of implant failure compared with non-smokers. Implementation of a smoking cessation protocol has been shown to improve chances of a successful outcome. The authors concluded that smoking should not be an absolute contraindication for implant therapy, rather patients should be informed that they are at a slightly greater risk of implant failure.

Review at 2 years

Patient concerns

The main concern was the 'lack of suction' of the maxillary complete denture – loss of retention and lack of stability.

Progressively over the past 12 months the patient felt the maxillary prosthesis became increasingly loose and would fall with chewing and speech. Mr T was satisfied with the mandibular RDP. The retention and stability of the soft tissue supported implant-retained mandibular complete RDP as described by the patient was adequate.

Medical status

Mr T is a diabetic controlled with medication and has hypercholesterolemia controlled with medication.

In the past 18 months Mr T has also begun smoking again and is currently smoking 5 cigarettes per day.

Mr T had been smoking intermittently over the past 30 years. Prior to implant surgery he ceased smoking but continued again 6 months later.

Inflammation of the lip commissures was diagnosed as angular cheilitis, which represents an opportunistic infection due to a combination of lowered immune status, multiple medications and smoking.

Oral health

Soft tissue health was satisfactory – cheeks, tongue, pharynx, palate, floor of the mouth and buccal sulcus were examined with no abnormalities detected.

Assessment of the complete RDP confirms lack of stability and retention.

Palpation of the underlying mucosa of the maxillary residual ridge did not indicate any fibrous tissue and the residual ridge was minimally resorbed. The maxillary complete denture was clean and free of stains despite the increased smoking. When viewed from the occlusal, there was little wear of the acrylic teeth.

The mandibular complete denture was retentive. The housing caps were intact and soft tissue health and hygiene around the ball abutments was excellent. The mandibular complete denture was very satisfactory. Note the change in the repeated OHRQL assessment.

The occlusion was checked for bilateral contacts in ICP and RCP. Multiple bilateral contacts on the posterior segments and light contact in the anterior segment were shown. Laterotrusive movements showed a balance occlusal scheme.

Additional treatment

A laboratory processed reline of the maxillary complete denture was provided.

Quality of life measure (2-year follow-up and pretreatment)

	Very good	Good	None	Bad	Very bad
Eating or enjoyment of food?	#			*	
Appearance?		#		*	
Speech?		#		*	
General health?		#	*		
Ability to relax or sleep?	#			*	
Social life?		#		*	
Romantic relationships?			# *		
Smiling or laughing?		#		*	
Confidence?		#		*	
Carefree manner (lack of worry)?		#		*	
Mood?		#	*		
Work or ability to do your usual jobs?		#	*		
Finances?		#	*		
Personality?		#	*		
Comfort?	#			*	
Breath odour?			# *		

*pretreatment; #, 2-year follow-up.

References

Awad, M.A., Lund, J.P., Dufresne, E. *et al.* (2003a) Comparing the efficacy of mandibular implant-retained overdentures and conventional dentures among middle-aged edentulous patients: satisfaction and functional assessment. *International Journal of Prosthodontics*, 16 (2), 117–122.

Awad, M.A., Lund, L.P., Shapiro, S.H. *et al.* (2003b) Oral health status and treatment satisfaction with mandibular implant overdentures and conventional dentures: a randomised trial in a senior population. *International Journal of Prosthodontics*, 6 (4), 390–396.

DeLuca, S., Habsha, E. & Zarb, G. (2006) The effect of smoking of osseointegrated dental implants. Part I: Implant survival. *International Journal of Prosthodontics*, 19 (5), 491–498.

Feine, J.S., Carlsson, G.E., Awad, M.A. *et al.* (2002) The McGill consensus statement on overdentures. Mandibular two-implant overdentures as first choice standard of care for edentulous patients. *International Journal of Oral & Maxillofacial Implants*, 17 (4), 601–602.

Fitzpatrick, B. (2006) Standard of care for the edentulous mandible: a systematic review. *Journal of Prosthetic Dentistry*, 95 (1), 71–78.

Kapur, K.K., Garrett, N.R., Hamada, M.O. *et al.* (1999) Randomized clinical trial comparing the efficacy of mandibular implant supported overdentures and conventional dentures in diabetic patients. Part III: comparisons of patient satisfaction. *Journal of Prosthetic Dentistry*, 82 (4), 416–427.

Case 12.2 Mr Atilla G

Michael Lewis

Patient: Mr Atilla G (date of birth 01/01/1959)

Presenting complaints

Date	16/06/2008
Chief complaint	'My bottom denture is not sitting properly'
Subsidiary complaints	'I have trouble eating because it doesn't sit properly'
History of complaints	Patient has had problems eating since the denture was issued 2 years ago
Patient's expectations	'I want my bottom dentures stable. I would like to try implants'

History
Medical history

Medical Practitioner	Dr E	
Respiratory	Nil	
Cardiovascular	Nil	
	Endocarditis	Nil
Gastrointestinal	Nil	
Neurological	Patient was dropped on head as a toddler and has been partially deaf in the left ear and completely deaf in the right ear since	
Endocrine	Nil	
Musculoskeletal	Patient had an accident in 1997 working as an industrial lifter. He has damaged lumbar vertebrae but has no pain at present	
Genitourinary	Nil	
Haematological	Nil	
	Bleeding	Nil
	Immune	Nil
Other	Allergies	NKA
	Smoking	0–5 cigarettes/day
	Infectious diseases	Nil
	Pregnancy	N/A
	Hospitalisation	2006 – cortisone injection in lumbar spine
	Medications	Nil

Social history

Marital status	Married		
Children	3 children (2 at home)		
Occupation	Medically retired since 1997. Previously an industrial lifter		
Smoking	Type	Tobacco	
	Frequency	0–5 cigarettes/day	
	Period	22 years	
Recreational drugs	Nil		
Diet	√	Soft drinks	2 cups/day
		Sports drinks	Nil
	√	Lemons	Patient sucks lemons
		Acidic foods	Nil
	√	Sweet foods	Patient occasionally has sweet foods
	√	Water	4–5 cups/day
	√	Tea	4 cups/day (no sugar)
	√	Coffee	2 cups/day (no sugar)
		Alcohol	Nil
	√	Hard/brittle foods	Sometimes has nuts
		Ice crunching	Nil
Habits/hobbies		Musical instrument	Nil
		Exercise	Nil
		Oral habits	Nil

Dental history

	Additional information		
Date of last examination	21/05/2008		
Oral hygiene	√	Brushing	Patient cleans denture once a day
		Flossing	N/A
	√	Mouthwash	Daily Listerine
		Toothpaste	N/A
Treatment		Restorations	N/A
		Endodontics	N/A
		Periodontics	N/A
		Orthodontics	N/A
	√	RDP	Complete maxillary RDP; complete implant-retained overdenture
		FDP	N/A
		TMD	N/A
	√	OMFS	2 implants in the mandibular second incisor region

Extraoral examination (Figures 12.2.1 & 12.2.2)
Aesthetics

Facial symmetry	Symmetrical	Nil
Profile	Straight	Nil
Nasolabial angle	90°	Nil
Facial folds	Nil	Nil
Midlines	Face/maxillary centrals	Maxillary dental midline 2 mm to right of facial midline
	Maxillary central alignment	
	Maxillary/mandibular centrals	Mandibular dental midline 1 mm to the left of maxillary dental midline
Lip posture	Symmetry	Symmetrical
	Upper lip	Thick
	Lower lip	Thick
	Competence	Yes
	Tooth display	Nil tooth display at rest
Occlusal plane	Parallel to ala tragus line	Yes
	Parallel to interpupillary line	No
	Over-eruption	Nil
Vertical	FWS	3.5 mm
	OVD assessment	Optimal
Smile assessment	Symmetry	Yes
	Lip line	Low
	Gingival display	Minimal
	Tooth display	90% maxillary incisal teeth, 50% mandibular incisal teeth
	Buccal corridor	Wide

Phonetics

	Normal	Abnormal
Labial (m)	√	
Labiodental (f/v)		√
Linguodontal (th)	√	
Interdental (s)		√
Linguopalatal (k/ng)		√

Temporomandibular assessment

TMJ		Further information
Click	Nil	
Crepitus	Nil	
Tenderness	Nil	

Muscle tenderness	Right	Left
Temporalis	Nil	Nil
Masseter	Nil	Nil
Posterior mandible	Nil	Nil
Anterior mandible	Nil	Nil
Glands	Nil	
Nodes	Nil	

Jaw movement	Measurement (corrected mm)	Reference points
Maximal opening	64	11–41 incisal edges
Right laterotrusion	12	Denture midlines
Left laterotrusion	13	Denture midlines
Midline deviation	1 mm to left	Denture midlines
Maximal protrusion	10	11–41 incisal edges
Opening pathway	Left corrected 'S' deviation	Frontal view
Overjet	2	11–41 incisal edges
Overbite	2	11–41 incisal edges
Further investigation required		No

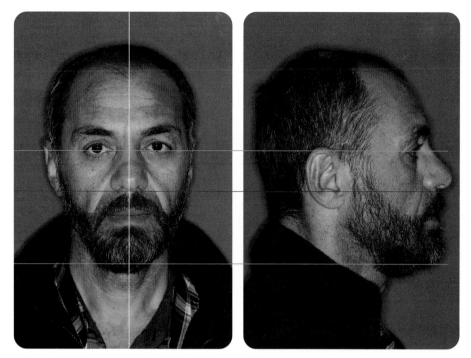

Figure 12.2.1 Extraoral examination. Note facial proportions.

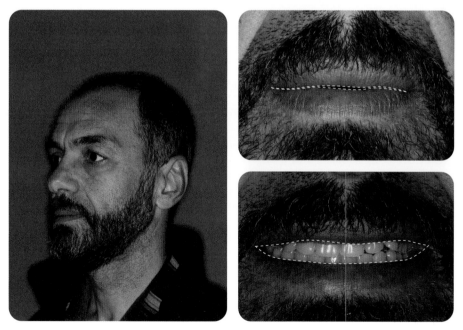

Figure 12.2.2 Extraoral examination – smile assessment. Note low smile line.

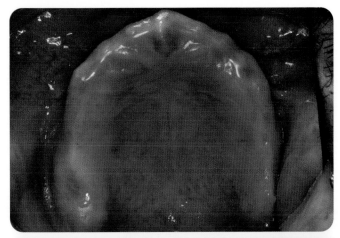

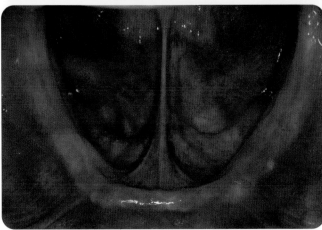

Figure 12.2.3 Intraoral examination. Note edentulous ridge form and contour.

Intraoral examination (Figure 12.2.3)
Soft tissues

Tissue	Healthy	Abnormal	Additional information
Lips	√		Nil
Labial vestibule	√		Nil
Cheeks	√		Nil
Palate	√		Nil
Oropharynx	√		Nil
Tongue	√		Nil
Floor	√		Nil
Frenal attachments	√		Nil

Ridges	Maxilla	Mandible
Arch shape	Square	Square
Resorption	Mild	Mild
Palatal vault	Shallow	
Tori	Nil	Nil
Frenal attachments	Midline and buccal	Buccal
Mucosa	Firm	Firm
Pathology	Nil	Mild keratinisation of mandibular ridge

Oral cleanliness

	Yes	No	
Plaque		√	
Calculus		√	
Food impaction	√		Patient reports food impaction under mandibular denture
Stains	√		Extrinsic stains on palatal of incisal teeth on complete dentures
Halitosis	√		

Saliva

Water intake	4 cups water/day
Quality	Good. Hydration from rest within 30 s of chewing. Resting saliva watery/clear and >5.0 ml stimulated saliva over a 5-minute period
Quantity	Good. Resting and stimulated salivary pH 6.8–7.8, and 10–12 points of buffering on the GC salivary test
Pathology	Nil
Medications affecting	Nil

Further investigation required   No

Occlusion

Skeletal classification	Class III				
Dental occlusion	Class I				
Angle right	Molar	Class I	Canine	Class I	
Angle left	Molar	Class I	Canine	Class I	
Anterior overbite	2 mm				
Anterior overjet	2 mm				
Cross-bites	Nil				
Open-bites	Teeth 22 and 23				
Curve of Spee	Undulating occlusal plane				
Curve of Wilson	Flat				
RP to IP slide	0 mm				
FWS	Close/M/swallow test		3.5 mm		

Tooth guidance

Right laterotrusion

Left laterotrusion

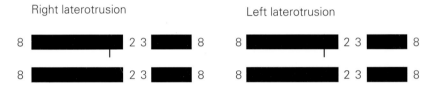

Protrusion

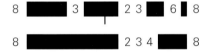

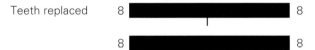

Previous dentures (Figure 12.2.4)

Teeth replaced

	Maxilla	Mandible
Age/number	10 months, set 1	10 months, set 1
Type	Acrylic base and teeth	Acrylic base and teeth
Kennedy classification	Complete	Complete
Appearance	Unaesthetic	Unaesthetic
LFH	Adequate	Adequate
Stability	Poor	Poor
Support	Poor	Fair
Retention	Poor	Poor
Hygiene	Fair. Patient sleeps with dentures every second night	Fair. Patient sleeps with dentures every second night
Patient opinion	Good	Poor. Patient feels mandibular denture is unretentive

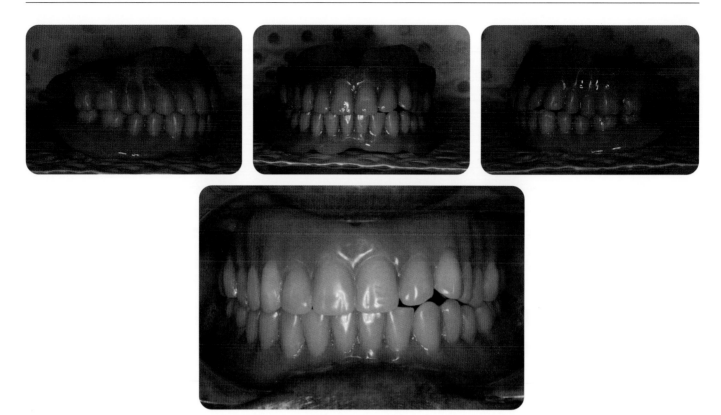

Figure 12.2.4 Presenting dentures.

Radiographs (Figure 12.2.5)
Orthopantomogram (22/04/2008)

Features	Radiographic data
TMJ	Not visible on OPG
Bone loss	Mild vertical maxillary and mandibular alveolar bone loss
Sinuses	Bilateral pneumatisation of maxillary sinus visible. Sinus radiopaque
Mandibular foramen and canal	Clear and patent. Distant from the mandibular alveolar crest
Mental foramen	Clearly visible. Distant from the alveolar crest
Retained roots	Nil
Pathology	Nil

Other radiographs

	Date	Radiographic data
OPG	06/03/2007	When teeth were present: teeth 38, 37, 36, 35, 34, 44, 45, 46, 47 showed moderate to severe horizontal bone loss, with severe bone loss localised to teeth 37, 36, 46
OPG	31/05/2006	When teeth were present teeth 14, 13, 12, 11, 23, 24, 27, 38, 37, 36, 35, 34, 44, 45, 46, 47 showed generalised moderate to severe horizontal bone loss, with severe bone loss localised to teeth 14, 13, 12, 11, 23, 24, 36, 46

Study casts

Articulation	Jaw position	RCP
	Face bow	Yes
Diagnostic wax-up	OVD change	0 mm
	Occlusal adjustment	N/A
	Crown lengthening	N/A

Problem list

Problem list	Details
Medical condition	Patient smokes 0–5 cigarettes/day
Aesthetics	Non-coincidence of facial and maxillary complete denture dental midline Maxillary and mandibular midlines on complete dentures are non-coincident Low smile line with wide buccal corridors
Speech	Patient is partially deaf and has an associated speech impairment Distortion of labiodental/interdental/linguopalatal sounds
TMD	Nil
Soft tissue	Nil
Oral hygiene	Inadequate denture hygiene on initial presentation
Saliva	Moderate water intake/high caffeine intake Adequate salivary quality and quantity
Periodontal	N/A
Edentulism	Completely edentulous in the maxilla and mandible Mild maxillary and mandibular residual ridge resorption
Occlusion	Class I dental occlusion on dentures Class II skeletal occlusion Optimal OVD
Tooth surface loss	N/A
Restorative	N/A
Prosthetic	Poor stability and retention of existing complete dentures
Endodontic	N/A

Treatment options (Figure 12.2.6)
Maxilla

Treatment option 1 (short treatment time: 1 month)
- Systemic and hygiene phase (see definitive treatment plan for details).
- Remake maxillary complete denture.

Treatment option 2 (medium to long treatment time: 6–9 months)
- Systemic and hygiene phase (see definitive treatment plan for details).
- Place four implants in the maxilla.
- Maxillary complete implant-retained overdenture.

Treatment option 3 (medium to long treatment time: 6–9 months)
- Systemic and hygiene phase (see definitive treatment plan for details).
- Place six implants in the maxilla.
- Maxillary complete FDP on six implants.

Mandible

Treatment option 1 (short treatment time: 1 month)
- Systemic and hygiene phase (see definitive treatment plan for details).
- Remake mandibular complete denture.

Treatment option 2 (medium treatment time: 3–4 months)
- Systemic and hygiene phase (see definitive treatment plan for details).
- Place two implants in the mandible.
- Mandibular complete implant-retained overdenture.

Treatment option 3 (medium to long treatment time: 6–9 months)
- Systemic and hygiene Phase (see definitive treatment plan for details).
- Place four implants in the mandible.
- Mandibular complete FDP on four implants.

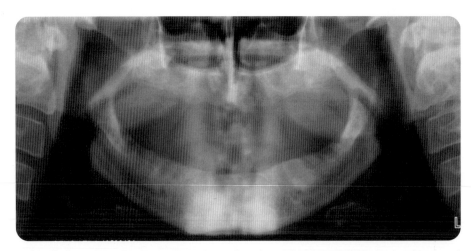

Figure 12.2.5 Radiographs. Orthopantomogram confirmed excellent bone in the mandible for implants and adequate bone in the maxilla.

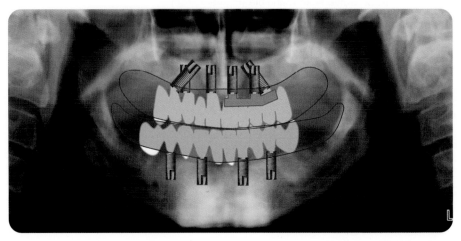

Figure 12.2.6 Treatment options.

Treatment plan

- Maxilla: treatment option 1.
- Mandible: treatment option 2.

Treatment phase	Detail	Time between phases
Systemic phase	Stop smoking counselling Dietary advice	Concurrent
Hygiene phase	Oral and denture hygiene instruction	Concurrent
Pre-prosthetic pretreatment: phase I	Provisional complete dentures to correct aesthetics and function Assess outcomes	
Pre-prosthetic pretreatment: phase II	NobelGuide scan of mandible Implants in 32 and 42 sites	
Prosthetic phase	Implant retained overdenture in mandible	3 months post-insertion
Maintenance	Review 6/12	

					Complete maxillary denture											
18	17	16	15	14	13	12	11	21	22	23	24	25	26	27	28	
48	47	46	45	44	43	42	41	31	32	33	34	35	36	37	38	
					Implant-retained mandibular overdenture											
						I			I							

Treatment sequence

Appointment no.	Procedure	Time (minutes)
1	Primary impressions of the edentulous maxilla and mandible	90
2	Secondary impressions of the edentulous maxilla and mandible Record post dam	90
3	Try-in processed clear bases Take MMR/face bow	90
4	Wax try-in F/F	60
5	Primary issue diagnostic F/F (Figure 12.2.7)	60
6	Secondary issue F/F	60
7	NobelGuide scan mandible (Figure 12.2.8)	60
8	Joint consult with implant surgeon	30
9	Implant surgery Viscogel reline of mandibular complete denture (Figure 12.2.9)	180
10	Pick up impression of mandibular implant positions	90
11	Try-in cast CoCr framework on clear processed base Record MM	90
12	Wax try-in -/F	90
13	Primary issue -/F	90
14	Secondary issue -/F Mill in occlusion on articulator (Figures 12.2 10 & 12.2.11)	120

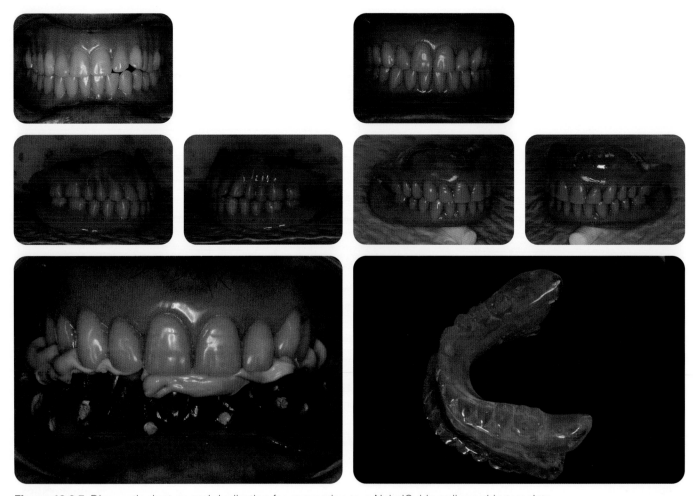

Figure 12.2.7 Diagnostic denture and duplication for conversion to a NobelGuide radiographic template.

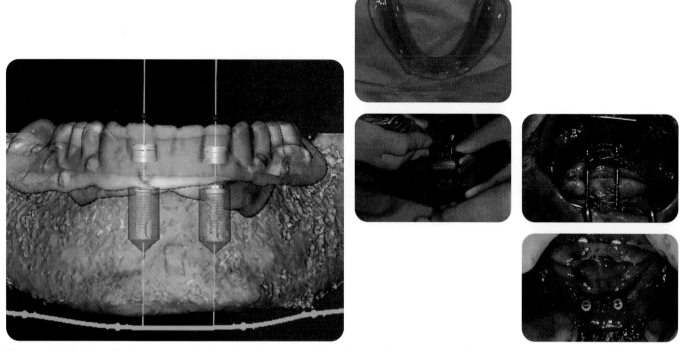

Figure 12.2.8 NobelGuide planning for implant locations with radiographic template and implant surgery to be guided by a surgical guide developed from the radiographic guide.

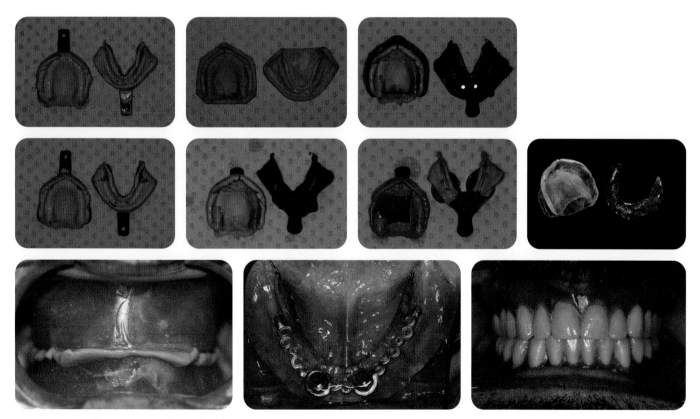

Figure 12.2.9 Construction of the definitive prosthesis.

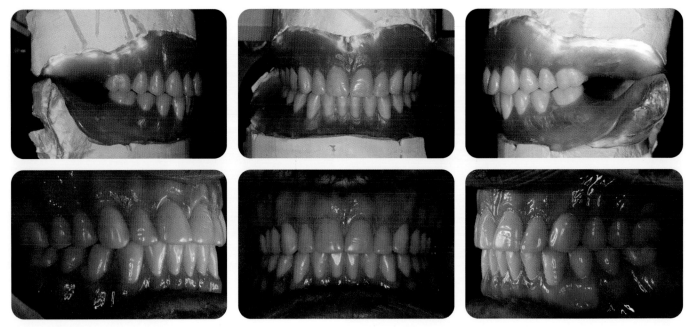

Figure 12.2.10 Definitive prosthesis and intraoral views of completed implant overdenture.

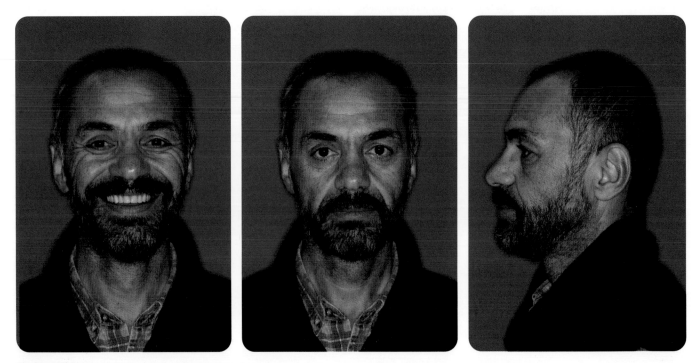

Figure 12.2.11 Extraoral view of completed treatment.

Treatment discussion

Mr G initially presented with the chief complaint that he was having trouble eating with his dentures and felt his mandibular complete denture 'didn't fit properly' and was unstable. Mr G was rendered edentulous due to advanced chronic periodontal disease and was issued an immediate F/F 6 months prior to presentation. He is a pensioner with limited funds and says he would be satisfied if we could stop his bottom denture from moving. Mr G is retired and is available to attend appointments when required. He is a casual smoker (0–5 cigarettes/day) and is not taking any medications.

Extraoral examination revealed a mild class III skeletal profile and symmetrical face. Intraoral examination showed mild residual ridge resorption in the maxilla and mandible. Mr G has adequate salivary quality and quantity. His presenting set of immediate complete dentures exhibit poor retention, aesthetics and stability. He cleans his dentures once a day and sleeps with his dentures every second night.

In order to address Mr G's concerns, it is important to consider the resorption pattern that follows full clearance. A 25-year longitudinal case series study (Tallgren 1972) on alveolar ridge resorption after full clearance and immediate denture issue, reported that the greatest amount of ridge resorption occurred within the first 9–12 months. The study found continual ridge resorption and remodelling for the remaining observation period, indicating that dentures require continual maintenance to the fitting surface to ensure optimal fit. In recognition of the drastic changes that occur in the initial 9–12 months post-issue, problems with stability and retention of tissue-borne prostheses are expected. At 12 months after the full clearance and after a 3-month trial of definitive complete dentures, Mr G advised that he still felt that his lower denture moves when eating.

Definitive rehabilitation of edentulism includes tissue-borne complete dentures, implant- and tissue-supported complete dentures and implant-borne FDPs.

A long-term, prospective case series (Jemt & Johansson 2006) followed 76 maxillary complete implant-borne FDPs over a 15-year period. The cumulative survival rate for implants and prostheses was 90.9% and 90.6%, respectively. A recent randomised control trial (Fischer et al. 2008) compared early (9–18 days) and conventional (2–3 months) loading of maxillary complete implant-borne FDPs and reported similar results between groups over 5 years. A randomised, cross-over trial (Heydecke et al. 2003) compared FDPs and implant-retained overdentures in the maxilla. At the end of the trial, 9/16 patients rated their general satisfaction, ability to speak and cleansability higher with the RDPs; however, it appears that there was strong individual preference. Mr G was satisfied with a complete denture in the maxilla.

Treatment options in the mandible include a remake of the existing complete mandibular denture, an implant-retained mandibular overdenture or an implant-borne FDP. A prospective randomised controlled trial (Awad et al. 2003) comparing patient-related outcomes with conventional and mandibular implant-retained overdentures indicated increased patient satisfaction and function with implant-retained overdentures. A 10-year prospective randomised controlled trial (Raghoebar et al. 2003) compared the outcomes of a conventional mandibular denture remake with vestibuloplasty and denture remake and implant-retained overdentures in a population who were dissatisfied with their mandibular complete dentures. Over a 10-year period, the implant-overdenture group was the most satisfied, with no significant differences between the conventional and vestibuloplasty groups. A prospective randomised controlled trial (Morais et al. 2003) comparing nutritional status of patients with conventional and mandibular implant-retained overdentures indicated improved nutritional status and general health with implant-retained overdentures. Ekelund et al. (2003) conducted a 20-year prospective case series study on the longevity of mandibular complete FDPs on implants and reported 97.5% success. Lindquist et al. (1996) reported a case series of 47 complete mandibular implant-borne FDPs and found a cumulative survival rate of 100% for all prosthesis.

The McGill Consensus (Feine et al. 2002) indicated that an implant-retained overdenture is the contemporary first choice in treatment of the mandibular arch. This statement does not take into account outcomes of FDPs on implants. A systematic review (Fitzpatrick 2006) indicated that there is no one 'standard' treatment for the edentulous mandible and individual patient preference exists. Mr G has a positive attitude towards RDPs and limited funds. A conventional denture remake was conducted at 9 months after extractions and on review 3 years later he was satisfied with his dentures; however, he felt that the mandibular complete denture was still unstable. As a result, an implant-retained overdenture was selected for the mandible.

Review at 1 year (Figure 12.2.12)

1. Oral health status
   - Oral hygiene. *Plaque control satisfactory, but some plaque-induced inflammation around implant abutments.*
   - Soft tissue health. *General soft tissues of ridge, palate and cheek firm and healthy.*
   - Home-care programme. *Brushes twice daily and uses Chlorhexidine mouth rinse, but needs reinforcement.*
   - Periodontal status. *Probing depth no change at implant at 43, but increased around implant at 33 where there is mobility of abutment and implant.*
2. Medical status. *No change in general health and no medications.*
3. Occlusion. *Bilateral contacts at ICP and lateral and protrusive excursive contacts provide stability for function. Patient requested heavier incisal contact to assist chewing of hard foods.*
4. Radiographs. *OPG radiograph indicates healthy bone status in general but appearance of bone loss at implant 33 position was confirmed with the periapical radiograph.*
5. Oral health related quality of life. *Comfort has been satisfactory and chewing of most foods apart from hard foods has been effective. The incisal contact with chewing of harder foods needs refinement of the quality of anterior tooth contact and revision of tooth arrangement. The overall aesthetic enhancement was an important contribution to self-confidence and social interaction.*
6. Additional comments about the treatment. *The patient confirmed that the discomfort associated with the placement of the two implants was minor and presented no problem; he would certainly undertake the process again if needed.*

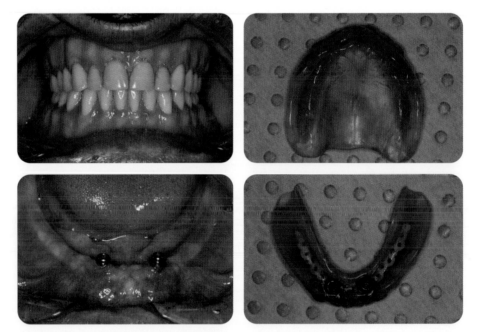

Figure 12.2.12 Review at 1 year. Patient was aware of movement with the mandibular implant overdenture and some discomfort with the 33 implant. Soft tissues were healthy but there was inflammation in peri-implant tissues with 33. Tissue surfaces of the prostheses indicates good denture hygiene.

References

Awad, M.A., Lund, J.P., Dufresne, E. *et al.* (2003) Comparing the efficacy of mandibular implant-retained overdentures and conventional dentures among middle-aged edentulous patients: satisfaction and functional assessment. *International Journal of Prosthodontics*, 16 (2), 117–122.

Ekelund, J.A., Lindquist, L.W., Carlsson, G.E. *et al.* (2003) Implant treatment in the edentulous mandible: a prospective study on Branemark system implants over more than 20 years. *International Journal of Prosthodontics*, 16 (6), 602–608.

Feine, J.S., Carlsson, G.E., Awad, M.A. *et al.* (2002) The McGill consensus statement on overdentures. Mandibular two-implant overdentures as first choice standard of care for edentulous patients. *International Journal of Oral & Maxillofacial Implants*, 17 (4), 601–602.

Fischer, K., Stenberg, T., Hedin, M. *et al.* (2008) Five-year results from a randomized, controlled trial on early and delayed loading of implants supporting full-arch prosthesis in the edentulous maxilla. *Clinical Oral Implants Research*, 19 (5), 433–441.

Fitzpatrick, B. (2006) Standard of care for the edentulous mandible: a systematic review. *Journal of Prosthetic Dentistry*, 95 (1), 71–78.

Heydecke, G., Boudrias, P., Awad, M.A. *et al* (2003) Within-subject comparisons of maxillary fixed and removable implant prostheses: patient satisfaction and choice of prosthesis. *Clinical Oral Implants Research*, 14 (1), 125–130.

Jemt, T. & Johansson, J. (2006) Implant treatment in the edentulous maxillae: a 15-year follow-up study on 76 consecutive patients provided with fixed prostheses. *Clinical Implant Dentistry & Related Research*, 8 (2), 61–69.

Lindquist, L.W., Carlsson, G.E. & Jemt, T. (1996) A prospective 15 year follow-up study of mandibular fixed prostheses supported by osseointegrated implants. Clinical results and marginal bone loss. *Clinical Oral Implants Research*, 7 (4), 329–336.

Morais, J.A., Heydecke, G., Pawliuk, J. *et al.* (2003) The effects of mandibular two-implant overdentures on nutrition in elderly edentulous individuals. *Journal of Dental Research*, 82 (1), 53–58.

Raghoebar, G.M., Meijer, H.J., van't Hof, M. *et al.* (2003) A randomized prospective clinical trial on the effectiveness of three treatment modalities for patients with lower denture problems. A 10 year follow-up study on patient satisfaction. *International Journal of Oral & Maxillofacial Surgery*, 32 (5), 498–503.

Tallgren, A. (1972). The continuing reduction of the residual alveolar ridges in complete denture wearers: a mixed-longitudinal study covering 25 years. *Journal of Prosthetic Dentistry*, 27(2), 120–132.

13

Developmental Complications: Cleft Lip and Palate

Introduction by Christine Wallace

Management of cleft lip and palate patients presents many challenges to the postgraduate student/clinician, not only from an anatomical perspective but also from the functional and aesthetic perspective of the patient. In the past, large bulky removable prostheses were often necessary, not only to replace missing teeth but also to correct the horizontal and/or vertical growth discrepancies or to provide an extension to separate the oronasal–pharyngeal space.

It is not unusual still to see in the older patient population people with only closure of the lip but not the alveolus, hard or soft palate. Conversely, other patients have had corrective surgeries performed at the appropriate time but still require grafting of the anterior maxilla to provide correct width and vertical height for prosthetic rehabilitation. Optimum patient management and coordination are the keys to successful patient outcomes.

Palatal development

Palatogenesis begins in the fifth week *in utero* and is complete by the twelfth week. The palate develops from two primordial structures: the primary and secondary palates. The primary palate (median palatine/nasal process) forms the premaxilla, which includes the incisor teeth and that portion of the hard palate anterior to the incisal foramen.

The secondary palate gives rise to the hard and soft palates, which develop from two horizontal mesodermal projections: the lateral palatine and nasal processes. The palatine shelves fuse in the midline to form the primary palate and the nasal septum. The fusion begins with the nasal septum anteriorly (ninth week) and is completed by the twelfth week posteriorly (the uvula region). The posterior portions of the palantine shelves do not become ossified and form the soft palate and uvula. The palatine raphe permanently indicates the line of fusion of the lateral palatine process. The incisal foramen remains the embryological border between the primary and secondary palate (Kernahan & Stark 1958).

Classification of clefts

Different classification systems have been proposed; however, a simple classification is preferred, based on embryology, which divides cleft lip and palate patients into three categories:

1. cleft lip and alveolus (primary palate);
2. cleft of the hard and soft palate (secondary palate);
3. a combination of primary and secondary palates (combination of 1 and 2).

Anterior clefts are caused by defective development of the primary palate due to a mesenchymal deficiency, whereas posterior clefts result from defective development of the secondary palate due to growth disturbances that interfere with fusion of the palatine shelves. Anterior clefts include cleft lip with or without a cleft of the alveolus. Posterior clefts involve the soft and/or hard palate up to the incisive foramen.

Cleft patients may also present with other anomalies. Syndromic forms of clefts are those with a medically or surgically relevant abnormality of an organ system beyond the anatomical cleft region and include developmental delay.

Incidence

The incidence of clefting varies in relation to the population studied. The generally accepted incident rate is that 1 in every 700 infants born has some form of clefting (CleftPALS NSW 2010). Left-sided unilateral clefts (70%) are more common than bilateral clefts of the lip and palate; right-sided clefts, as in this case presentation, are the least common (Berkowitz 1994, 2005).

Clefts of the upper lip, with or without cleft palate, occur in approximately 1 in 1000 births, with varying frequency among ethnic groups (Thompson & Thompson 1980, Vanderas 1987, Nussbaum *et al*. 2007). Male clefts are twice as frequent as female clefts. Clefts of the primary palate may be unilateral or bilateral; it is most commonly found on the left in patients with unilateral cleft lip.

Cleft palate, with or without cleft lip, occurs in approximately 1 in 2500 births. Isolated cleft palate is more common in females (Burdi & Silvey 1969). The embryological basis of cleft palate is failure of the mesenchymal masses of the lateral palatine processes to meet and fuse with each other, the nasal septum and/or the posterior margins of the primary palate. This could result in a cleft of the primary palate, cleft of the primary and secondary palates, or cleft of the secondary palates only. Clefts of the secondary palate may involve both the hard or soft palates or may be limited to the soft palate only.

Aetiology

Clefts can be caused by a number of factors that affect the pregnant mother in the first trimester. These include infections and toxicity, poor diet, hormonal imbalances and genetic factors. Most clefts are caused by multiple genetic and non-genetic factors. Evaluation of twins indicates that genetic factors play a greater role in cleft lip, with or without cleft palate, compared with cleft palate only. Complete clefts involving the lip, alveolus and palate are usually transmitted through a male sex-linked gene (Thompson & Thompson 1980).

Rehabilitation/management

Multidisciplinary management of cleft palate patients provides the best comprehensive care. However, the optimal management of the cleft palate patient from birth to completion of treatment continues to present formidable challenges for each team member. Additionally, an inter-disciplinary review by Bardach and Morris (1990) of the global multidisciplinary team approach in the management of the cleft lip and palate illustrates the diversity of treatment strategies and techniques available throughout the world for the management of these cases.

Treatment challenges possibly encountered in the older patient include:

- the reduced size of the maxilla;
- excessive interarch space;
- lack of bony palate;
- poor alveolar ridge development;
- shallow palatal vault;
- scarring from lip closure;
- increased caries;
- over-eruption of teeth;
- medication-induced xerostomia;
- long-term speech-related issues.

References

Bardach, J. & Morris, H.L. (1990) *Multidisciplinary Management of Cleft Lip and Palate*. Saunders, Philadelphia.

Berkowitz, S. (1994) *The Cleft Palate Story*. Quintessence, Chicago.

Berkowitz, S. (2005) *Cleft Lip and Palate*. Springer, New York.

Burdi, A.R. & Silvey, R.G. (1969) Sexual differences in closure of the human palatal shelves. *Cleft Palate Journal*, 6, 1–7.

CleftPALS NSW: The Cleft Palate and Lip Society of New South Wales (2010) *About CleftPALS* (http://www.cleftpalsnsw.org.au/cleft.html, accessed 5 November 2010)

Kernahan, D.A. & Stark, R.B. (1958). A new classification for cleft lip and palate. *Plastic & Reconstructive Surgery & the Transplantation Bulletin*, 22 (5), 435–441.

Nussbaum, R.L., McInnes, R.R. & Willard, H.F. (2007) *Thompson & Thompson Genetics in Medicine*, 7th edn. Saunders/Elsevier, Philadelphia.

Thompson, J.S. & Thompson, M.W. (1980) *Genetics in Medicine*, 3rd edn. Saunders, Philadelphia.

Vanderas, A.P. (1987) Incidence of cleft lip, cleft palate and cleft lip and palate among races: a review. *Cleft Palate Journal*, 24 (3), 216–225.

Case 13.1 Mr Louis S

Agnes Lai

Patient: Mr Louis S (date of birth 29/03/1937)

Presenting complaints

Date	31/08/2007
Chief complaint	Pain on eating. Only eating porridge and mash
	Progressive loss of teeth
	Wish to be able to eat properly and have improved appearance
Subsidiary complaints	Traumatic deep bite
	Fractured fillings
	Dry mouth – more since wearing P/-
History of complaints	Debilitated mouth
	Multiple root remnants from recurrent dental caries
	High caries risk
	Multiple restorations: heavily restored and failing periodontal conditions
	Localised periodontitis associated with 13, 22, 23, 42-32 bridge
	RDP P/- CoCr – temporary for aesthetic only (January 2008)
Patient's expectations	Eat better
	Look normal
	Comfortable mouth without pain

History
Medical history

Medical Practitioner		
Congenital	Cleft lip and palate – closed surgically when young	
Cardiovascular	Hypertension	
	Endocarditis	Nil
Gastrointestinal	Nil	
Respiratory	Nil	
Neurological	Nil	
Endocrine	Nil	
Musculoskeletal	Nil	
Genitourinary	Nil	
Haematological	Nil	
	Bleeding	Nil
	Immune	Nil
Other	Allergies	Nil
	Smoking	Nil
	Infectious diseases	Nil
	Pregnancy	N/A
	Hospitalisation	Nil
	Medications	Coversyl 5 mg

Social history

Marital status	Married		
Children	1 daughter (married)		
Occupation	Retired, looking after family Wife recently diagnosed with breast cancer Son-in-law recently diagnosed with terminal gastrointestinal cancer		
Smoking	Nil		
Recreational drugs	Nil		
Diet	3 meals a day + tea		
		Soft drinks	Nil
		Sports drinks	Nil
		Lemons	Nil
		Acidic foods	Nil
		Sweet foods	Biscuit with tea
		Water	5 glasses
		Tea	1 cup
		Coffee	1 cup/day (milk, no sugar)
		Alcohol	Nil
		Hard/brittle foods	Nil
		Ice crunching	Nil
Habits/hobbies		Musical instrument	Nil
		Exercise	Nil
		Oral habits	Nil

Dental history

			Additional information
Date of last examination			
Oral hygiene	√	Brushing	Twice daily
		Flossing	Nil
		Mouthwash	Nil
	√	Toothpaste	Colgate
Treatment	√	Restorations	
		Endodontics	Nil
	√	Periodontics	
		Orthodontics	Nil
	√	RDP	
	√	FDP	
		TMD	Nil
	√	OMFS	

Extraoral examination (Figure 13.1.1)
Aesthetics

Facial form	Oval, dolicofacial	
Facial symmetry	Nose slightly to the left and Z-plasty and chin to the right	
Profile	Straight	
Nasolabial angle	90°	
Facial folds	Cheeks are sunken	
Midlines	Face/maxillary centrals	Face midline to the right of maxillary centrals
	Maxillary central alignment	Missing
	Mandibular centrals	Coincident with chin midline
Lip posture	Symmetry	Asymmetry – pull to the right by Z-plasty
	Upper lip	Thick in the middle and tapers to thin laterally
	Lower lip	Thin
	Competence	Good
	Tooth display	Nil at rest
Occlusal plane	Parallel to ala tragus line	Does not exist
	Parallel to interpupillary line	Cant to the right
	Over-eruption	Overeruption of 22 and 23, 43 and 44
Vertical	FWS	5 mm
	OVD assessment	P/- VD = 74 mm, OVD = 69 mm
Smile assessment	Symmetry	Lower lip, upper lip asymmetrical
	Lip line	High
	Gingival display	Undulated
	Tooth display	100% upper and lower anterior
	Buccal corridor	Less wide

Phonetics

All sounds have nasal resonance due to partial repair with cleft of soft palate.
Mr S is not concerned about this.

Temporomandibular assessment

TMJ	No present symptoms or history of joint sounds or tenderness
Muscle tenderness	No tenderness to palpation bilaterally of temporalis and masseter muscles, posterior and anterior mandible
Glands and nodes	NAD

Jaw movement	Measurement (corrected mm)	Reference points
Maximal opening	60	Corrected, ref 22
Right laterotrusion	15	Estimate
Left laterotrusion	15	Estimate
Midline deviation	N/A	
Maximal protrusion	10	
Opening pathway	Straight	
Overjet	180% 10 mm with P/-	
Overbite	10	

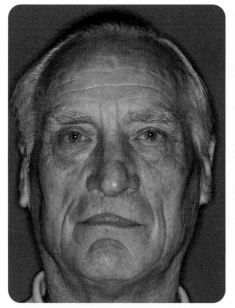
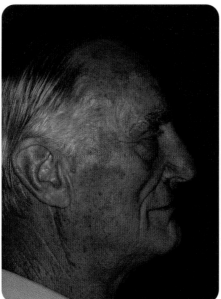
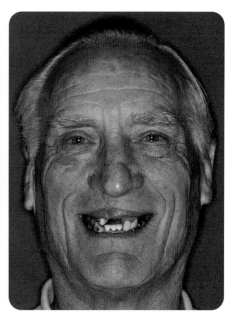
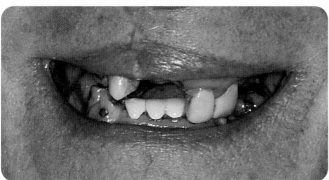

Figure 13.1.1 Extraoral examination. Full face and profile views and smile without existing maxillary prosthesis.

Intraoral examination (Figure 13.1.2)
Soft tissues

Tissue	Healthy	Abnormal	Additional information
Lips		√	Z-plasty
Labial vestibule		√	Post-surgical mucosal healing Soft swelling in anterior maxillary labial vestibule
Cheeks	√		Unsupported by missing teeth
Palate		√	Partial cleft closure – opening of labial sulcus at site 13 Anterior palate, soft palate
Oropharynx		√	Asymmetrical uvula and pharyngeal muscles
Tongue	√		
Floor	√		
Frenal attachments	√		

Ridges	Maxilla	Mandible
Arch shape	U-shape	U-shape
Resorption	Moderate	Moderate
Palatal vault	Flat, oro–antral fistula	
Tori	Nil	Nil
Frenal attachments	High	Medium
Mucosa	Thick	Thick
Pathology	Cleft	

Oral cleanliness

Condition	Yes	No			
Plaque	√		Generalised	Severe	Supragingival
Calculus	√		Generalised	Mild	Supragingival and subgingival
Food impaction	√		Under denture and around abutments		
Stains	√		Around margins of restorations		
Halitosis		√			

Saliva

Water intake	Low
Quality	Good
Quantity	Good
Pathology	Nil
Medications affecting	Coversyl
Further investigation required	No

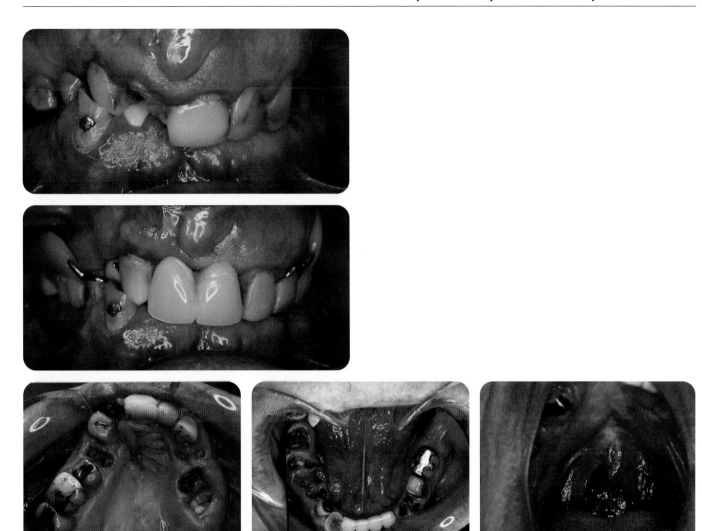

Figure 13.1.2 Intraoral examination. Upper images are anterior views when the patient initially presented with a broken down dentition showing the deep bite with and without the existing maxillary prosthesis. The lower images show occlusal views of the maxilla (note the surgical repair of the cleft defect) and mandible and indicate the degree of tooth breakdown and the extent of oral rehabilitation required. The lower right image shows the oropharynx where uvula asymmetry illustrates the velopharyngeal deficit.

Occlusion

Skeletal classification	Class III			
Dental occlusion	Class II division I			
Angle right	Molar class	N/A	Canine	Class II
Angle left	Molar class	N/A	Canine	Class II
Anterior overbite	180%		10 mm	
Anterior overjet	10 mm			
Cross-bites	15			
Open-bites				
Curve of Spee	RHS -		LHS -	
Curve of Wilson				
RP to IP slide	0 mm			
TWS	Close/M/swallow test		5 mm	

Tooth guidance

Right laterotrusion

```
  5  3    |2 3
 4 3 2 1 1|2 3  5 6
```

Left laterotrusion

```
   5  3    |2 3
 4 3 2 1  1 2 3 |5 6
```

Protrusion

```
  5  3    |2 3
 4 3 2 1 1|2 3   5 6
```

Tooth surface loss

General

```
  5  3 2   |2 3
 4 3 2 1 1|2 3   5 6
```

Attrition

```
  5  3 2   |2 3
 4 3 2 1 1|2 3  5 6
```

Erosion

```
   5  3 2   |2 3
 4 3 2 1  1 2 3 |5 6
```

Abrasion

```
  5  3 2   |2 3
 4 3 2 1 1|2 3  5 6
```

Bruxofacets

```
   5  3 2   |2 3
 4 3 2 1  1 2 3 |5 6
```

Periodontium

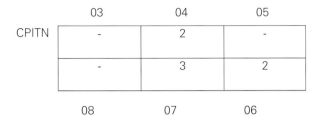

	03	04	05
CPITN	-	2	-
	-	3	2
	08	07	06

Diagnosis	Chronic generalised gingivitis, localised periodontitis 31 and 41		
Gingiva	Biotype	Thick	
	Colour	Pink	
	Contour		
	Consistency		
Papillae	Colour	Pink	
	Contour	Normal, blunted	
Symmetry	Undulated		

Periodontal charting

Facial upper

Tooth no.	18	17	16	15	14	13	12	11	21	22	23	24	25	26	27	28
Recession				111		800				300	101					
Pocket				323		1510				223	311					
Bleeding				√√√		√√√				√√√	√--					
Suppuration																
Buccal furcation																
Distal furcation																
Mobility																

Palatal upper

Tooth no.	18	17	16	15	14	13	12	11	21	22	23	24	25	26	27	28
Recession				200		530				110	000					
Pocket				313		329				224	323					
Bleeding				---		√√√				--√	√√√					
Suppuration																
Mesial furcation																

Lingual lower

Tooth no.	48	47	46	45	44	43	42	41	31	32	33	34	35	36	37	38
Recession					000	343	111	131	121	000	000		000	000		
Pocket					111	113	213	113	314	212	233		233	333		
Bleeding					---	---	---	--√	√√√	---	---		---	---		
Suppuration																
Furcation																
Mobility																

Facial lower

Tooth no.	48	47	46	45	44	43	42	41	31	32	33	34	35	36	37	38
Recession					231	231	000	000	000	111	000		111	121		
Pocket					113	314	424	335	535	423	222		111	121		
Bleeding					---	--√	√-√	√-√	√√√	---	---		---	---		
Suppuration																
Furcation																
Mobility																

Dental charting

Tooth no.	Clinical findings	Comments
18	Absent	Nil
17	Absent	Nil
16	Absent	Nil
15	Moderate MOD amalgam	Nil
14	Absent	Nil
13	Mesially tilted; uprighted by composite	Pseudopocket; poor gingival health, secondary caries
12	Absent	Nil
11	Absent	Nil
21	Absent	Nil
22	Large composite labially held by pins	Requires replacement
23	Large composite labially held by pins	Amalgam restoration under composite
24	Absent	Nil
25	Absent	Nil
26	Absent	Nil
27	Absent	Nil
28	Absent	Nil
38	Absent	Nil
37	Absent	Nil
36	Large MOD amalgam	Nil
35	Large composite resin held by pins	Nil
34	Absent	Nil
33	Severe wear	Nil
32	Splinted crowns	PAL at apex
31	splinted crowns	Nil
41	Splinted crowns	Nil
42	Splinted crowns	Nil
43	Severe wear	Nil
44	Large amalgam	Caries and pulpal involvement – PAL present
45	Absent	Nil
46	Absent	Nil
47	Absent	Nil
48	Unerupted	Nil

Previous dentures

Teeth replaced | 7 6   4   1 | 1   4   6 7

	Maxilla	Mandible
Age/number	1 since January 2008	Nil
Type	P/- CoCr	Nil
Kennedy classification	I mod II	Nil
Appearance	Patient satisfied	Nil
LFH	Good	Nil
Stability	Good	Nil
Support	Good	Nil
Retention	Good	Nil
Hygiene	Poor	Nil
Patient opinion	Positive	Nil

Special tests

Test	Performed	Additional information
Percussion	√	32 and 44 TTP
Palpation	√	32 labial TTP, soft lump NAD
Vitality	√	Only 44, 43, 33, 36, 37 are positive

Periapical films (13/02/2008)

15 _____

13 Secondary caries

22 _____

23 _____

36 _____

35 _____

33 _____

32 _Palatal_____

31 _____

41 _____

42 _____

43 _____

44 _____

48 Unerupted_____

Radiographs (Figure 13.1.3)
Orthopantomogram (13/02/2008)

General bone loss	Moderate vertical bone loss
Sinuses	NAD
Retained roots	NAD
Pathology	5 × 4 mm calcific body superimposed on right ascending rami – further investigation needed
Caries	15 distal
Restorations	15, 13, 22, 23, 36, 35, 33, 32, 31, 41, 42, 43, 44
Other	Nil

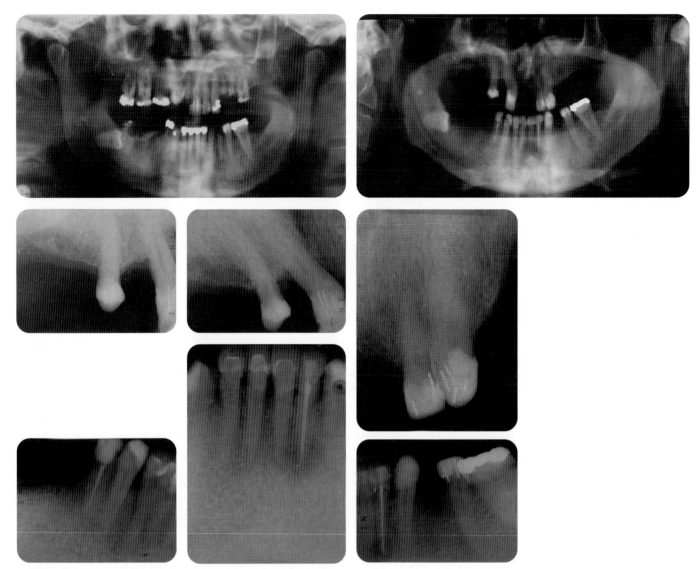

Figure 13.1.3 Radiographs. The left orthopantomogram (OPG) shows the presenting oral status. The right OPG indicates the status of teeth and bone after extraction of hopeless teeth. Periapical views when patient presented for work up of treatment plan and confirms minimal alveolar bone loss around remaining teeth.

Study casts

Articulation	Jaw position	RCP
	Face bow	Yes
Diagnostic wax-up	OVD change	3mm
Occlusal plane	Undulated	

Provisional diagnosis

- Chronic gingivitis.
- 31 and 41 localised periodontitis.
- 32 and 44 apical periodontitis.
- 13 secondary caries.
- Kennedy class I mod II in the maxilla.
- Kennedy class II mod I in the mandible.
- Partial closure of hard and soft cleft palate.
- Unerupted 48.

Problem list
Patient perceived

- Abnormal appearance.
- Lacks teeth for function.

Dentist perceived

- High lip line.
- Poor oral hygiene.
- Uneven ridge display.
- Transition zone goes from high to low.
- Malpositioned and malaligned maxillary dentition.
- Undulated occlusal plane.

Treatment goals
Short-term

- Disease control.
- Improve aesthetic.
- Improve function.

Long-term

- Maintainable prosthesis that provides reasonable longevity, acknowledging patient's lifestyle, eating pattern, general health and oral hygiene ability.
- Increase patient knowledge and awareness of oral health and regular dental visits, as well as ongoing maintenance.

Provisional phase (Figure 13.1.4)

- Oral hygiene instruction.
- Scale and clean.
- Endodontic treatment for 44 and 32.
- Provisional P/P acrylic.
- OVD change by composite, amalgam and provisional crowns for 42–32.

Reassessment phase

- Review periodontal status – improved oral hygiene and bleeding on probing.
- Review endodontic status – 32 and 44 both showed resolution in bone.
- Review aesthetic and functional satisfaction of P/P acrylic RDP – patient is satisfied with improvement from provisional prosthesis. RDP lacks retention.

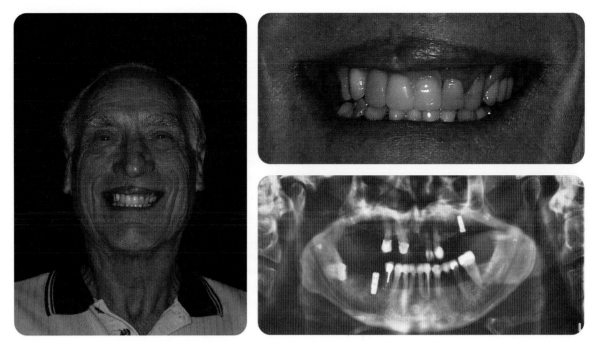

Figure 13.1.4 Control phase. Provisional maxillary removable prosthesis to restore occlusal vertical dimension and dental aesthetics. Orthopantomogram shows provisionalisation phase for implant overdenture support.

Treatment options
Maxilla

Option 1
- Telescopic crowns on remaining four abutment teeth. Single tooth implant in 26 position for implant telescopic abutment. Telescopic denture F/- over 15 and 13 with built out flange, 22 and 23 double crowns and 26 telescopic on implant.
- Advantage: correction of arch form, easy to control OVD, more aesthetic, load more evenly distributed, easy to clean.
- Higher cost and treatment time.

Option 2
- Single milled crowns on remaining four abutments, P/- CoCr.
- Advantage: lower cost, least treatment time.
- Less aesthetic, distal extension denture, less retentive.

Option 3
- Surgical augmentation and full fixed implant-supported prosthesis.

Mandible
- Post-core 44, single crowns 44 to 33 bridge, 34 to 36 bridge.
- Single tooth implant 46.

Treatment plan
Patient has chosen option 1 due to cost, but it also allows preservation of remaining vital dentition.

Further diagnostic phase (Figure 13.1.5)
After discussion with patient for maxillary options, patient chose option 1:
- provisional crowns in mandible;
- provisional crowns in maxilla;
- iCAT for maxilla with overdenture stent and mandibular radiographic stent.

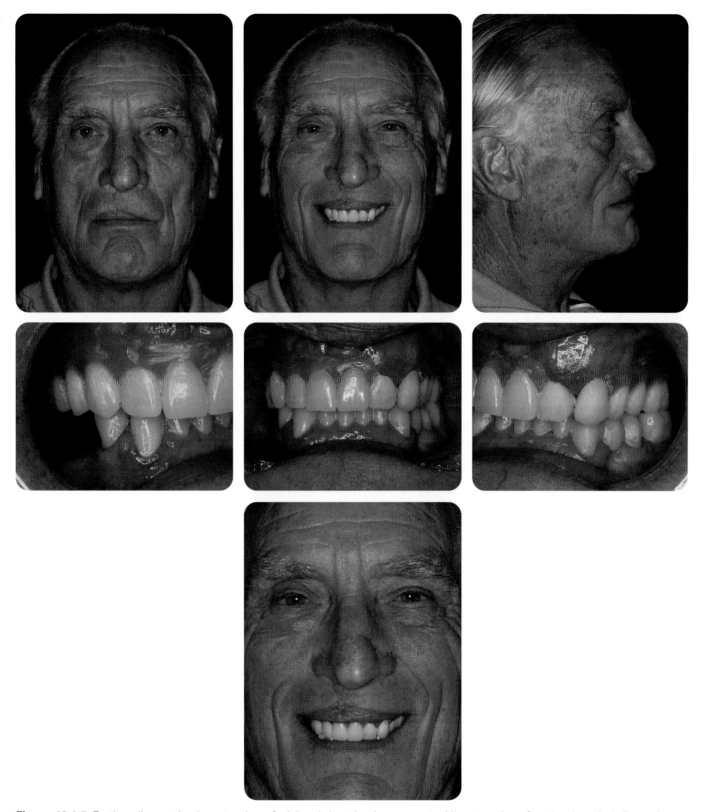

Figure 13.1.5 Further diagnostic phase to show facial and dental enhancement with restoration of occlusal vertical dimension and dental arch form.

Treatment discussion

Aesthetics

- Mr S is pleased with the harmony of the dental arch at time of try-in.
- The limitation of design was discussed, given the anatomy and tooth arrangement such that the dental midline does not coincide with the facial midline; the tooth proportion of lateral incisor and canine do not mirror those on the left. Mr S understands and recognises these factors; however, he is pleased with the overall harmony and the variation is of no concern. He is happy with overall aesthetic improvement.

Function

- Mr S is aware of the difference and advantage of a flat occlusal plane at try-in.
- Mr S is happy with the number of occlusal units around the arch provided throughout the provisional stage.

Cost

- Mr S has indicated that he can contribute to costs and has agreed for the laboratory work to be completed in-house.

Maintenance

- Mr S is aware of ongoing maintenance and responsibility including daily meticulous oral hygiene, 6-monthly prophylaxis privately and annual recall at the hospital. These are important to reduce biological risks and complications such as secondary caries and gingivitis.
- Mr S understands that future maintenance cost will be required for a remake. Minor frequent maintenance will include tightening of implant screws and denture reline.

Treatment sequence

- Preparation of 15, 13, 22, 23 (Figure 13.1.6).
- Impression and die preparation for maxilla.
- Construct first coping for telescopic abutment and construct surgical guide for the 26 implant.
- Surgery for 26 and 46 implant (Figure 13.1.7).
- Reline maxillary provisional denture fortnightly for 4 months:
  ○ Fixture – mandibular level impression.
- Continue with finalising preparations (Figure 13.1.8).
- Impressions for dies.
- Pick up impression.
- Provisional crown for 46 constructed (Figure 13.1.9).
- External laboratory – customised 26 telescopic abutment and galvano – second copings x 5.
- Maxillary –try-in of casting and wax against mandibular provisional prosthesis.
- Issue of definitive prosthesis (Figure 13.1.9).

Review at 15 months (Figures 13.1.10 & 13.1.11)

1. Oral health status – oral hygiene and plaque control – soft tissue health – check home-care programme and advise on frequency of brushing, use of dental floss and mouth rinses.
   Patient was more motivated and maintained excellent oral hygiene and prosthesis hygiene.
   Note recurrent dental caries associated with restorations or new carious lesions; note periodontal status – check probing depths and record changes; new PA radiographs to check alveolar bone levels.
   - *No periodontal issues and soft tissue health was excellent.*
   - *The maxillary denture was stained and there were wear marks on the palatal surfaces of the maxillary anterior teeth where the lower anteriors contacted in function. The flange around 22/23 had been designed to be thin but had chipped away. It was not causing irritation and did not affect aesthetics. As a result the outer surface was polished.*
   - *The telescopic crowns and lower crowns were excellent and no chipping, open margins or chipped margins were detected.*
2. Medical status – change in general health and implications for oral health.
   An improved diet was possible with improved distribution of teeth and jaw support.
3. Occlusion – check tooth contacts with GHM foil at ICP, RCP, lateral and protrusive excursive contacts.
   Bilateral balanced contacts on ICP and RCP. Protrusion was guided by central incisors; laterotrusion was guided by canines.
4. Radiographs – PA views for specific details of the status of crowns on teeth and implants.
   Radiographs showed good support around the teeth and implants.
5. Discuss oral health related quality of life – comfort, appearance, function – chewing and speech; whether there has been a change in confidence, social interaction and relationships.
   The patient commented that his rehabilitation provided marked improvement in appearance, speech, social life, smiling/laughing, self-confidence; and marked increased satisfaction with eating and enjoyment of food, improved general health, ability to sleep and work and improved mood.
6. Additional comments about the treatment and whether they would undertake the process again if needed.
   - *The patient was very happy with the results and enjoys the retention of the telescopic denture and can even bite into an apple.*
   - *He reported in general a great increase in comfort and function with the increase in OVD and fixed rehabilitation of the mandibular dentition.*
   - *He also reported that oral hygiene was more manageable and that he would undertake the process again if needed.*

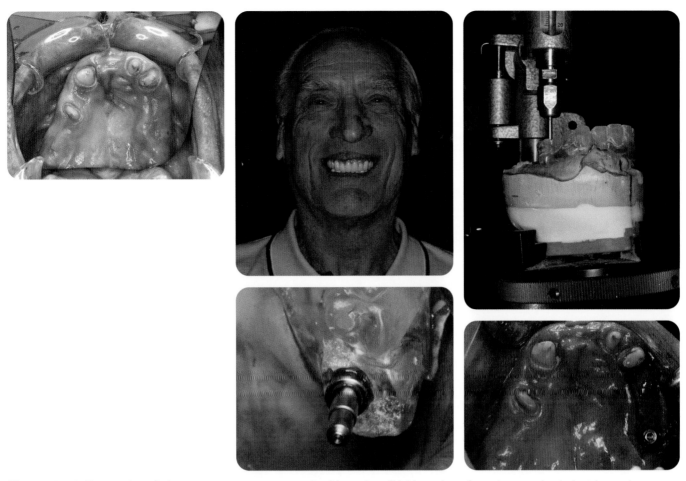

Figure 13.1.6 Preparation of abutments to a common path of insertion. Trial insertion of overlay prosthesis (set in wax). Preparation of radiographic guide for implant alignment to conform with the path of insertion determined in the tooth preparation. Axial image of potential implant site indicating available bone height and width. Surgical placement of implant using the surgical guide. Occlusal view of implant and its alignment relative to the tooth preparations.

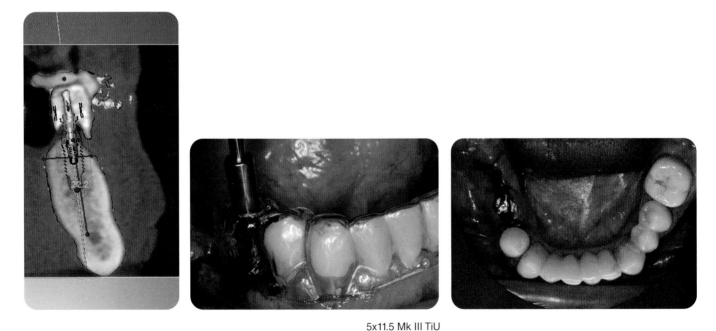

5x11.5 Mk III TiU

Figure 13.1.7 Axial image of potential mandibular implant site indicating height and width measurements of available bone. Implant surgery using surgical guide. Occlusal view of implant position.

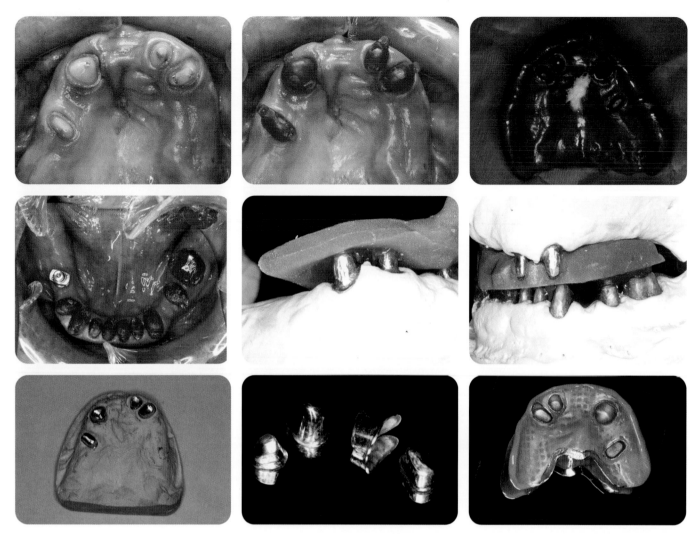

Figure 13.1.8 The upper images show the bonnet pick-up impression. Middle images the transfer record procedure and using Duralay resin and Moyco wax to verify the accuracy of the transfer record. Lower images show the primary gold copings constructed with the milled secondary copings incorporated within the chrome design of the overlay prosthesis.

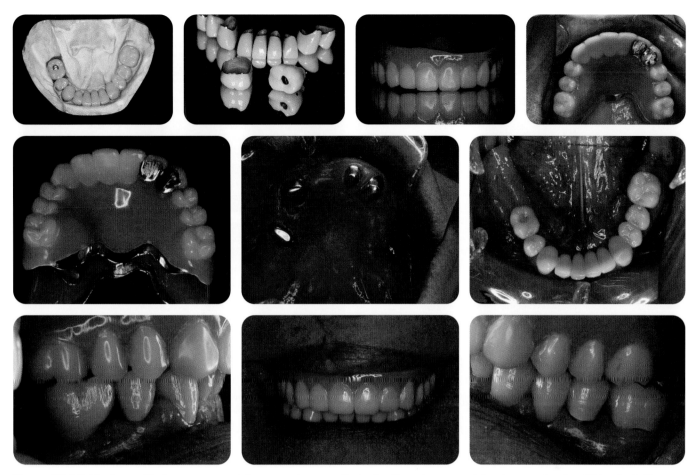

Figure 13.1.9 Final mandibular ceramo-metal crowns for mandibular teeth and screw-retained crown for the 46 implant. The overlay maxillary prosthesis is retained by frictional fit with the milled copings and the implant at 27 position. Final prosthesis in position with restoration of facial soft tissues and aesthetics.

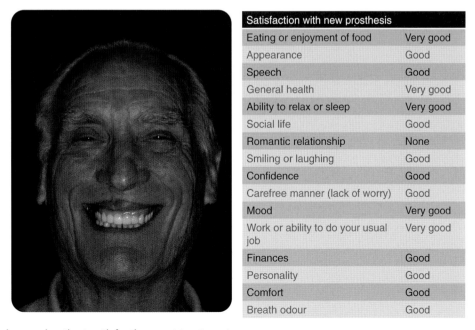

Satisfaction with new prosthesis	
Eating or enjoyment of food	Very good
Appearance	Good
Speech	Good
General health	Very good
Ability to relax or sleep	Very good
Social life	Good
Romantic relationship	None
Smiling or laughing	Good
Confidence	Good
Carefree manner (lack of worry)	Good
Mood	Very good
Work or ability to do your usual job	Very good
Finances	Good
Personality	Good
Comfort	Good
Breath odour	Good

Figure 13.1.10 Review and patient satisfaction post-treatment.

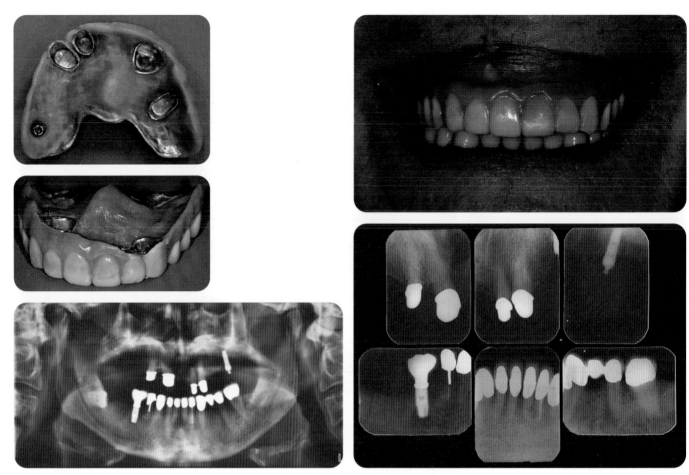

Figure 13.1.11 Review at 15 months. Note the broken flange on the upper-left images which has been repaired in the clinical view; there was evident patient satisfaction and wellbeing. The orthopantomogram indicated no measurable change in bone levels and PA views confirm the individual tooth and implant bone status is unchanged.

Reading list

Bergman, B., Hugoson, A. & Olsson, C-O. (1982) Caries, periodontal and prosthetic findings in patients with removable partial dentures: a ten year longitudinal study. *Journal of Prosthetic Dentistry*, 48 (5), 506–514.

Brägger, U., Karoussis, I., Person, R. *et al.* (2005) Technical and biological complications/failures with single crowns and fixed partial dentures on implants: a 10 year prospective cohort study. *Clinical Oral Implants Research*, 16 (3), 326–334.

Goodacre, C.J., Bernal, G. & Rungcharassaeng, K. (2003) Clinical complications in fixed prosthodontics. *Journal of Prosthetic Dentistry*, 90 (1), 31–41.

Klineberg, I, Kingston, D. & Murray, G. (2007) The bases for using a particular occlusal design in tooth and implant-borne reconstructions and complete dentures. *Clinical Oral Implants Research*, 18 (Suppl.3), 151–167.

Krennmair, G., Krainhöfner, M., Waldenberger, O. *et al.* (2007) Dental implants as strategic supplementary abutments for implant-tooth-supported telescopic crown-retained maxillary dentures: a retrospective follow-up study for up to 9 years. *International Journal of Prosthodontics*, 20 (6), 617–622.

Lang, N.P., Pjetursson, B.E., Tan, K. *et al.* (2004) A systematic review of the survival and complication rates of fixed partial dentures (FPDs) after an observation period of at least 5 years - II. Combined tooth–implant-supported FPDs. *Clinical Oral Implants Research*, 15 (6), 643–653.

Manhart, J., Chen, H.Y., Hamm, G. *et al.* (2004) Buonocore Memorial Lecture. Review of clinical survival of direct and indirect restorations in posterior teeth of permanent dentition. *Operative Dentistry*, 29 (5), 481–508.

Tan, K., Pjetursson, B.E., Lang, N.P. *et al.* (2004) A systematic review of the survival and complication rates of fixed-partial dentures (FPDs) after an observation period of 5 years. *Clinical Oral Implants Research*, 15 (6), 654–666.

Walton, T.R. (1999) A 10-year longitudinal study of fixed prosthodontics: clinical characteristics and outcome of single unit metal ceramic crowns. *International Journal of Prosthodontics*, 12 (6), 519–526.

Walton, T.R. (2002) An up to 15 year longitudinal study of 515 metal-ceramic FPDs: Part 1: outcomes. *International Journal of Prosthodontics*, 15 (5), 439–445.

Wöstmann, B, Balkenhol, M,, Weber, A. *et al.* (2007) Long-term analysis of telescopic crown retained removable partial dentures: survival and need for maintenance. *Journal of Dentistry*, 35 (12), 939–945.

Wöstmann, B., Balkenhol, M., Andrea, K. *et al.* (2008) Dental impact on daily living of telescopic crown-retained partial dentures. *International Journal of Prosthodontics*, 21 (5), 419–421.

14

Congenital Malformations (Tooth Agenesis)

Introduction by Alan Yap

Tooth agenesis is the term used to denote the failure of tooth development resulting in one or more missing teeth. Failure of tooth development is caused by dysplasia of the ectoderm or ectodermal dysplasia. Ectodermal dysplasia is a group of hereditary disorders involving an absence or deficiency of tissues and structures derived from the embryonic ectoderm (Dorland 2003). Clinical signs include trichodysplasia (abnormal hair) in 91% of cases, tooth agenesis in 80%, onychondysplasia (abnormal nails) in 75%, and dyshidrosis (abnormal sweat glands) in 42% (Holbrook 1988). There has been a wide variation in reports on the birth prevalence of ectodermal dysplasia, ranging from 1:10000 to 1:100000 (Myrianthopolous 1985). The prevalence of tooth agenesis does appear to be increasing, likely due to greater dental awareness, earlier diagnoses and possibly a greater number of carriers who do not display symptoms.

Hypodontia is the term denoting the absence of six or less teeth in the secondary dentition, excluding the third molars. When more than six teeth are missing, the term oligodontia is used; anodontia is the term used when all teeth are missing. Tooth agenesis has been shown to have a significant impact on oral health related quality of life of patients aged 11–15 years (Wong et al. 2006). The congenital absence of teeth may affect aesthetics, speech and masticatory function. Furthermore, tooth agenesis may result in reduced alveolar bone growth, which has implications in the development of lower facial height, support and stability for removable prostheses and the placement of dental implants. The principal aims of treatment are to restore missing teeth and bone, establish an acceptable vertical dimension and provide support for facial soft tissues.

The planning and treatment of patients with tooth agenesis is complex. Oral rehabilitation of patients with tooth agenesis has historically involved partial or complete removable prostheses supported by tissue or teeth (overdentures). The development and acceptance of osseointegrated dental implants has provided an additional treatment modality. Implant survival rates in these patients have been reported to be generally high, ranging between 88.5% and 100% (Yap & Klineberg 2009). However, a high percentage of these patients experienced one or more implant failures with reports ranging between 16.7% and 35.7% in ectodermal dysplasia patients and between 4.3% and 38.5% in oligodontia patients (Yap & Klineberg 2009). These data raise questions concerning treating these patients: whether there should be a plan for failure; should more implants be placed to allow for implant failure; or should dentists design prostheses to allow for implant failures? The answer is no, because 93–100% of implant failures occurred before prosthesis insertion (Kearns et al. 1999, Guckes et al. 2002, Sweeney et al. 2005). Thus, implant number and position, and prosthesis design, should be idealised in the planning phase. When treatment planning for these patients, dentists have a duty of care to inform patients and their parents that approximately one in every 3–4 patients will have failure of one or more implants and that, should implant failure occur, cost will increase as will treatment time. An extended period of provisionalisation is recommended.

Although rate of implant failure was relatively high, all patients eventually received implant-borne prostheses (Kearns et al. 1999, Guckes et al. 2002, Sweeney et al. 2005). Prosthesis complications, including screw loosening and sore spots, have also been reported to be significant in patients with tooth agenesis (Öczakir et al. 2005, Poggio et al. 2005, Sweeney et al. 2005). As a result, it is important for patients to understand that there is a high level of prosthesis maintenance required. The expense of dental treatment has been estimated to be high, which correlates with the severity of tooth agenesis and the need for orthodontic or implant treatment (Murdock et al. 2005). The majority of these patients have been shown to require multidisciplinary treatment, including orthodontics, oral maxillofacial surgery and prosthodontics, with protracted treatment periods (Murdock *et al.* 2005, Poggio *et al.* 2005, Worsaae *et al.* 2007).

Despite these shortcomings, quality of life has been shown to improve in oligodontia patients receiving implant and prosthodontic treatment (Finnema *et al.* 2005). The following cases illustrate the treatment-planning process and treatment outcomes in patients with tooth agenesis in an interdisciplinary environment.

References

Dorland's Illustrated Medical Dictionary (2003), 30th edn. Saunders, Philadelphia.

Finnema, K.J., Raghoebar, G.M., Meijer, H.J. *et al.* (2005). Oral rehabilitation with dental implants in oligodontia patients. *International Journal of Prosthodontics*, 18 (3), 203–209.

Guckes, A.D., Scurria, M.S., King, T.S. *et al.* (2002). Prospective clinical trial of dental implants in persons with ectodermal dysplasia. *Journal of Prosthetic Dentistry*, 88 (1), 21–25.

Holbrook, K.A. (1988) Structural abnormalities of the epidermally derived appendages in skin from patients with ectodermal dysplasia: insight into developmental errors. In: *Recent Advances in Ectodermal Dysplasias* (eds C.F. Salinas, J.M. Optiz & N.W. Paul), pp. 15–44. Liss, New York.

Kearns, G., Sharma, A., Perrott, D. *et al.* (1999) Placement of endosseous implants in children and adolescents with hereditary ectodermal dysplasia. *Oral Surgery Oral Medicine Oral Pathology Oral Radiology & Endodontics*, 88 (1), 5–10.

Murdock, S., Lee, J., Guckes, A. *et al.* (2005) A cost analysis of dental treatment for ectodermal dysplasia. *Journal of the American Dental Association*, 136 (9), 1273–1276.

Myrianthopolous, N.C. (1985) *Malformations in Children from One to Seven Years: A Report from the Collaborative Perinatal Project*. Liss, New York.

Öczakir, C., Balmer, S. & Mericske-Stern, R. (2005) Implant-prosthodontic treatment for special care patients: a case series study. *International Journal of Prosthodontics*, 18 (5), 383–389.

Poggio, C.E., Salvato, M. & Salvato, A. (2005) Multidisciplinary treatment of agenesis in the anterior and posterior areas: a long term retrospective analysis. *Progress in Orthodontics*, 6 (2), 262–269.

Sweeney, I.P., Ferguson, J.W., Heggie, A.A. *et al.* (2005) Treatment outcomes for adolescent ectodermal dysplasia patients treated with dental implants. *International Journal of Paediatric Dentistry*, 15 (4), 241–248.

Wong, A.T., McMillan, A.S. & McGrath, C. (2006) Oral health-related quality of life and severe hypodontia. *Journal of Oral Rehabilitation*, 33 (12), 869–873.

Worsaae, N., Jensen, B.N., Holm, B. *et al.* (2007) Treatment of severe hypodontia-oligodontia – an interdisciplinary concept. *International Journal of Oral & Maxillofacial Surgery*, 36 (6) 473–480.

Yap, A.K. & Klineberg, I. (2009) Dental implants in patients with ectodermal dysplasia and tooth agenesis: A critical review of the literature. *International Journal of Prosthodontics*, 22 (3), 268–276.

Case 14.1 Mr Grant H

Johnson P.Y. Chou

Patient: Mr Grant H (date of birth 16/05/1987)

Presenting complaints

Date	31/7/2008
Chief complaint	'Can't smile with my teeth'
Subsidiary complaints	Small teeth; missing teeth; retained deciduous teeth
History of complaints	Since 15 years old
Patient's expectations	'Have normal teeth'

History
Medical history

Medical Practitioner		
Respiratory	Nil	
Cardiovascular	Nil	
Endocarditis	Nil	
Gastrointestinal	Nil	
Neurological	Nil	
Endocrine	Nil	
Musculoskeletal	Three bulging discs of lower back diagnosed by GP 24/4/2008	
Genitourinary	Nil	
Haematological	Nil	
	Bleeding	Nil
	Immune	Nil
Other	Allergies	Nil
	Genetics	Mild ectodermal dysplasia (clinical diagnosis with no genetic testing): oligodontia. Course dry hair, slow-growing nails, minimal sweating
	Smoking	Nil
	Infectious diseases	Nil
	Pregnancy	Nil
	Hospitalisation	Nil
	Medications	Mobic 15 mg capsules

Social history

Marital status		Single	
Children		0	
Occupation		Air conditioning technician	
Smoking		Nil	
Recreational drugs		Nil	
Diet	√	Soft drinks	2 cokes/week
	√	Sports drinks	1/week
		Lemons	Nil
		Acidic foods	Nil
		Sweet foods	Nil
	√	Water	4–5 glasses/day
		Tea	Nil
		Coffee	Nil
	√	Alcohol	5–10 beers on Saturday nights
		Hard/brittle foods	Nil
		Ice crunching	Nil
Habits/hobbies		Musical instrument	Nil
	√	Exercise	Soccer
	√	Oral habits	Nail biting

Dental history

		Additional information	
Date of last examination			
Oral hygiene	√	Brushing	Twice daily
		Flossing	Nil
		Mouthwash	Nil
	√	Toothpaste	Colgate
Treatment	√	Restorations	Nil
		Endodontics	Nil
		Periodontics	Nil
	√	Orthodontics	July 2005 – July 2008: fixed appliance in the mandible to move 43 distal to create space for dental implant
		RDP	Nil
		FDP	Nil
		TMD	Nil
		OMFS	Nil

Extraoral examination (Figures 14.1.1 & 14.1.2)
Aesthetics

Facial symmetry	Asymmetrical	
Profile	Concave	
Nasolabial angle	>90°	
Facial folds	Mentalis	
Midlines	Face/maxillary centrals	Coincides
	Maxillary/mandibular centrals	4mm to the RHS of facial midline
Lip posture	Symmetry	Symmetrical
	Upper lip	Thin
	Lower lip	Thin
	Competence	Yes
	Tooth display	Nil at rest
Occlusal plane	Parallel to ala tragus line	Yes
	Parallel to interpupillary line	No
	Over-eruption	Nil
Vertical	FWS	3mm
	OVD assessment	Optimal
Smile assessment (Figure 14.1.2)	Symmetry	Yes
	Lip line	Moderate
	Gingival display	None
	Tooth display	50%
	Buccal corridor	Moderate

Phonetics

	Normal	Abnormal
Labial (m)	√	
Labiodental (f/v)	√	
Linguodental (th)	√	
Interdental (s)	√	
Linguopalatal (k/ng)	√	

Temporomandibular assessment

TMJ		Additional information
Click	Nil	
Crepitus	Nil	
Tenderness	Nil	

Muscle tenderness	Right	Left
Temporalis	Nil	Nil
Masseter	Nil	Nil
Posterior mandible	Nil	Nil
Anterior mandible	Nil	Nil
Glands	Nil	
Nodes	Nil	

Jaw movement	Measurement (mm)	Reference points
Maximal opening	43	Tooth 11
Right laterotrusion	12	Maxillary dental midline
Left laterotrusion	12	Maxillary dental midline
Midline deviation	No	
Maximal protrusion	13	
Opening pathway	Straight	
Overjet	5	
Overbite	−3	
Further investigation required	No	

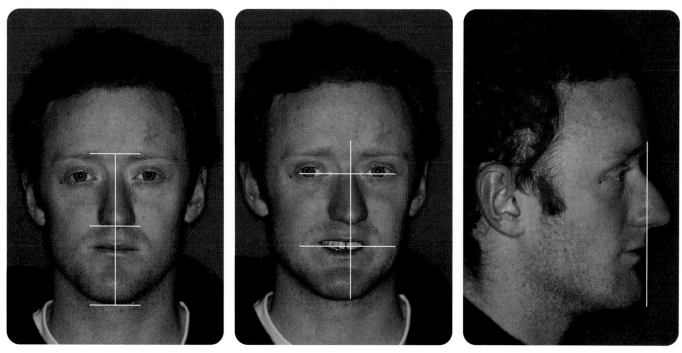

Figure 14.1.1 Extraoral examination.

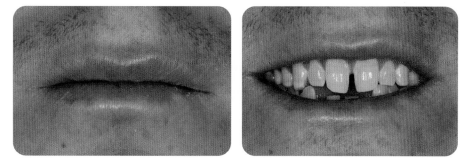

Figure 14.1.2 Extraoral examination. Smile assessment.

Intraoral examination (Figure 14.1.3)
Soft tissues

Tissue	Healthy	Abnormal	Additional information
Lips	√		Nil
Labial vestibule	√		Nil
Cheeks	√		Nil
Palate	√		Nil
Oropharynx	√		Nil
Tongue	√		Nil
Floor	√		Nil
Frenal attachments	√		Nil

Oral cleanliness

Condition	Yes	No			
Plaque	√		Localised	Mild	Supragingival
Calculus	√		Localised	Moderate	Supragingival
Food impaction		√	Nil		
Stains		√	Nil		
Halitosis		√	Nil		

Saliva

Water intake		4–5 glasses/day
Quality		Satisfactory
Quantity		Satisfactory
Pathology		Nil
Medications affecting		Nil
Further investigation required	Yes	Saliva testing
Resting saliva	Hydration	30–60 seconds
	Viscosity	Frothy/bubbly pH: 6.8–7.8
Stimulated saliva	Quantity	3.5–5.0 ml
	Buffering	10–12 points

Periodontium

CPITN

1	0	1
1	0	1

Gingiva	Biotype	Medium
	Colour	Pink
	Contour	Normal
	Consistency	Firm
Papillae	Colour	Pink
	Contour	Normal

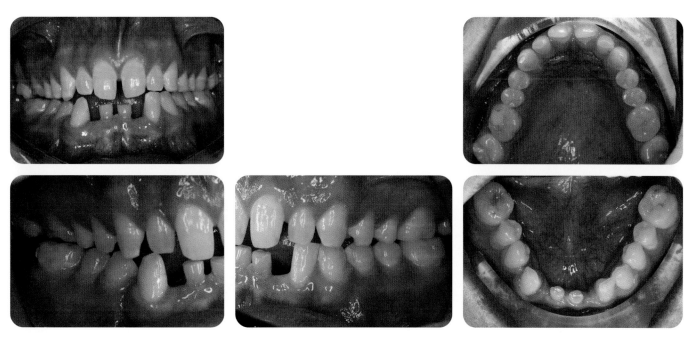

Figure 14.1.3 Intraoral examination. Note horizontal ridge deficiency in the congenitally missing 31–42 region.

Periodontal charting

Maxillary buccal

Tooth no.	18	17	16	15	14	13	12	11	21	22	23	24	25	26	27	28
Pocket		212	211	112	111	111	111	111	111	112	212	212	212	212	212	
Bleeding													√		√	
Suppuration																
Recession																
Buccal furcation																
Distal furcation																
Mobility																

Maxillary palatal

Tooth no.	18	17	16	15	14	13	12	11	21	22	23	24	25	26	27	28
Pocket		212	212	212	211	111	111	111	111	111	111	212	212	212	212	
Bleeding												√	√	√		
Suppuration																
Recession																
Mesial furcation																

Mandibular lingual

Tooth no.	48	47	46	45	44	43	42	41	31	32	33	34	35	36	37	38
Pocket			212	212	212	212				111	111	212	212	212		
Bleeding			√	√									√			
Suppuration																
Recession										5						
Furcation																

Mandibular buccal

Tooth no.	48	47	46	45	44	43	42	41	31	32	33	34	35	36	37	38
Pocket			222	211	112	212				212	212	122	212	212		
Bleeding													√			
Suppuration																
Recession																
Furcation																
Mobility																

Occlusion

Skeletal classification	Class II	
Dental occlusion	Class II	
Angle right	Molar II	Canine I
Angle left	Molar II	Canine II
Anterior overbite	–3 mm	
Anterior overjet	5 mm	
Cross-bites	Yes – 16, 46	
Open-bites	Yes – anterior	
Curve of Spee	RHS +	LHS +
Curve of Wilson	+	
RP to IP slide	1 mm anterior	
FWS	Close/M/swallow test	3 mm

Tooth guidance

Right laterotrusion   Left laterotrusion

<u>8 7 6 5 4 3 2 1| 1 2 3 4 5 6 7 8</u>   <u>8 7 6 5 4 3 2 1| 1 2 3 4 5 6 7 8</u>

8 7 6 5 4 3 2 1 1 2 3 4 5 6 7 8   8 7 6 5 4 3 2 1 1 2 3 4 5 6 7 8

Protrusion

<u>8 7 6 5 4 3 2 1| 1 2 3 4 5 6 7 8</u>

8 7 6 5 4 3 2 1 1 2 3 4 5 6 7 8

Tooth surface loss

Caries

<u>8 7 6 5 4 3 2 1| 1 2 3 4 5 6 7 8</u>

8 7 6 5 4 3 2 1 1 2 3 4 5 6 7 8

Attrition   Erosion (specify surface)

<u>8 7 6 5 4 3 2 1| 1 2 3 4 5 6 7 8</u>   <u>8 7 6 5 4 3 2 1| 1 2 3 4 5 6 7 8</u>

8 7 6 5 4 3 2 1 1 2 3 4 5 6 7 8   8 7 6 5 4 3 2 1 1 2 3 4 5 6 7 8

Abrasion (specify surface)   Abfraction (specify surface)

<u>8 7 6 5 4 3 2 1| 1 2 3 4 5 6 7 8</u>   <u>8 7 6 5 4 3 2 1| 1 2 3 4 5 6 7 8</u>

8 7 6 5 4 3 2 1 1 2 3 4 5 6 7 8   8 7 6 5 4 3 2 1 1 2 3 4 5 6 7 8

Dental charting

Tooth no.	Clinical findings	Comments
18	Missing	Congenitally missing
17	Unrestored	Nil
16	Composite: small OB	Nil
15	Unrestored	Nil
14	Unrestored	Nil
13	Unrestored	Nil
12	Unrestored	Nil
11	Unrestored	Nil
21	Unrestored	Nil
22	Unrestored	Nil
23	Unrestored	Nil
24	Unrestored	Nil
25	Unrestored	Nil
26	Unrestored	Nil
27	Unrestored	Nil
28	Missing	Congenitally missing
38	Missing	Congenitally missing
37	Missing	Congenitally missing
36	Composite: small occlusal Caries: DO Retained orthodontic cement: B	Nil
35	Unrestored	Nil
34	Retained orthodontic cement: B	Nil
33	Retained orthodontic cement: B	Nil
32	Root distally angulated Recession: 5 mm on the lingual side	Nil
31	Missing	Congenitally missing
71	Moderate attrition	Retained deciduous tooth
81	Moderate attrition	Retained deciduous tooth
41	Missing	Congenitally missing
42	Missing	Congenitally missing
43	Retained orthodontic cement: B	Nil
44	Retained orthodontic cement: B	Nil
45	Retained orthodontic cement: B	Nil
46	Composite: small occlusal Caries: occlusal Retained orthodontic cement: B	Nil
47	Missing	Congenitally missing
48	Missing	Congenitally missing

Special tests

Test	Performed	Additional information
Percussion	√	All negative to percussion test
Vitality	√	All positive to cold test

Radiographs (Figure 14.1.4)
Orthopantomogram (19/12/2008)

Features	Radiographic data
TMJ	No pathology
Bone loss	No
Sinuses	No pathology
Mandibular canal	Visible
Mental foramen	–
Retained roots	No
Pathology	No

Periapical films (19/12/2008) (Figure 14.1.5)

Tooth no.	Information	Tooth no.	Information
18	Missing	38	Missing
17	Present	37	Missing
16	Present	36	Caries: occlusal
15	Present	35	Present
14	Present	34	Present
13	Present	33	Present
12	Present	32	Present
11	Present	31	Missing
	Present	71	Present
	Present	81	Present
21	Present	41	Missing
22	Present	42	Missing
23	Present	43	Present
24	Present	44	Present
25	Present	45	Present
26	Present	46	Caries: occlusal
27	Present	47	Missing
28	Missing	48	Missing

Study casts (Figures 14.1.6 & 14.1.7)

Articulation	Position	RCP
	Face bow	Yes
Diagnostic wax-up (Figure 14.1.7)	OVD change	–0.5 mm
	Occlusal adjustment	Yes
	Crown lengthening	No

Diagnosis

Medical	Three bulging discs of lower back, taking Mobic 15 mg capsules Ectodermal dysplasia
Periodontal	Recession
Biomechanical	Dental caries
Functional	Mild generalised attrition Abnormal neuromuscular habits: nail biting Missing teeth: 37, 31, 41, 42, 47 Straight 1 mm asymptomatic anterior–posterior CR-CO slides Anterior open-bite
Aesthetic	Incisal length: long Diastema: 12D, 11M+D, 21M+D, 22M, 23D Tooth to tooth proportions: small maxillary anterior teeth Tooth form not ideal: long central incisors Gingival outline not ideal: mild gingival asymmetry

Problem list

Problem	Details
Medical condition	Three bulging discs of lower back, taking Mobic 15 mg capsules Ectodermal dysplasia
Aesthetics	Small teeth: 12, 11, 21, 22 Missing teeth: 31, 41, 42 Retained deciduous teeth: 71 and 81
Speech	None
TMD	None
Soft tissue	None
Oral hygiene	None
Saliva	Low water intake: 4–5 glasses water/day
Periodontal	Recession: 5 mm on the lingual side of tooth 32
Edentulism	None
Occlusion	Angle's classification: II Straight 1 mm anterior–posterior asymptomatic CR-CO slide Nail biting habits Anterior open bite
Tooth surface loss	Generalised mild attrition on remaining dentition
Restorative	Caries: 36DO, 46O
Prosthetic	None
Endodontic	None

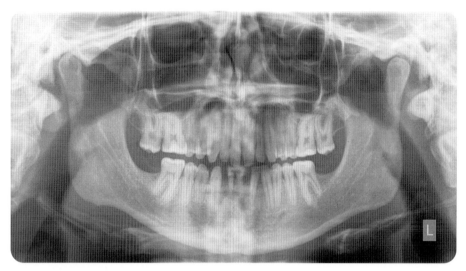

Figure 14.1.4 Preoperative radiograph. Panoramic radiograph.

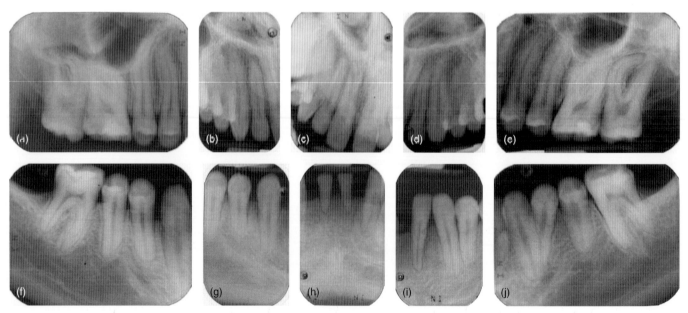

Figure 14.1.5 Preoperative radiograph. Periapical radiographs.

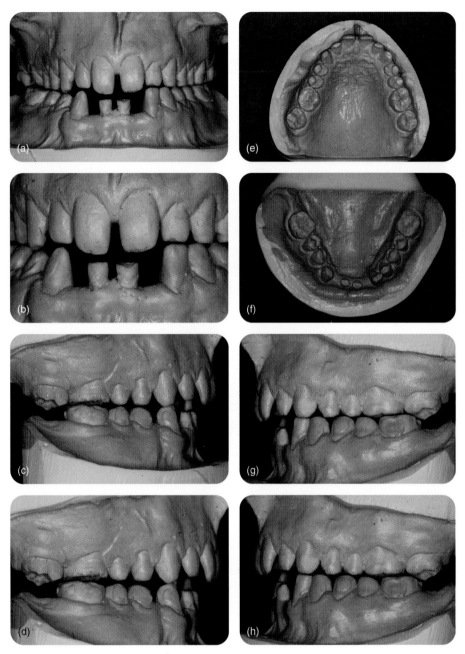

Figure 14.1.6 Preoperative study casts.

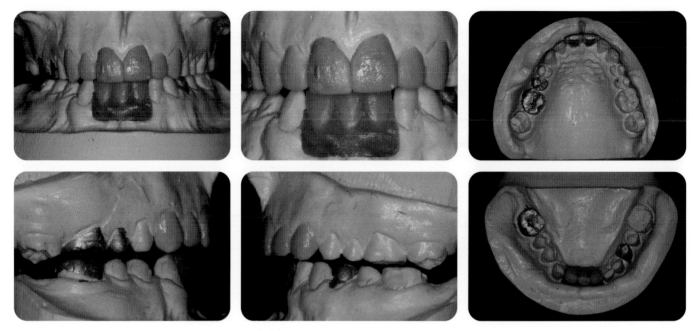

Figure 14.1.7 Diagnostic wax-up. Note occlusal adjustments to stabilise occlusal contact and reduce anterior open-bite.

Treatment goals

Short-term goals
- Disease control/stability:
  - caries control;
  - behavioural control:
    - education to stop nail biting habits;
    - diet counselling (increase water intake).

Long-term goals
- Improve facial aesthetics.
- Improve function.
- Replace missing teeth.
- Modify occlusal plane.
- Protect remaining tooth structure.

Treatment options

Option 1
- Extraction of retained deciduous teeth 71 and 81 + replace missing teeth 31, 41 and 42 with removable partial denture + direct composite/indirect porcelain veneer restorations for teeth 13–23.

- Removable partial denture to replace missing teeth 31, 41 and 42.

Option 2
- Extraction of retained deciduous teeth 71 and 81 + replace missing teeth 31, 41, 42 with dental implants + direct composite/indirect porcelain veneer restorations for tooth 13–23.
- Dental implants: 41 and 42.
- Implant-supported FDPs: 31–42 cantilevered implant-supported FDPs.

Option 3
- Extraction of retained deciduous teeth 71 and 81and permanent tooth 32 + replace missing teeth 32, 31, 41, 42 with dental implants + direct composite/indirect porcelain veneer restorations for teeth 13–23.
- Dental implants: 32 and 42.
- Implant-supported FDPs: 32–42 implant-supported FDPs.

Advantages and disadvantages of different options to replace missing teeth

Removable dental prostheses

Advantages	Disadvantages
Replace multiple teeth in multiple sites	Removable prostheses may not be liked by patient and may reduce self-confidence
Support obtained from mucosa and/or teeth	Connectors cover soft tissue such as the palate and gingival
The least expensive restorations	In subjects with less than ideal oral hygiene they may compromise the health of the periodontal tissues and promote caries around abutment teeth
Generally do not require extensive preparation of abutment teeth	Retentive elements such as clasps may spoil aesthetics
May be designed to accommodate future tooth loss	Maintenance requirements and durability
Can be used to replace missing soft tissue	
Can provide good lip support by incorporating labial flanges	
Aesthetics may be very good	

Fixed dental prostheses

Advantages	Disadvantages
Fixed	Involve considerable tooth preparation which sometimes result in pulpal sequela
Improved aesthetics, including that of abutment tooth if they need to be improved/harmonised	Failure due to decementation and caries of abutment teeth may lead to further tooth loss
Medium term predictability is good for short span bridges	Moderately expensive
Improved occlusion and guidance possible	Highly operator-dependent requiring exacting techniques both clinically and technically
Minimally compromise oral hygiene	Require lengthy clinical time and temporary restorations
	Irreversible

Dental implants

Advantages	Disadvantages
Fixed or removable	Dependent upon presence of adequate bone quantity and quality
Independent of natural teeth – can provide fixed restoration where no abutment teeth exist	Involve surgical procedure(s)
Immune to dental caries	Highly operator/technique-dependent
High level of predictability	High initial expense and lengthy treatment time
Good maintenance of supporting bone	Maintenance requirements especially for removable or extensive fixed prostheses

Treatment plan and discussion

Patient chose option 3 with direct composite veneer restorations for the following reasons:

- maxillary and mandibular dentition have good prognoses;
- dental implants for long-term outcome;
- age of the patient: young.

Treatment planning for dental implants

Dental implants are used to replace missing teeth and not healthy or compromised teeth. There were no comparative studies identified to evaluate the outcomes of implant single crowns, tooth-supported FDPs, restored endodontically treated tooth and extraction without tooth replacement. The term 'success' was defined in different ways both within and among different treatment modes, complications were largely not reported and psychosocial outcomes were incompletely addressed. There were no significant differences in survival between restored RCT teeth, tooth-supported conventional FDPs (3 and 4 units) and single-tooth implants. The decision to treat a tooth endodontically or replace it with an implant must be based on factors other than the treatment outcomes of the procedures themselves (prognostic risk factors: medical history, smoking, caries; patient preferences; and economics). Limited data suggest that extraction without replacement in visible areas results in inferior psychosocial outcomes compared with alternatives of retention or replacement.

Natural teeth versus periodontally or endodontically compromised teeth

Holm-Pederson et al. (2007) conducted a systematic review to compare the longevity of healthy teeth, periodontally compromised, endodontically compromised and oral implants; 49 articles were included. The longevity for teeth with healthy periodontal tissues was up to 99.5% over 50 years, periodontally compromised was 92–93%, and high survival and success rate for endodontically compromised and dental implants was 82–94%. They concluded that oral implants, when evaluated after 10 years of service, do not surpass the longevity of even compromised but successfully treated natural teeth. Tomasi et al. (2008) conducted a systematic review to compare the loss rate of teeth and dental implants. They found in clinically well-maintained patients, the loss rate at teeth was lower than at implant. They also acknowledge that comparisons of longevity of teeth and dental implants are difficult due to heterogeneity of data.

Endodontics versus dental implants versus fixed dental prosthesis

Torabinejad et al. (2007) conducted a systematic review to compare the outcomes, benefits and harms of endodontic care and restoration compared to extraction and placement of implant single crowns, FDPs (short span of

3–4 units and also includes cantilever, resin-bonded and conventional ceramo-metal and all-ceramic) and extraction without tooth replacement. A total of 143 studies were included and only five studies were randomised clinical trials. There were no comparative studies and success was defined in very different ways, both within and between different treatment modes, complications were largely not reported and psychosocial outcomes were incompletely addressed. They concluded that the limited data suggested that extraction without replacement in visible areas resulted in inferior psychosocial outcomes compared with the alternatives of retention or replacement. Implant and endodontic treatments (on a per tooth basis) for periodontally sound teeth resulted in superior long-term survival, compared with FDPs.

Salinas and Eckert (2007) conducted a systematic review to compare implant single crowns and tooth-supported FDPs. A total of 51 articles were identified in the implant literature and 41 in the tooth-supported dental prostheses literature. There were no comparative studies. They found differences at 5 years between the survival of implant-supported single crowns and natural tooth-supported FDPs when resin-bonded and conventionally retained FDPs were grouped. The difference disappeared when implant-supported single crowns were compared with conventionally tooth-supported FDPs.

Iqbal and Kim (2007) conducted a systematic review to compare implant single crowns and endodontically restored teeth. A total of 55 studies related to single-tooth implants and 13 studies related to restored RCT teeth were included. The term 'endodontically treated teeth' encompasses a broad range of treatment categories that are associated with different treatment outcomes. Ideally, the outcome of each of these categories (initial treatment without apical periodontitis, initial treatment with apical periodontitis, non-surgical and surgical retreatment of failing RCTs) needs to be individually compared with implants. However, at present the survival rates of these categories of endodontic therapy with coronal restorations are not available in the literature. They found no significant differences in survival between restored RCT teeth and single-tooth implants. The results of this systematic review indicate that the decision to treat a tooth endodontically or replace it with an implant must be based on factors other than the treatment outcomes of the procedures themselves (prognostic risk factors: medical history, smoking, caries; patient preferences and economics).

Outcomes of removable partial dentures

Patient cooperation and oral hygiene are the most important factors influencing disease status on teeth adjacent to treated and untreated edentulous spaces.

Bergman et al. (1982) conducted a 10 and 25 years prospective longitudinal study on 30 patients treated with removable partial denture. They followed up 27 and 23 patients out of 30 patients at 10 and 25 years, respectively. Patients were recalled yearly and most of the removable partial dentures were mandibular bilateral distal-extension dentures. They found patient cooperation was excellent, and no significant deterioration of periodontal status of the remaining teeth was found. In addition, there was a low increase in the frequency of decayed and filled tooth surfaces during follow-up.

Aquilino *et al.* (2001) conducted a retrospective study and found a significant difference in 10-year survival rates of teeth adjacent to treated and untreated posterior bounded edentulous spaces: FDPs > untreated > removable partial dentures. However, the authors acknowledged that there was a bias in allocating FPDs to teeth with good prognosis.

Incisal edge position assessment

Fradeani (2006) in his review discussed the use of following parameters to assess incisal edge position assessment:

- dentolabial: exposure of maxillary teeth at rest (range of 1–5 mm) + incisal curve (parallel with the lower lip);
- phonetics: 's' sound (buccolingual direction) + 'f' and 'v' sounds (inside the vermilion border of the lower lip);
- tooth: OB/OJ (to allow anterior guidance).

Outcomes of direct versus indirect veneers

There is no reliable evidence to show a benefit of one type of veneer restoration over the other with regard to the longevity of the restoration.

Wakiaga *et al.* (2004) conducted a Cochrane review on the effectiveness of direct versus indirect laminate veneer restorations. They included one study and concluded that there is no reliable evidence to show a benefit of one type of veneer restoration over the other with regard to the longevity of the restoration.

Meijering *et al.* (1997) conducted a prospective clinical trial to measure the satisfaction of patients with respect to aesthetics of veneer restorations. A total of 180 veneer restorations of three different types (direct composite, indirect composite and porcelain) were placed on anterior teeth. Patients were asked to fill in questionnaires at baseline and at 1- and 2-year recalls. They found no dif-ference on satisfaction between the three different types of veneer restorations at 1-year follow-up. Patients with porcelain veneers had greater satisfaction at 2-year follow-up.

Outcomes of tooth replacement options

Pjetursson *et al.* (2007) conducted a systematic review and found 10-year survival of conventional tooth-supported FDPs was 89.2%, the figure for cantilever FDPs was 80.3%, implant-supported FDPs 86.7%, combined tooth-implant-supported FDPs 77.8% and implant-supported single crowns (SCs) 89.4%. Despite high survival rates, 38.7% of patients with implant-supported FDPs had some complications after the 5-year observation period, compared with 15.7% for conventional FDPs and 20.6% for cantilever FDPs, respectively. For conventional tooth-supported FDPs, the most frequent complications were biological complications such as caries and loss of pulp vitality. Compared with tooth-supported FDPs, the incidence of technical complications was significantly higher for the implant-supported reconstructions. The most frequent technical complications were fractures of the veneer material (ceramic fractures or chipping), abutment or screw loosening and loss of retention.

Pjetursson *et al.* (2008) conducted a systematic review with inclusion of 17 studies and found an estimated survival of resin bonded bridges of 87.7% after 5 years. The most frequent complication was de-bonding (loss of retention) 19.2%, and biological complications (caries on abutments and resin-bonded bridges lost due to periodontitis) occurred in 1.5% of abutments and 2.1% of resin-bonded bridges.

Type of prostheses	Survival rates (%)	
	5 year	10 year
Conventional FDP	93.8	89.2
Implant-supported FDPs	95.2	86.7
Implant-supported SCs	94.5	89.4
Tooth-implant supported FDPs	95.5	77.8
Cantilever FDPs	91.4	80.3
Resin-bonded FDPs	87.7	

Treatment sequence

Initial therapy

- Preventive advice:
  - diet counselling: increase water intake;
  - stop nail biting habits.
- Scaling, root planning, oral hygiene instructions:
  - mechanical debridement of plaque and calculus deposits adherent to the clinical crowns and roots of teeth;
  - oral hygiene instruction;
  - removal of orthodontic cements on mandibular teeth.
- Operative dentistry:
  - restoration and conservative control of dental caries: 36DO + 46O;
  - restoration and conservative control of dental caries: 36DO + 46O.
- Fabrication of interim provisional restoration:
  - fabrication of radiographic guide for planned implant sites;
  - extraction of retained deciduous teeth 71 and 81 and permanent tooth 32;
  - removable partial denture to replace missing teeth 32, 31, 41 and 42.
- Imaging for surgical and corrective therapy (Figure 14.1.8).
- Placement of endosseous implants: 32 and 42 (Figure 14.1.9).
- Transitional implant-supported restoration:
  - allow for soft tissue maturation;
  - fabrication of implant-retained provisional restoration 32–42.

Prosthetic phase (Figure 14.1.10)

- Placement of direct composite veneer restorations on teeth 13–23.
- Placement of implant-supported FDPs 32–42:
  - check the individual and collective fit of the restorations;
  - adjust the contact point or contact areas, occlusion and aesthetics.
- Installation and adjustment of an occlusal splint.
- Maintenance.

Informed consent

Benefits	Control of disease Improvement of aesthetics Replace missing teeth Protect remaining tooth structure
Alternatives	No treatment Removable partial denture Tooth-supported FDPs
Advised	Treatment time Provisional restorations will be made during treatment Longevity of the restorations Cost of the treatment
Complications	Implant supported crown and bridges: • biological: soft tissue complications, loss of peri-implant bone, suboptimal aesthetics • technical: loss of retention, fracture of materials, fracture of the framework, abutment or occlusal screw loosening, fracture of occlusal screws, fracture of implants Implant surgery: • oral soft tissue: haemorrhage, neurosensory disturbances, tissue emphysema, infections, wound dehiscence, aspiration or ingestion of surgical instruments, postoperative pain • hard tissue: periapical implant pathosis and endodontic considerations, lack of primary implant stability, inadvertent penetration into the maxillary sinus or nasal fossa, sinus lift predicaments, mandibular fracture
Maintenance	Regular dental visits on a 4–6 monthly basis

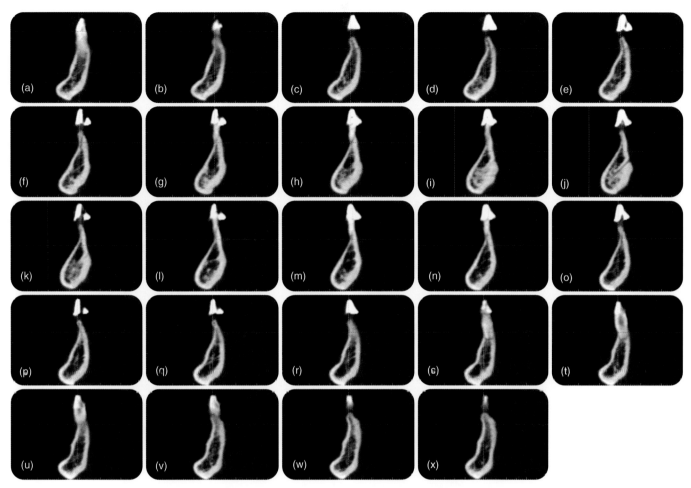

Figure 14.1.8 Preoperative iCAT radiograph of 42–32 region. Note the horizontal ridge deficiency in the buccal region.

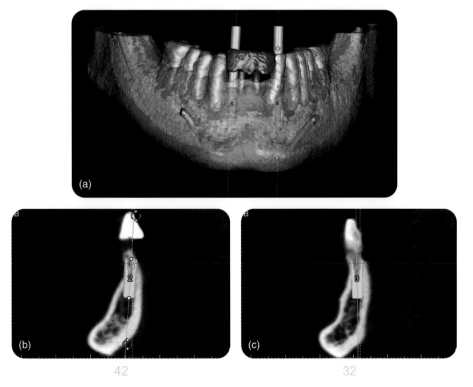

Figure 14.1.9 Simplant surgical planning. Note planned extraction 32 and placement of implant in the 32 and 42 region.

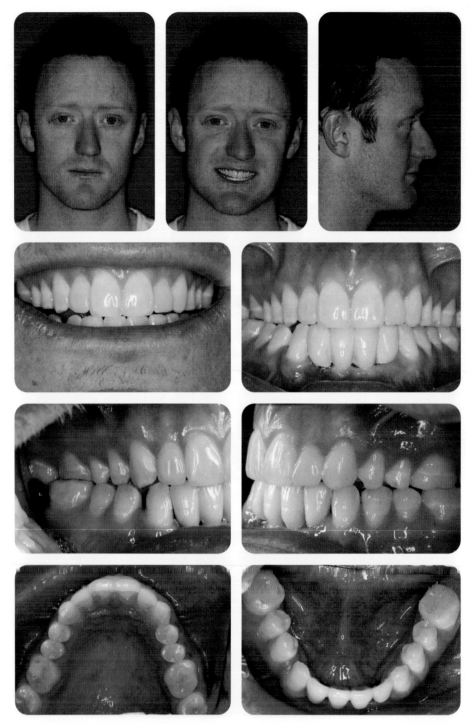

Figure 14.1.10 Extraoral and intraoral photos of completed treatment. Note direct composite build-up of teeth 13–23.

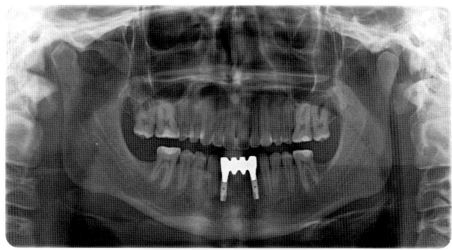

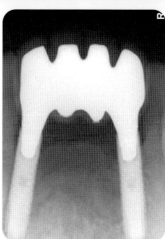

Figure 14.1.11 One-year postoperative radiographs after repair of 11+23 composite.

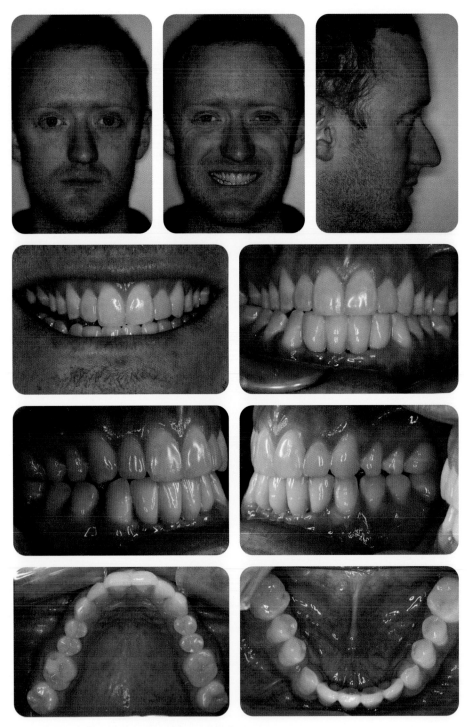

Figure 14.1.12 One-year postoperative extraoral and intraoral photos.

Review at 1 year (Figures 14.1.11 and 14.1.12)

1. Oral health status:
   - Oral hygiene and plaque control: *good.*
   - Soft tissue health: *no gingival inflammation.*
   - Check on home-care programme and advise on frequency of brushing, use of dental floss and mouth rinses: *flosses once a day and brushes twice daily.*
   - Note and record recurrent dental caries associated with restorations or new carious lesions: *no new carious lesions.*
   - Note periodontal status – check probing depths and record changes; new PA radiographs to check alveolar bone levels (see 3 below): *no changes in periodontal status.*

2. Occlusion:
   - Check tooth contacts with GHM foil at ICP, RCP, lateral and protrusive excursive contacts – note lateral contact details: *right and left canine guidance.*
   - Especially where there is a fracture of restorative material – record, photograph fracture and contact details with GHM foil and comment on reason for fracture: *heavy protrusive contacts.*

3. Radiographs (Figure 14.1.11):
   - 1-year review PA views for specific details of the status of crowns on teeth and implants. Check crown margins and alveolar bone levels; measure thread exposure to bone crest around implants and correlate with clinical details as in 1 above: *new OPG taken and PA of 32-42; no change noted.*

4. Discuss oral health related quality of life – comfort, appearance, function – chewing and speech; whether there has been a change in confidence, social interaction and relationships. *Main change is the improved appearance and improved chewing function. Definitely more confident with smiling and social interaction.*

5. Seek any additional comments from the patient about the treatment and whether they would undertake the process again if needed. *Patient would definitely undertake the process again if needed.*

References

Aquilino, S.A., Shugars, D.A., Bader, J. *et al.* (2001) Ten-year survival rates of teeth adjacent to treated and untreated posterior bounded edentulous spaces. *Journal of Prosthetic Dentistry*, 85 (5), 455–460.

Bergman, B., Hugoson, A. & Olsson, C.O. (1982) Caries, periodontal and prosthetic findings in patients with removable partial dentures: a ten-year longitudinal study. *Journal of Prosthetic Dentistry*, 48 (5), 506–514.

Fradeani, M. (2006) Evaluation of dentolabial parameters as part of a comprehensive esthetic analysis. *European Journal of Esthetic Dentistry*, 1 (1), 62–68.

Holm-Pedersen, P., Lang, N.P. & Muller, F. (2007) What are the longevities of teeth and oral implants? *Clinical Oral Implants Research*, 18 (Suppl. 3), 15–19.

Iqbal, M.K. & Kim, S. (2007) For teeth requiring endodontic treatment, what are the differences in outcomes of restored endodontically treated teeth compared to implant-supported restorations. *International Journal of Oral & Maxillofacial Implants*, 22 (Suppl.), 96–116.

Meijering, A.C., Roeters, F.J., Mulder, J. *et al.* (1997) Patients' satisfaction with different types of veneer restorations. *Journal of Dentistry*, 25 (6), 493–497.

Pjetursson, B.E., Bragger, U., Lang, N.P. *et al.* (2007) Comparison of survival and complication rates of tooth-supported fixed dental prostheses (FDPs) and implant-supported FDPs and single crowns. *Clinical Oral Implants Research*, 18 (Suppl. 3), 97–113.

Pjetursson, B.E., Tan, W.C., Tan, K. *et al.* (2008) A systematic review of the survival and complication rates of resin-bonded bridges after an observation period of at least 5 years. *Clinical Oral Implants Research*, 19 (2), 131–141.

Salinas, T.J. & Eckert, SE. (2007) In-patients requiring single-tooth replacement, what are the outcomes of implant as compared to tooth-supported restorations? *International Journal of Oral & Maxillofacial Implants*, 22 (Suppl.), 71–95.

Tomasi, C., Wennstrom, J.L. & Berglundh, T. (2008) Longevity of teeth and implants – a systematic review. *Journal of Oral Rehabilitation*, 35 (Suppl. 1), 23–32.

Torabinejad, M., Anderson, P., Bader, J. *et al.* (2007) Outcomes of root canal treatment and restoration, implant-supported single crowns, fixed partial dentures, and extraction without replacement: a systematic review. *Journal of Prosthetic Dentistry*, 98 (4) 285–311.

Wakiaga, J.M., Brunton, P., Silikas, N. *et al.* (2004) Direct versus indirect veneer restorations for intrinsic dental stains. *Cochrane Database of Systematic Reviews*, Issue 1 viewed online. www.thecochranelibrary.com.

Case 14.2 Mr Tobiah J

Michael Lewis

Patient: Mr Tobiah J (date of birth 08/02/1985)

Presenting complaints

Chief complaint	'The missing teeth on either side (points to maxillary lateral incisors) replaced first'
Subsidiary complaints	'The missing ones down the bottom (points to mandibular incisors) replaced, but that doesn't matter as much'
History of complaints	'I've grown quite used to the situation . . . no problems eating or speaking'
	'I've been missing teeth my whole life'
Patient's expectations	'It's more of a looks thing'

History
Medical history

Medical Practitioner	Dr R	
Respiratory	Asthma	
Cardiovascular	NAD	
	Endocarditis	Nil
Gastrointestinal	NAD	
Neurological	NAD	
Endocrine	NAD	
Developmental	X-linked hypohidrotic ectodermal dysplasia	
Musculoskeletal	NAD	
Genitourinary	NAD	
Haematological	NAD	
	Bleeding	Nil
	Immune	Nil
Other	Allergies	NKA
	Smoking	Nil
	Infectious diseases	Nil
	Pregnancy	N/A
	Hospitalisation	Nil
	Medications	Seretide prn

Social history

Marital status	Unmarried		
Children	None		
Occupation	Construction Industry as a boat builder		
Smoking	Nil		
Recreational drugs	Nil		
Diet		Soft drinks	Nil
		Sports drinks	Nil
		Lemons	Nil
	√	Acidic foods	2–3 pieces of fruit/day
		Sweet foods	Nil
	√	Water	At least a few litres of water/day
		Tea	Nil
	√	Coffee	6 cups coffee/day
		Alcohol	Nil
	√	Hard/brittle foods	Sometimes chews nuts
	√	Ice crunching	Sometimes crunches ice between teeth
Habits/hobbies		Musical instrument	Nil
	√	Exercise	Soccer and boxing (sparring only)
	√	Oral habits	Might put a nail between teeth when working

Dental history

		Additional information	
Date of last examination 19/03/2008			
Oral hygiene	√	Brushing	1–2/day
	√	Flossing	1–2/day
		Mouthwash	Nil
	√	Toothpaste	Colgate
Treatment	√	Restorations	Replace/reshape restorations on maxillary and mandibular canines.
	√	Endodontics	Endodontic consult re teeth 23 and 33
	√	Periodontics	Crown lengthening surgery on teeth 13 and 23
		Orthodontics	Nil
		RDP	Nil
	√	FDP	Tooth-borne crown on teeth 13 and 23
			FDP on implants in 12 and 22 sites
			FDP on implant 33 and tooth 43
		TMD	Nil
	√	OMFS	Extract teeth 11, 21, 33, 42
			Implant fixtures in 12, 22 and 33 sites

Extraoral examination
Aesthetics (Figures 14.2.1 & 14.2.2)

Facial symmetry	Symmetrical	
Profile	Convex	
Nasolabial angle	90°	
Facial folds	Deep labiomental fold	
Midlines	Face/maxillary centrals	Coincident
	Maxillary central alignment	Parallel to facial midline
	Maxillary/mandibular centrals	N/A
Lip posture	Symmetry	Symmetrical
	Upper lip	Thick
	Lower lip	Thick
	Competence	Yes
	Tooth display	80% maxillary incisal display/40% mandibular incisal display at repose
Occlusal plane	Parallel to ala tragus line	Yes
	Parallel to interpupillary line	Yes
	Over-eruption	Nil
Vertical	FWS	1 mm
	OVD assessment	Optimal
Smile assessment	Symmetry	Yes
	Lip line	High
	Gingival display	High
	Tooth display	5 mm gingival display above maxillary incisors, 40% mandibular incisal display
	Buccal corridor	Narrow

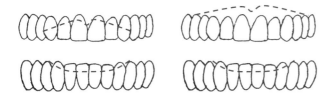

| At rest | Broad smile |

Phonetics

	Normal	Abnormal
Labial (m)	√	
Labiodental (f/v)		√
Linguodental (th)	√	
Interdental (s)	√	
Linguopalatal (k/ng)	√	

Temporomandibular assessment

TMJ		Additional information
Click	Nil	NAD
Crepitus	Nil	NAD
Tenderness	Nil	NAD

Muscle tenderness	Right	Left
Temporalis	Nil	Nil
Masseter	Nil	Nil
Posterior mandible	Nil	Nil
Anterior mandible	Nil	Nil
Glands	Nil	
Nodes	Nil	

Jaw movement	Measurement (mm)	Reference points
Maximal opening	45	11 and 42 incisal edges
Right laterotrusion	8	11 mesial – 43 mesial incisal edges
Left laterotrusion	12	11 mesial – 43 mesial incisal edges
Midline deviation	Not assessable	N/A
Maximal protrusion	10	11 and 42 incisal edges
Opening pathway	Straight	Frontal view
Overjet	13	11 and 42 incisal edges
Overbite	3	11 and 42 incisal edges
Further investigation required	No	

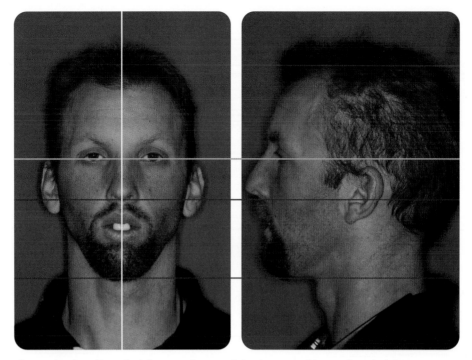

Figure 14.2.1 Extraoral examination. Note facial proportions and the increased lower face height.

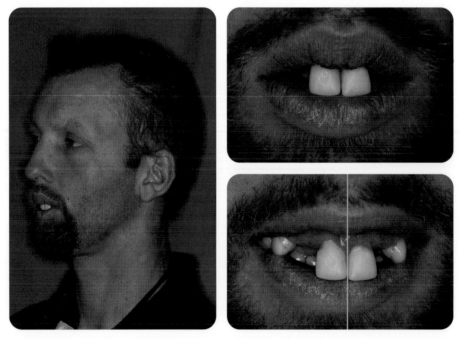

Figure 14.2.2 Extraoral examination. Smile assessment. Note short upper lip and incisor tooth visibility with lips at rest.

Intraoral examination (Figure 14.2.3)
Soft tissues

Tissue	Healthy	Abnormal	Additional information
Lips	√		NAD
Labial vestibule	√		NAD
Cheeks	√		NAD
Palate		√	Slight redness on soft palate
Oropharynx		√	3 mm in diameter, smooth raised area on tongue
Tongue	√		NAD
Floor	√		NAD
Frenal attachments		√	Maxillary midline frenal attachment is red and inflamed

Ridges	Maxilla	Mandible
Arch shape	U-shaped	U-shaped
Resorption	Mild	Severe
Palatal vault	Moderate	N/A
Tori	NAD	NAD
Frenal attachments	Midline and buccal	Midline
Mucosa	Flabby/firm	Flabby/firm
Pathology	Nil	Nil

Oral cleanliness

Condition	Yes	No	
Plaque		√	
Calculus		√	
Food impaction	√		Self-report
Stains	√		Microleakage around CR restorative margins 13, 23, 33, 42, 43
Halitosis		√	

Saliva

Water intake	At least a few litres of water/day
Quality	Watery/clear resting saliva, pH 6.8–7.8, stimulated saliva has pH of 6.8–7.8, with 10–12 points of buffering capacity
Quantity	Hydration from rest <30 seconds, 3.5–5.0 ml stimulated salivary flow over 5 minutes
Pathology	NAD
Medications affecting	NAD
Further investigation required	No

Periodontium

CPITN

1	1	3
1	1	1

Gingiva	Biotype	Thick
	Colour	Deep pink
	Contour	Knife-edge around unrestored teeth – rolled and receded around composite resin restorations
	Consistency	Firm around unrestored teeth – swollen and puffy around composite resin restorations
Papillae	Colour	Fiery-red between maxillary central incisors, elsewhere coral pink
	Contour	Enlarged between maxillary central incisors, elsewhere normal

Periodontal charting (Figure 14.2.4)

Maxillary buccal

Tooth no.	18	17	16	15	14	13	12	11	21	22	23	24	25	26	27	28
Pocket		223	223		222	222		223	221		222	222		433	221	
Bleeding					+			+++	++							
Suppuration																
Recession		120	111		110	002		311	124		200	010		001	111	
Buccal furcation																
Distal furcation																
Mobility		I	I		I	I		II	II		I	I		I	I	

Maxillary palatal

Tooth no.	18	17	16	15	14	13	12	11	21	22	23	24	25	26	27	28
Pocket		232	223		333	323		122	322		223	333		323	321	
Bleeding			++		++			+	++		+	+		+	+	
Suppuration																
Recession		111	101		110	112		420	025		310	001		111	110	
Mesial furcation																

Mandibular lingual (Figure 14.2.5)

Tooth no.	48	47	46	45	44	43	42	41	31	32	33	34	35	36	37	38
Pocket		333	222	323	323	312	211				111	112	223	323	323	
Bleeding			+									+		+		
Suppuration																
Recession		000	010	000	000	010	014				310	020	020	010	000	
Furcation																

Mandibular buccal

Tooth no.	48	47	46	45	44	43	42	41	31	32	33	34	35	36	37	38
Pocket		323	322	213	213	211	111				212	212	213	323	223	
Bleeding			+									+		+		
Suppuration																
Recession		021	110	010	020	011	124				310	020	020	010	000	
Furcation																
Mobility		I	I	I	I	I	I				I	I	I	I	I	

Occlusion

Skeletal classification	Class II				
Dental occlusion	Class II division 1				
Angle Right	Molar	Class II	Canine	Class II
Angle left	Molar	Class II	Canine	Class II
Anterior overbite	3 mm				
Anterior overjet	13 mm				
Cross-bites	NAD				
Open-bites	Anterior open bite				
Curve of Spee	RHS flat		LHS flat	
Curve of Wilson	+				
RP to IP slide	1 mm vertical, forward and left				
FWS	M test		1 mm	

Tooth guidance

Right laterotrusion   Left laterotrusion

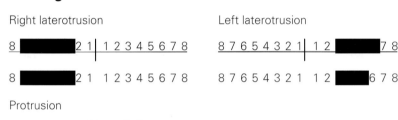

Protrusion

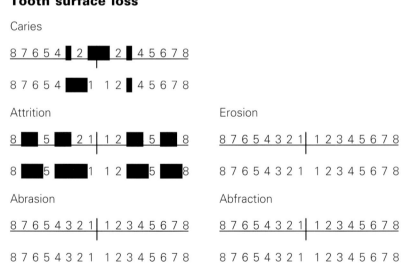

Tooth surface loss

Caries

Attrition   Erosion

Abrasion   Abfraction

Dental charting

Tooth no.	Clinical findings	Comments
18	Not present	
17	Tooth present. Enamel hypoplasia. No restorations detected	Staining in fissures. No probable decay
16	Tooth present. Enamel hypoplasia. No restorations detected	Staining in fissures. No probable decay
15	Not present	Space closed orthodontically
14	Tooth present. Enamel hypoplasia. No restorations detected	Staining in fissures. No probable decay
13	Tooth present. Enamel hypoplasia. Composite resin reshaping of tooth	Microleakage around mesiopalatal margin of restoration
12	Not present	Space comparable to the size of the central incisors present. Minimal horizontal alveolar resorption
11	Tooth present. Enamel hypoplasia. Composite resin reshaping of tooth	Microleakage around cervical portion of restoration. Excessive proclination and recession associated with maxillary central incisors
21	Tooth present. Enamel hypoplasia. Composite resin reshaping of tooth	Microleakage around cervical portion of restoration. Excessive proclination and recession associated with maxillary central incisors
22	Not present	Space comparable to the size of the central incisors present. Minimal horizontal alveolar resorption.
23	Tooth present. Enamel hypoplasia. Composite resin reshaping of tooth	Microleakage around palatal margin of restoration
24	Tooth present. Enamel hypoplasia. No restorations detected	Staining in fissures. No probable decay
25	Not present	Space closed orthodontically
26	Tooth present. Enamel hypoplasia. Occlusal fissure sealant present	No probable decay
27	Tooth present. Enamel hypoplasia. No restorations detected	Staining in fissures. No probable decay
28	Not present	
38	Not present	
37	Tooth present. Enamel hypoplasia. No restorations detected	Staining in fissures. No probable decay
36	Tooth present. Enamel hypoplasia. No restorations detected	Staining in fissures. No probable decay
35	Tooth present. Enamel hypoplasia. No restorations detected	Staining in fissures. No probable decay
34	Tooth present. Enamel hypoplasia. No restorations detected	
33	Tooth present. Enamel hypoplasia. Composite resin reshaping of tooth	Significant leakage around cervical margin of restoration. Invasive cervical resorption
32	Not present	
31	Not present	
41	Not present	
42	Tooth present. Enamel hypoplasia. Composite resin reshaping of tooth	Microleakage around cervical margin of restoration
43	Tooth present. Enamel hypoplasia. Composite resin reshaping of tooth	Significant leakage around distobuccal margin of restoration
44	Tooth present. Enamel hypoplasia. No restorations detected	
45	Tooth present. Enamel hypoplasia. No restorations detected	Staining in fissures. No probable decay
46	Tooth present. Enamel hypoplasia. No restorations detected	Staining in fissures. No probable decay
47	Tooth present. Enamel hypoplasia. No restorations detected	Staining in fissures. No probable decay
48	Not present	

Previous dentures

Teeth replaced   <u>8 7 6 5 4 3 ▉ 1 | 1 ▉ 3 4 5 6 7 8</u>

                       8 7 6 5 4 3 2 1   1 2 3 4 5 6 7 8

	Maxilla	**Mandible**
Age/number	Present	Absent
Type	Essix appliance	Cast metal framework
Kennedy classification	Class IV mod 1	Class IV
Appearance	Unsatisfactory	N/A
LFH	N/A	N/A
Stability	Stable	N/A
Support	Tooth-borne	N/A
Retention	Retentive	N/A
Hygiene	Fair	N/A
Patient opinion	'It doesn't look all that good . . . I mainly wear it as a retainer'	'It was quite irritating . . . I got rid of it!'

Special tests

Test	Performed	Additional information
Percussion	√	No tooth tested tender to percussion
Vitality	√	23 non-responsive to carbon dioxide testing. Remaining dentition tested positive

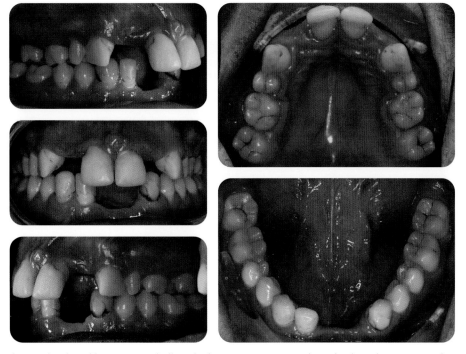

Figure 14.2.3 Intraoral examination. Note congenitally missing permanent teeth and edentulous space size.

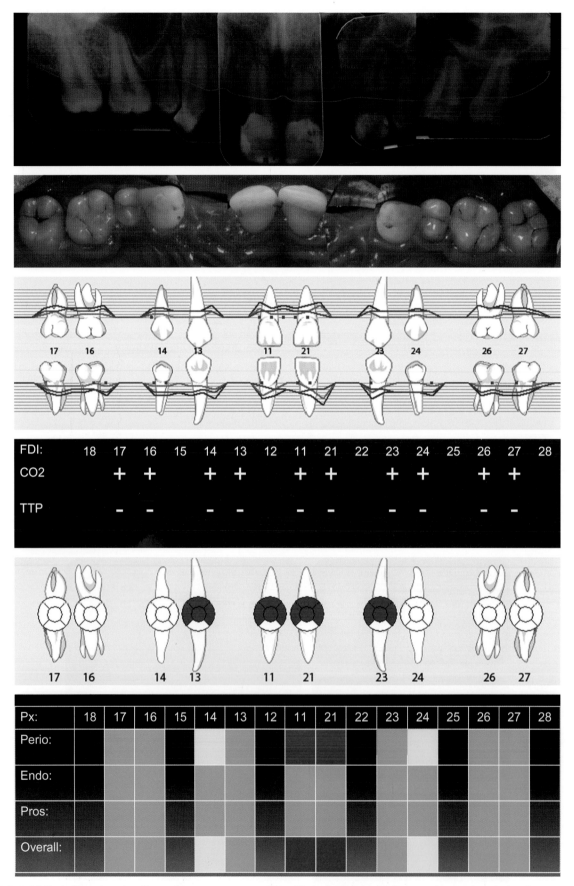

FDI:	18	17	16	15	14	13	12	11	21	22	23	24	25	26	27	28
CO2		+	+		+	+		+	+		+	+		+	+	
TTP		−	−		−	−		−	−		−	−		−	−	

Px:	18	17	16	15	14	13	12	11	21	22	23	24	25	26	27	28
Perio:																
Endo:																
Pros:																
Overall:																

Figure 14.2.4 (a) Periodontal and radiographic assessment of maxillary dentition. (b) Restorative and endodontic assessment of maxillary dentition.

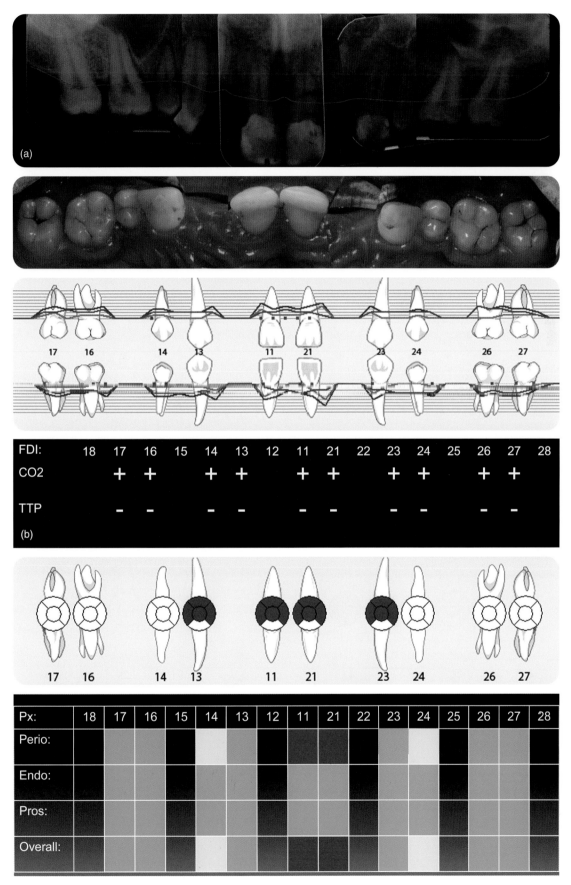

FDI:	18	17	16	15	14	13	12	11	21	22	23	24	25	26	27	28
CO2		+	+		+	+		+	+		+	+		+	+	
TTP		−	−		−	−		−	−		−	−		−	−	

(b)

Px:	18	17	16	15	14	13	12	11	21	22	23	24	25	26	27	28
Perio:																
Endo:																
Pros:																
Overall:																

Figure 14.2.4 (*Continued*)

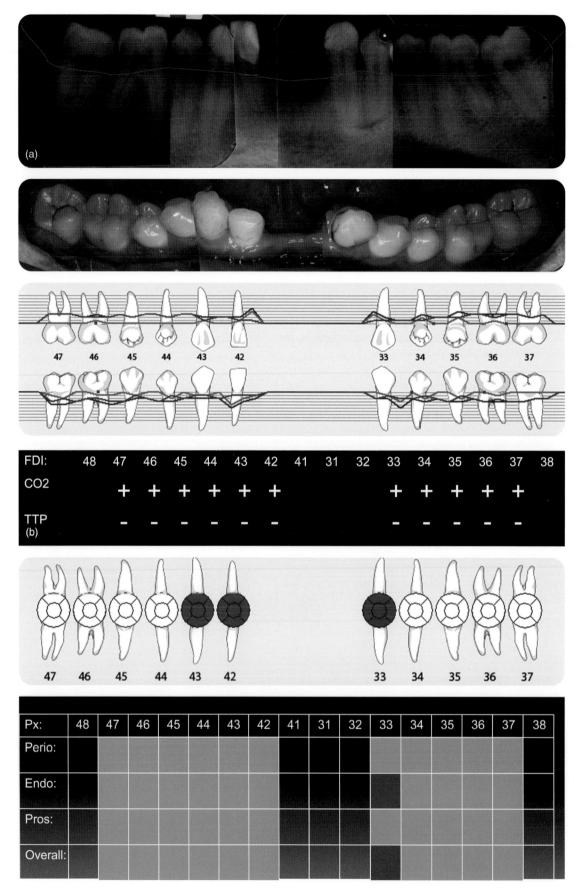

Figure 14.2.5 (a) Periodontal and radiographic assessment of mandibular dentition. (b) Restorative and endodontic assessment of mandibular dentition.

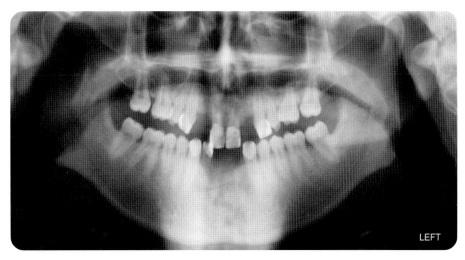

Figure 14.2.6 Radiograph – orthopantomogram.

Radiographs (Figure 14.2.6)
Orthopantomogram (03/04/2008)

Features	Radiographic data
TMJ	NAD
Bone loss	Mild to moderate horizontal bone loss around the maxillary anterior teeth
Sinuses	Maxillary and nasal sinus clear and patent. Pneumatised over the maxillary fist molars
Mandibular foramen and canal	Clear and patent. Distant for the roots of the mandibular teeth
Mental foramen	Not visible on OPG
Retained roots	Nil
Pathology	Mild to moderate generalised external root resorption

Periapical films

Tooth no.	Information	Tooth no.	Information
18	Tooth not present	38	Tooth not present
17	Tooth present. No horizontal bone loss. Sinus floor close to tooth roots. No visible periapical pathology. No restorations present on tooth	37	Tooth present. No horizontal bone loss. No visible periapical pathology. No restorations present on tooth
16	Tooth present. No horizontal bone loss. Sinus floor traces around alveolus. Mild external root resorption. Tapered root form. No restorations present on tooth	36	Tooth present. No horizontal bone loss. Mild external root resorption. No visible periapical pathology. No restorations present on tooth
15	Tooth not present	35	Tooth present No horizontal bone loss. Mild external root resorption. No visible periapical pathology. No restorations present on tooth
14	Tooth present. Mild horizontal bone loss. Sinus close to tooth roots. Moderate to severe external root resorption. Tapered root form. No restorations present on tooth	34	Tooth present. No horizontal bone loss. Mild external root resorption. No visible periapical pathology. No restorations present on tooth
13	Tooth present. Mild horizontal bone loss. Mild to moderate external root resorption. Composite resin restoration present, with visible marginal breakdown	33	Tooth present. No horizontal bone loss. Mild external root resorption. No visible periapical pathology. Mild internal root resorption noted in the middle portion of the root. Composite resin restoration present, with visible marginal breakdown
12	Tooth not present	32	Tooth not present
11	Tooth present. Moderate horizontal bone loss. Wide incisal canal present between maxillary central incisors. Mild to moderate external root resorption. Composite resin restoration present, with visible marginal breakdown	31	Tooth not present
21	Tooth present. Moderate horizontal bone loss. Wide incisal canal present between maxillary central incisors. Mild to moderate external root resorption. Composite resin restoration present, with visible marginal breakdown	41	Tooth not present
22	Tooth not present	42	Tooth present. No horizontal bone loss. Mild to moderate external root resorption. No visible periapical pathology. Composite resin restoration present
23	Tooth present. Mild horizontal bone loss. Mild to moderate external root resorption. Composite resin restoration present	43	Tooth present. No horizontal bone loss. No visible periapical pathology. Composite resin restoration present
24	Tooth present. Mild horizontal bone loss. Moderate external root resorption. No restorations present on tooth	44	Tooth present. No horizontal bone loss. No visible periapical pathology. No restorations present on tooth
25	Tooth not present	45	Tooth present. No horizontal bone loss. Mild-moderate external root resorption. No visible periapical pathology. No restorations present on tooth.
26	Tooth present. No horizontal bone loss. Sinus floor traces around alveolus. Mild external root resorption. Tapered root form. No restorations present on tooth	46	Tooth present. No horizontal bone loss. No visible periapical pathology. No restorations present on tooth
27	Tooth present. No horizontal bone loss. Sinus floor traces around alveolus. Mild external root resorption. Tapered root form. No restorations present on tooth	47	Tooth present. No horizontal bone loss. No visible periapical pathology. No restorations present on tooth
28	Tooth not present	48	Tooth not present

Other radiographs

Other radiographs	Date	Radiographic data (Figures 14.2.4 & 14.2.5)
OPG	27/03/2001	Teeth present include 17, 16, 55, 14, 13, 11, 21, 23, 24, 65, 26, 27, 37, 36, 35, 34, 33, 73, 42, 43, 44, 45, 46, 47 No restorations present Large midline diastema between teeth 11 and 21
Lat ceph	27/03/2001	Excessively proclined maxillary central incisors Retrognathic mandible Competent lips
OPG	29/04/2005	No change in teeth present since 2001 Teeth 13, 11, 21, 23, 33, 73, 42, 43 have been restored with composite
Lat ceph	29/04/2005	Maxillary central incisors have been retroclined Competent lips

Study casts

Articulation	Position	ICP
	Face bow	Yes
Diagnostic wax-up	OVD change	Not required
	Occlusal adjustment	
	Crown lengthening	Teeth 13, 23

Problem list

Problem list	Details
Medical condition	X-linked hypohidrotic ectodermal dysplasia
Aesthetics	Poor aesthetic arrangement of skeletal and dental structures High lip line Excessive proclination of maxillary incisor teeth Excessively large space in the maxillary lateral incisor sites Small, malformed incisor teeth
Speech	Distortion of labiodental sounds
TMD	NAD
Soft tissue	NAD
Oral hygiene	Fair oral hygiene Patient reports insufficient oral hygiene practices
Saliva	NAD
Periodontal	Generalised mild horizontal bone loss Advanced horizontal bone loss localised to the maxillary central incisors
Edentulism	Maxilla: • Kennedy classification class III mod 1 • mild residual ridge resorption Maxilla: • Kennedy classification class IV • severe residual ridge resorption
Occlusion	Moderate to severe class II skeletal classification Severe class II division 1 dental occlusion Molar guidance on excursive movements Posterior teeth only in contact
Tooth surface loss	Mild generalised attrition
Restorative	Poorly contoured composite resin restorations on maxillary and mandibular teeth with leakage at the margins
Prosthetic	Wide arch form in maxilla, with excessive maxillary intercanine width Excessive space for maxillary anterior teeth
Endodontic	Mild generalised external root resorption, with moderate to severe resorption associated with maxillary first premolars Invasive cervical resorption on tooth 33

Treatment options (Figure 14.2.7)
Maxilla

Treatment option 1 (1 month)
- Systemic and hygiene phase (see definitive treatment plan for details).
- Replace composite resin restorations on teeth 13, 23.
- Extract maxillary central incisors.
- RPD replacing teeth 12, 11, 21, 22.

Treatment option 2 (2 months)
- Systemic and hygiene phase (see definitive treatment plan for details).
- Refer tooth 23 to endodontist for opinion on vitality.
- Extract maxillary central incisors.
- FDP on teeth 13, 23.

Treatment option 3 (6–9 months)
- Systemic and hygiene phase (see definitive treatment plan for details).
- Refer tooth 23 to endodontist for opinion on vitality.
- Extract maxillary central incisors.
- Single crowns on teeth 13, 23.
- FDP on implants in 12 and 22 sites.

Treatment option 4 (2–3 years)
- Systemic and hygiene phase (see definitive treatment plan for details).
- Refer tooth 23 to endodontist for opinion on vitality.
- Refer to oral surgery – consider orthognathic surgery.

- Extract maxillary central incisors.
- Single crowns on teeth 13, 23.
- FDP on implants in 12 and 22 sites.

Mandible

Treatment option 1 (2–3 months)
- Systemic and hygiene phase (see definitive treatment plan for details).
- Extract tooth 33.
- Replace CR on teeth 42, 43.
- RDP replacing teeth 33, 32, 31, 41.

Treatment option 2 (6 months)
- Systemic and hygiene phase (see definitive treatment plan for details).
- Extract teeth 33, 42.
- Implant in 33 site.
- FDP on implant 33 and tooth 43.

Treatment option 3 (6 months)
- Systemic and hygiene phase (see definitive treatment plan for details).
- Extract teeth 33, 42, 41.
- Place implants in 33 and 43 sites.
- FDP on implants in the 33 and 43 sites.

Treatment plan
- Maxilla: treatment option 3.
- Mandible: treatment option 2.

Treatment phase	Detail	Timeline
Hygiene phase	Preventative strategy: • oral hygiene instruction • debridement • remineralisative protocols (nightly tooth mousse)	0
Pre-prosthetic pretreatment: phase I	Refer to an endodontist for teeth 23, 33 Extract teeth 11, 21, 33, 42 Provisional acrylic FDP for 13, 23 Provisional acrylic RPD replacing teeth 33, 32, 31, 41, 42	After endodontic consultation
Pre-prosthetic pretreatment: phase II	Crown lengthening for teeth 13, 23 Implant placement in 12, 22, 33 sites	2 months postextraction
Prosthetic phase	ACC single crowns on teeth 13, 23 ACC FDP on implants in 12 and 22 sites MCC FDP on implant 33 and tooth 34	2–3 months post-implant placement
Maintenance	Occlusal splint Issue mouth guard Review at 6 months	

					ACC	ACC---P---P---ACC		ACC						
						I		I						
18	17	16	15	14	13	12	11 / 21	22	23	24	25	26	27	28
48	47	46	45	44	43	42	41 / 31	32	33	34	35	36	37	38
									I					
					MCC----P----P----P----MCC									

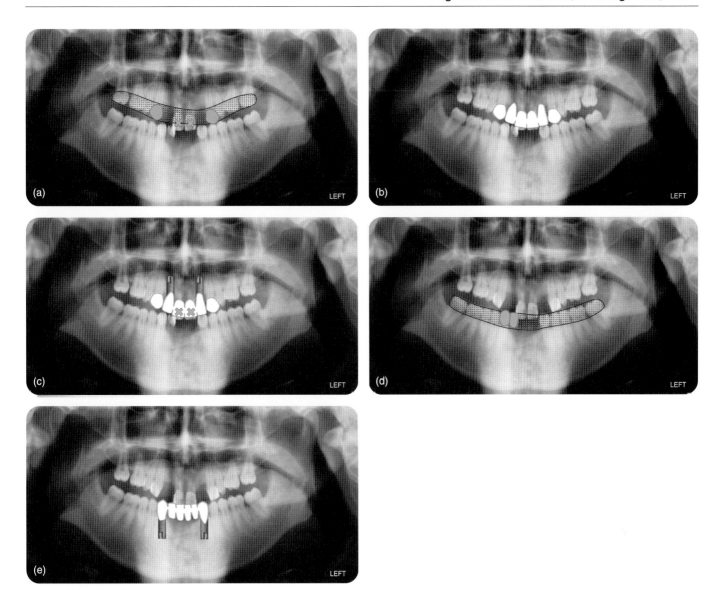

Figure 14.2.7 NobelGuide treatment options a, b, c, d, e.

Treatment sequence

Appointment	Procedure	Time (minutes)
1	Present treatment options to patient Oral hygiene instruction using disclosing solution Remineralisative protocol (tooth mousse nightly) Debridement Refer teeth 23, 33 to an endodontist for assessment Dress tooth 33 with calcium hydroxide	180
2	Review oral hygiene Consolidate definitive treatment plan	90
3	Crown preparation on teeth 13, 23 Extract teeth 13, 23 Impression of teeth 13, 23 Provisional FDP on teeth 13, 23	240
4	Extract tooth 33, 42 Issue provisional -/P replacing teeth 33, 32, 31, 41, 42	120
5	Issue Artglass FDP on teeth 13, 23	120
6	Issue radiographic guide for implants in sites 12, 22, 33	90
7	Joint consultation with surgeon (Figure 14.2.8)	60
8	Implant placement in sites 12, 22, 33 Adjust provisional FDP and RPD (Figure 14.2.9)	180
9	Review implant placement 1/52 postoperatively	30
10	Review implant placement 1/12 postoperatively	30
11	Definitive crown preparation teeth 13, 23 Impression	180
12	Definitive crown preparation tooth 43 Impression	120
13	Pick up impression for maxillary and mandibular arches	180
14	Verify impressions (Figure 14.2.10) Face bow/MMR/tooth shade	
15	Issue crowns for teeth 13, 23 Issue FDP on implants in 12 and 22 sites Issue FDP on tooth 43 and implant in 33 site Impressions for occlusal splint	180
16	RV 1/52 post-issue Issue occlusal splint	120
17	RV 3/52 post-issue Review oral hygiene	60
18	RV 5/52 post-issue (Figure 14.2.11)	30

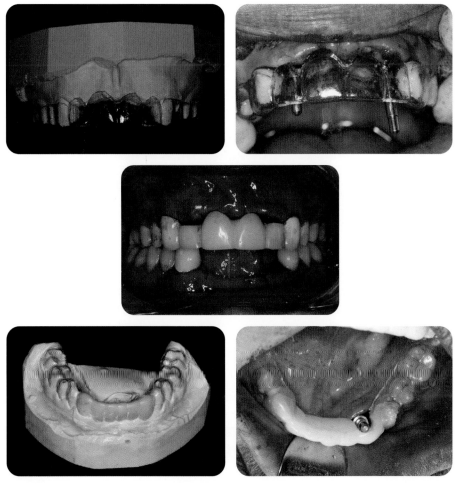

Figure 14.2.8 Implant surgery was determined with NobelGuide for implant locations and a surgical guide was developed from a diagnostic wax-up. See surgical guide and diagnostic preparations.

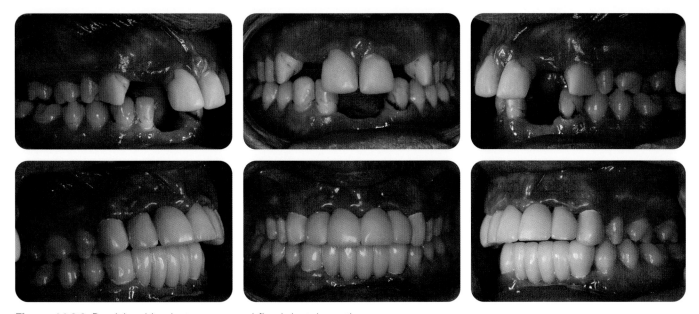

Figure 14.2.9 Provisional implant crowns and fixed dental prostheses.

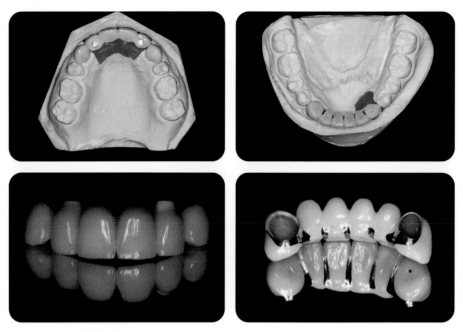

Figure 14.2.10 Construction of the definitive prosthesis.

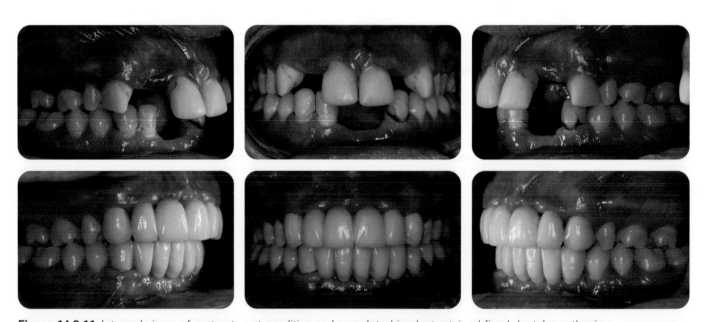

Figure 14.2.11 Intraoral views of pretreatment condition and completed implant-retained fixed dental prosthesis.

Treatment discussion

Mr J presented with the chief complaint that he wanted 'his missing teeth replaced'. He had no problems with eating or speaking and his desire for tooth replacement was to improve his appearance. Mr J reported an extensive history of dental treatment, beginning 10 years before, he has had two courses of orthodontic treatment as well as restorative and removable prosthodontic treatments. Mr J was diagnosed in 2000 with X-linked hypohidrotic ectodermal dysplasia, a condition associated with absence of structures of ectodermal origin. Dental manifestations may include multiple missing teeth, fine sparse hair, dry skin, maxillary hypoplasia and eversion of the lips. Teeth are small and conical, often with a large diastema.

Extraoral examination revealed a marked class II skeletal profile, with lip incompetence and a deep labiomental fold. There were excessively proclinated maxillary central incisors, which formed a lip trap against the lower lip. Mr J has a high smile line, with narrow buccal corridors and no mandibular incisal display. Intraoral examination revealed gingival inflammation around large composite resin restorations on teeth 13, 11, 21, 23, 33, 42 and 42. Teeth 11 and 22 were excessively proclined, exhibited class II mobility and deep periodontal probing depths. The interincisal space created by orthodontics was excessive for the missing maxillary lateral incisors and the residual ridge in the mandibular anterior region was knife-edge in cross-section. Radiographic examination revealed a moderate to large internal resorption defect on tooth 33 at the mid-root level. The patient requested replacement of teeth 12, 22, 32, 31 and 41. He had no success in the past with wearing partial dentures and preferred a fixed solution. Mr J declined treatment options involving orthognathic surgery or further orthodontic treatment.

Teeth 11 and 21 have a poor periodontal and prosthetic prognosis. In order to replace teeth 12, 11, 21 and 22 with a fixed solution, we can use a tooth-borne or implant-borne approach. A systematic review by Pjetursson et al. (2007a) reported the 5- and 10-year survival data for FDP on implants to be 95.2% and 86.7%, respectively. Comparable values were found when FDP were supported by teeth (93.8% and 89.5%, respectively). In a retrospective, cross-sectional study, Walton et al. (1986) found that the canine-to-canine bridge had the highest level of service of all tooth-borne bridges, with an average lifespan of 10.4 years; however, subject numbers were low and the study was retrospective. Cone-beam CT scans demonstrated substantial bone in the 12 and 22 sites. In light of the wide span and the good clinical service offered by an FDP on implants, Mr J elected to replace the missing maxillary incisors with an FDP on implants in the 12 and 22 sites.

In order to replace teeth 32, 31 and 41 with a FDP, tooth-borne or implant-borne options are possible. Cone-beam CT scan revealed insufficient bone in 32, 31 and 41 sites. Tooth 33 was examined by an endodontist who diagnosed untreatable grade IV invasive cervical resorption. Tooth 42 is of little value to support a long-span FDP, hence would be extracted if fixed treatment is sought. This leaves the treatment options of extraction of teeth 33 and 42 and an FDP on and implant in the 33 site and tooth 43, or further extraction of teeth 33, 42 and 43 and an FDP on implants in 33 and 43 sites.

In the systematic review by Pjetursson et al. (2007a), the authors concluded that the 5- and 10-year survival data on implant–implant FDPs was 95.2% and 86.7%, respectively. When the support was a combination of implant and tooth, the respective values were 95.5% at 5 years and 77.4% at 10 years. Both the implant–implant and implant–tooth connections were characterised by similar prosthetic and biological outcomes at 5 years. Pjetursson and colleagues concluded that FDPs should preferentially include solely implant-supported FDPs and only for reasons of anatomical structures or patient-centred preferences, and as a second option should FDPs on teeth and implants be chosen. This information was presented to the patient and he elected to preserve tooth 43. The edentulous space in the mandibular arch was restored with an FDP on an implant in the 33 site and tooth 43, and was chosen for anatomical and patient-centred preferences, both of which comply with the reported data.

The restorations on teeth 13 and 23 will require replacement due to poor aesthetics and caries. Several approaches are available to restore lost tooth structure, including a direct and indirect approach. A direct approach allows the use of composite resin, while an indirect approach allows use of all-ceramic or metal–ceramic materials. Limited evidence is available on the long-term clinical service of large composite resin reconstruction of anterior teeth. Poyser et al. (2007) conducted a case series on 168 composite resin build-ups at an increased OVD, over a 2.5-year follow-up period where 6% required replacement. Hemmings et al. (2000) conducted a randomised control trial to test the clinical service of microfill and microhybrid composite resin restorations used to restore anterior teeth at an increased OVD. A total of 89.4% of restorations were successful after 30 months, with substantially better results when a microhybrid composite resin was used. The systematic review by Pjetursson et al. (2007b) reported 5-year survival rates for metal–ceramic restorations and all-ceramic restorations of 95.6% and 93.3%, respectively. When Procera copings were used, results were comparable. In a large prospective case series (Walton et al. 1999) of up to 10-year follow-up of tooth supported metal-ceramic crowns, 94% were surviving at 10 years, with a 3% repair and failure rate respectively. As the literature shows, extracoronal restorations demonstrate excellent longevity and aesthetics, and the FDPs on implants restored in ceramic, and teeth 13 and 23 restored with ceramo-metal.

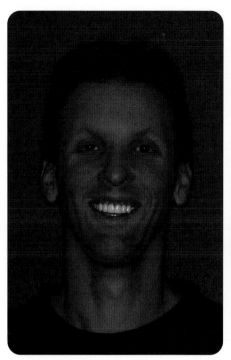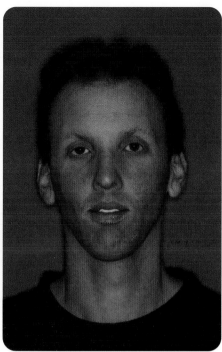

Figure 14.2.12 Extraoral views of completed treatment – note high smile line.

Review at 1 year (Figure 14.2.12)

1. Oral health status - oral hygiene and plaque control – soft tissue health – check home-care programme and advise on frequency of brushing, use of dental floss and mouth rinses; note recurrent dental caries associated with restorations or new carious lesions; note periodontal status – check probing depths and record changes; new PA radiographs to check alveolar bone levels

   Intraoral examination of soft and hard tissues did not reveal any significant abnormalities. Oral hygiene was fair, with mild interproximal soft deposits. The patient reported adequate oral hygiene practices: brushing twice a day with a medium tooth brush and flossing once a day. Periodontal probing depths were 3mm or less, with absence of bleeding on probing. The patient developed moderate gingival recession, with 1mm buccal gingival recession around the crown margins on teeth 13, 23 and 43 and the titanium abutment in site 33. The patient reported some sensitivity on tooth 43; however, restorative margins remain intact and no new carious lesions were noted. Neither the teeth nor prosthesis had developed mobility.

2. Medical status – change in general health and implications for oral health

   There were no changes in medical status.

3. Occlusion – check tooth contacts with GHM foil at ICP, RCP, lateral and protrusive excursive contacts – note lateral contact details, especially where there is a fracture of restorative material – record, photograph fracture and contact details with GHM foil and comment on reason for fracture.

   Neither the prosthesis nor the crowns showed any signs of material fracture. The prostheses were in shim stock clearance, with canine guidance on excursive movements. The teeth showed mild to moderate wear facets; however, the patient was not aware of any parafunctional habits.

4. Radiographs – 1-year review PA views for specific details of the status of crowns on teeth and implants. Check crown margins and alveolar bone levels; measure thread exposure to bone crest around implants and correlate with clinical details as in 1 above; at 2 years an OPG may add global information.

   Periapical radiographs demonstrated consistent bone levels around the teeth as well as the implants. No change in the apical periodontal ligament was recorded. Implant prosthesis did not demonstrate an opening between the implant–prosthetic junction.

5. Discuss oral health related quality of life – comfort, appearance, function – chewing and speech; whether there has been a change in confidence, social interaction and relationships.

   The patient reported improvement in comfort, appearance and function since initial examination and remarked 'It is 100% on what it was'. The patient advised that he is still cautious in using his front teeth to 'rip into crusty bread'.

6. Seek any additional comments from the patient about the treatment and whether they would undertake the process again if needed.

   The patient responded positively that he would proceed with treatment again.

References

Hemmings, K.W., Darbar, U.R. & Vaughan, S. (2000) Tooth wear treated with direct composite restorations at an increased vertical dimension: results at 30 months. *Journal of Prosthetic Dentistry*, 83 (3), 287–293.

Pjetursson, B.E., Bragger, U., Lang, N.P. *et al.* (2007a) Comparison of survival and complication rates of tooth-supported fixed dental prostheses (FDPs) and implant-supported FDPs and single crowns (SCs). *Clinical Oral Implants Research*, 18 (Suppl. 3), 97–113.

Pjetursson, B.E., Sailer, I., Zwahlen, M. *et al.* (2007b) A systematic review of the survival and complication rates of all-ceramic and metal-ceramic reconstructions after an observation period of at least 3 years. Part I: Single crowns. *Clinical Oral Implants Research*, 18 (Suppl. 3), 73–85.

Poyser, N.J., Briggs, P.F., Chana, H.S. *et al.* (2007) The evaluation of direct composite restorations for the worn mandibular anterior dentition - clinical performance and patient satisfaction. *Journal of Oral Rehabilitation*, 34 (5), 361–376.

Walton, J.N., Gardner, F.M. & Agar, J.R. (1986) A survey of crown and fixed partial denture failures: length of service and reasons for replacement. *Journal of Prosthetic Dentistry*, 56 (4), 416–421.

Walton, T.R. (1999) A 10-year longitudinal study of fixed prosthodontics: clinical characteristics and outcome of single-unit metal-ceramic crowns. *International Journal of Prosthodontics*, 12 (6) 519–526.

15

Rehabilitation after Tumour Surgery

Introduction by Christine Wallace

A multidisciplinary team is the key to success in the management of this select patient cohort. The ultimate goals are: to remove the cancer and prevent its recurrence; to preserve or restore form and function; to minimise the postoperative sequelae; and to try to maintain patient morale. Currently, the therapeutic modalities that are available include surgery, radiation treatment, chemotherapy, combined modality treatment, as well as different strategies aimed at lifestyle changes and hence prevention.

The optimal rehabilitation of the patient treated for tumour of the oral cavity begins at the time of diagnosis and requires extensive preoperative planning to allow:

- optimal surgical reconstruction to minimise large deficits and loss of form and function without prior warning;
- utilisation of surgical templates and proformers where applicable to allow communication and deglutition as quickly as possible post-surgery;
- postoperative assessment of the patient's deficits and limitations to allow further surgical or prosthodontic rehabilitation in order to provide the patient with the best quality of life possible.

A discussion on the aetiology, histology and staging of the tumours of the head and neck region is outside the realm of this synopsis. However, it is important to understand some of the general characteristics of these tumours and how these influence treatment. For example:

1. Certain primary sites are considered high risk since they have a higher risk for nodal metastasis compared to other sites in the oral cavity. The more posteriorly located lesion will require consideration of elective treatment of the clinically negative neck in initial treatment planning.
2. The size of the primary tumour impacts significantly on the decision to:

- either close the defect surgically or prosthetically, or
- whether to treat the tumour surgically or primarily by radiation.

3. Whether the tumour has invaded bone will impact on the need for surgical resection of either the maxilla or mandible. A decision will be required as to whether primary closure can be achieved or if a free tissue transfer is required. Obviously, this treatment procedure comes with increased risk and morbidity at the donor site.
4. Clinically palpable lymph nodes will mandate the need for comprehensive neck dissection as part of the surgical protocol necessitating postoperative physiotherapy for improved cervical movements.
5. History of previous treatment influences the selection of therapy for a subsequent tumour. For example, patients who have previously received radiation therapy are not considered candidates for further radiation therapy if they develop a second oral cancer.

Additionally, confounding treatment modalities are patient factors that include the person's age, general medical condition and tolerance to extensive time-consuming surgical treatment, as well as their lifestyle choices and proximity to care. Patients in the older category are not necessarily precluded from complex and long-term treatment options but they may require ongoing assistance with keeping appointments as well as help with accepting the outcome of their treatment (Piccirillo 1995, Singh *et al.* 1997).

Ultimately, the treatment choice is patient and surgeon specific. It is decided in a multidisciplinary team environment where all the factors can be examined and discussed with the patient and their family. Unfortunately, even in this environment patients do experience side-effects of treatment, including issues with mastication, deglutition, speech, oral competence, tongue mobility, cosmesis and self-image. Prosthodontists are able to best manage many of these issues prosthetically either

---

Oral Rehabilitation: A Case-Based Approach, First Edition. Edited by Iven Klineberg, Diana Kingston.
© 2012 Blackwell Publishing Ltd. Published 2012 by Blackwell Publishing Ltd.

with a fixed or removable appliances. Working in conjunction with speech pathologists, many devices can be made quite simply that can be modified for individual patient specifics to address many of the patient's needs and provide an excellent functional result. There are times when a removable appliance will not be successful and it is in these circumstances that a surgical solution may be required; in severe situations maybe nothing more can be done for the patients.

References

Piccirillo, J.F. (1995) Inclusion of comorbidity in a staging system for head and neck cancer. *Oncology (Williston Park)*, 9 (9), 831–836.

Singh, B., Bhaya, M., Stern, J. *et al.* (1997) Validation of the Charleston comorbidity index in patients with head and neck cancer; a multi-institutional study. *Laryngoscope*, 107 (11), 1469–1475.

Case 15.1 Mrs Beryl K

Max Guazzato

Patient: Mrs Beryl C (date of birth 09/05/1926)

Presenting complaint

Description	'I would like to replace some of the missing maxillary teeth to support the lip and be able to talk'
Onset	'In September 2005 I lost a molar without any apparent reason. I was seen by a local dentist who thought I had gum disease and neglected the situation for a few months. Later I joined A service and saw a dentist and had another tooth extracted and a denture made to replace the missing teeth. The gum was still inflamed (red patch) and I was then finally referred to an oncologist at a B hospital' 'A surgical procedure was completed in August 2006. I was diagnosed with squamous cell carcinoma (SCC) which was low grade but invasive. As a result I had a hemimaxillectomy, and my salivary glands and lymph nodes were removed. A skin graft covered the deficiency. Since then I have been waiting for a prosthesis to replace my missing teeth' Official diagnosis from hospital documents: 'well-differentiated invasive SCC'
Frequency	N/A
Duration	N/A
Intensity	N/A
Triggering	N/A
Aggravating	N/A
Alleviating	N/A
Treatment received	See above
Medication	Nil
Allergies	Nil
Trauma	N/A

Other complaints

Function	'Normal before the SCC, limited to the left side. Talking is a problem I have to focus. I've always had malocclusion'
TMD	Nil
Headaches	Nil
Parafunction	Nil
Habits	Nil
Cervical	Nil
Dental	Currently being seen in the general dentistry clinic at the Centre for Oral Health for minor dental treatment
Periodontal	History of periodontitis currently seen by specialist clinic at the Centre for Oral Health
Dentures	Did not like the aesthetics of the partial denture (saw the wires)
Splint	Nil
Saliva	'Sometimes I feel my mouth is dry'
Breathe	Nose breather
Cosmetic	Nil
Others	Loss of hearing and pressure in the right ear (fluid built up) and nerve damage

Patient's expectations

- 'I would like to have a prosthesis to support my lip and be able to talk properly.'
- 'I would like to improve my appearance.'
- 'I know that function would be still limited, but I would like to increase my confidence.'

History
Medical history

General Practitioner		
Cardiovascular	Endocarditis	
	Cerebrovascular accident (stroke) in 1981 and 1991 that did not cause residual deficits – most likely a transient ischaemic attack. There is currently 75% blockage of some arteries. Ms K had an angina episode during the surgical procedure for SCC	
	Hyperlipidaemia	
	Recently, Ms K has been hospitalised for 1 day (mid October) with symptoms such as irregular heartbeat and fatigue. She was prescribed Digoxin and released the day after (suspected congestive heart failure)	
Respiratory	Nil	
Gastrointestinal	Nil	
Neurological	Nil	
Endocrine	Nil	
Haematological	Nil	
Integumentary	Nil	
Genitourinary	Nil	
Musculoskeletal	Osteoarthritis	
Immune system	Nil	
Allergies	Antibiotics (patient is not sure about this and no tests have been done)	
Operations	Lost finger in an accident; endartectomy, SCC	
Trauma	Nil	
Others	Carcinoma (SCC of the maxilla)	
Medication	Naprosyn 500 mg/day (naproxen) alternated with Inza 500 mg/day (naproxen)	Osteoarthritis (increases risk of heart attack; interacts and neutralises aspirin)
	Aspirin 100 mg every 2 days	To prevent transient ischaemic attack (may cause severe bleeding)
	Lipitor 40 mg/day	Hypercholesterolaemia
	Premarin 30 mg/day	Hormone replacement therapy
	Tofranil 25 mg/day	Depression (may cause dry mouth)
	Digoxin 10 mg/day	Congestive heart failure

Social history

Marital status	Divorced		
Children	4		
Occupation	Retired registered nurse		
Recreational drugs	Nil		
Smoking	Nil		
Diet			
		Soft drinks	Nil
		Sports drinks	Nil
		Lemons	Nil
		Acidic foods	Nil
		Sweet foods	Nil
	√	Water	1–2 L/day
		Tea	Nil
	√	Coffee	1 cup coffee/day
		Alcohol	Nil
		Hard/brittle foods	Nil
		Ice crunching	Nil
Habits/hobbies	Gardening		

Dental history

Date of last examination	Seen at B hospital since 2006
Oral hygiene routine	Brushes 2–3 times a day and flosses regularly
TMD	Nil
Splint	Nil
OMFS	Diagnosed with SCC of the right maxilla in 2006. In September 2005 Ms K lost a molar without any apparent reason. She saw a dentist who confused the lesion with periodontal disease and neglected it for a few months. In 2006, Ms K joined A service where she had another tooth extracted and a denture made to replace the missing teeth. The gum was still inflamed (red patch) and she was finally referred to an oncologist at B hospital In August 2006 she was diagnosed with SCC, which was low grade but invasive. She therefore had a hemimaxillectomy, and salivary glands and lymph nodes were removed. A skin graft covered the deficiency. The official diagnosis from hospital documents is 'well-differentiated invasive SCC'
Extractions	Numerous maxillary teeth (only 23, 24, 25, 26, 27 are present) and some mandibular posterior teeth (38, 37, 36, 35, 45, 48 have been extracted)
Dentures	Mandibular partial denture fitted in 1980 and still functional Maxillary partial denture fitted in 2006 and never worn
Orthodontics	Nil
Periodontics	Regularly seen by periodontist after the removal of the SCC for periodontal maintenance
Endodontics	Nil
Crown and bridge	FGC 46
Implants	Nil
Cosmetic	Nil
Other	Extensive restorative work

Extraoral examination (Figure 15.1.1)
Aesthetics

Head and neck	Muscles and lips pull to the right as a result of surgical removal of the maxilla (right side only), parotid gland and the lymph nodes	
Facial symmetry	Asymmetric due to the surgical procedure for the SCC and removal of the right maxilla, salivary gland and the regional lymph nodes	
Profile	Concave due to lack of teeth from 18 to 23, lack of support for the upper lip, skeletal class III, loss of OVD	
Nasolabial angle	80° (loss of vertical dimension)	
Facial folds	Deep and asymmetric nasolabial folds	
Midlines	Face/maxillary centrals	N/A
	Maxillary/mandibular centrals	Mandibular midline deviated on the right side by some millimetres (difficult to assess without teeth)
Lip posture	Symmetry	Asymmetric
	Upper lip	Short and incompetent
	Lower lip	Normal
	Competence	No
	Tooth display	Up to 25, high lip line
Occlusal plane	Parallel to ala tragus line	No
	Parallel to interpupillary line	No
	Over-eruption	Slightly anterior lower teeth
Vertical	FWS	7 mm
	OVD assessment	OVD reduced
Smile assessment	Symmetry	No
	Lip line	High
	Gingival display	Nil
	Tooth display	From 23 to 25
	Buccal corridor	N/A

Phonetics

	Normal	Abnormal
Labial (m)		√
Labiodental (f/v)		√
Linguodental (th)		√
Interdental (s)		√
Linguopalatal (k/ng)		√

Temporomandibular assessment

TMJ		Additional information
Click	Nil	NAD
Crepitus	Nil	NAD
Tenderness	Nil	NAD

Muscle tenderness	Right	Left
Temporalis	Nil	Nil
Masseter	Nil	Nil
Posterior mandible	Nil	Nil
Anterior mandible	Nil	Nil
Glands	Nil	
Nodes	Nil	

Jaw movement	Measurement (mm)	Reference points
Maximal opening	45	Tooth 23
Right laterotrusion	WNL	
Left laterotrusion	WNL	
Midline deviation	N/A	
Maximal protrusion	N/A	
Opening pathway	Slightly deviated right side	
Overjet	−2 (assessed on previous photographs)	
Overbite	2 (assessed on previous photographs)	

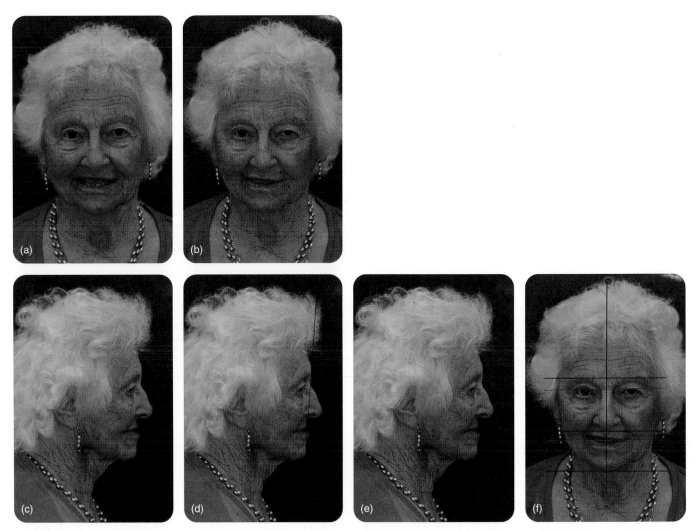

Figure 15.1.1 Extraoral examination. Patient attempting to smile (a), nerve and muscle damage caused by the hemimaxillectomy resulted in poor control of facial muscles and facial expression. Patient in intercuspal position showing concave profile and an acute nasolabial angle (b–e). Facial symmetry but reduced lower third facial height (f).

Intraoral examination (Figure 15.1.2)
Soft tissues

Tissue	Healthy	Abnormal	Additional information
Lips		√	Angular cheilitis
Labial vestibule		√	Not present on the right
Cheeks	√		
Palate		√	Not present on the right
Oropharynx	√		
Tongue	√		
Floor	√		
Frenal attachments	√		

Ridges	Maxilla	Mandible
Edentulous areas	18–22 included	38–33 and 45
Arch shape	N/A	V-shaped
Resorption	Severe in the region of 11–22	Moderate in quadrant 3
Palatal vault	N/A	N/A
Tori	Nil	Nil
Frenal attachments	Average	Average
Mucosa	Flabby in the region of 11–22	Normal
Pathology	No	No

Oral cleanliness

Condition	Yes	No			
Plaque	√		Generalised	Moderate	Supragingival + subgingival
Calculus	√		Localised	Mild	Supragingival + subgingival
Food impaction	√		23–24		
Stains	√		Generalised		
Halitosis		√			

Saliva

Water intake	1–2 L water/day and 1 cup coffee/day
Quality	Slightly low: watery; pH 6.6; buffering capacity 7 (low)
Quantity	Low: 4.0 ml in 5 minute test
Pathology	Nil
Medications affecting	Tofranil

Periodontium

CPITN

–	–	2
2	2	2

Gingiva	Biotype	Medium
	Colour	Pink with localised areas of inflammation and redness
	Contour	Normal
	Consistency	Firm
Papillae	Colour	Pink with localised areas of inflammation and redness
	Contour	Normal

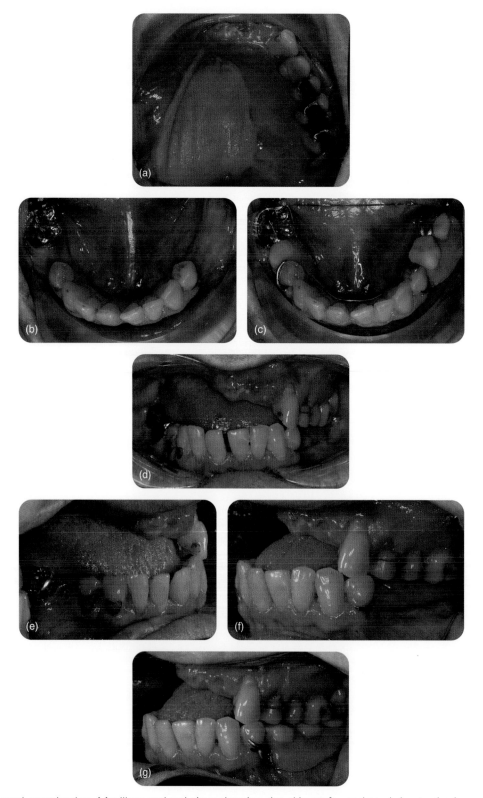

Figure 15.1.2 Intraoral examination. Maxillary occlusal view showing the skin graft used to obdurate the large maxillary deficiency on the right (a). Mandibular occlusal view with (c) and without (b) removable dental prosthesis. Frontal view with teeth in intercuspal position; the only occlusal contact was between tooth 23 and 34 (d); lateral view without (e,f) and with the denture (g).

Periodontal charting

Maxillary arch

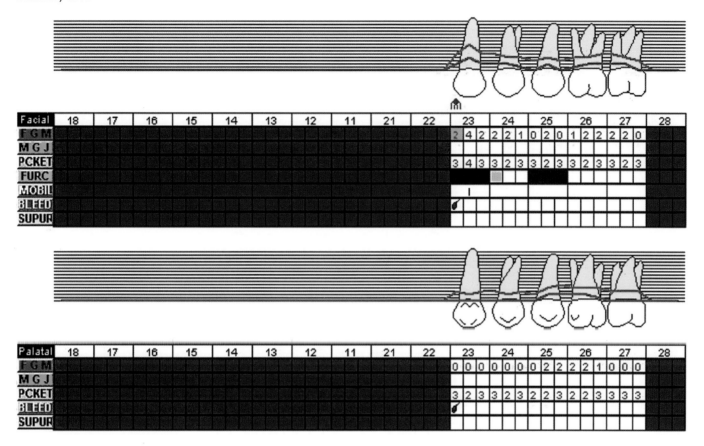

Facial	18	17	16	15	14	13	12	11	21	22	23		24		25		26		27		28
F G M											2 4	2 2	2 1	0 2	0 1	2 2	2 2	0			
M G J																					
PCKET											3 4	3 3	2 3	3 2	3 3	2 3	3 2	3			
FURC																					
MOBIL											I										
BLEED											✔										
SUPUR																					

Palatal	18	17	16	15	14	13	12	11	21	22	23		24		25		26		27		28
F G M											0 0	0 0	0 0	0 2	2 2	2 1	0 0	0			
M G J																					
PCKET											3 2	3 3	2 3	2 2	3 2	2 3	3 3	3			
BLEED											✔										
SUPUR																					

Mandibular arch

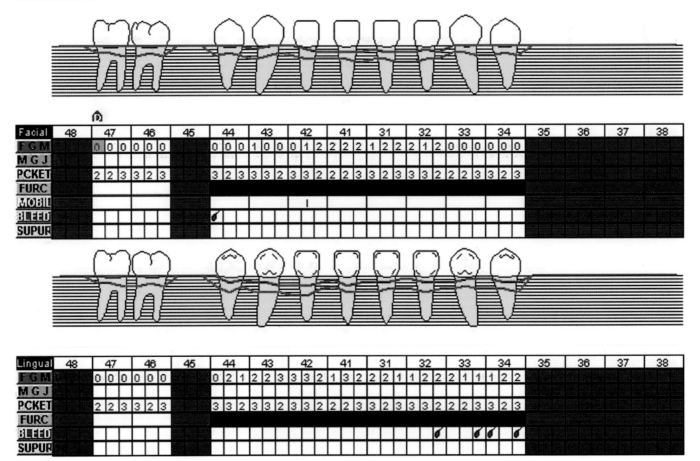

Facial

	48	47	46	45	44	43	42	41	31	32	33	34	35	36	37	38
FGM		0 0 0	0 0 0		0 0 0	1 0 0	0 1 2	2 2 2	1 2 2	2 2 1	2 0 0	0 0 0				
MGJ																
PCKET		2 2 3	3 2 3		3 2 3	3 3 2	3 3 2	2 2 3	3 2 3	3 3 2	2 2 3	3 2 3				
FURC																
MOBIL							I									
BLEED					●											
SUPUR																

Lingual

	48	47	46	45	44	43	42	41	31	32	33	34	35	36	37	38
FGM		0 0 0	0 0 0		0 2 1	2 2 3	3 3 2	1 3 2	2 2 1	1 2 2	2 1 1	1 2 2				
MGJ																
PCKET		2 2 3	3 2 3		3 3 2	3 3 2	3 3 2	2 2 3	3 2 3	3 3 2	2 2 3	3 2 3				
FURC																
BLEED										●	● ●	●				
SUPUR																

Occlusion

Arch compatibility	Fairly compatible arches, compatibility compromised by skeletal class III relationship			
Occlusal plane	Curve of Spee	N/A		
	Curve of Wilson	N/A		
Posterior support	Nil			
Skeletal class classification	Class III (assessed with clinical examination)			
Angle right	Molar	Class II	Canine	Class I
Angle left	Molar	Class II	Canine	Class I
Anterior overbite	N/A			
Anterior overjet	N/A			
Cross-bites	Nil			
Open-bites	Nil			
RP to IP slide	0 mm			
FWS	Close/M/swallow test	7 mm		

Tooth guidance

Right laterotrusion

```
              3 4 5 6 7 8
  7 6   4 3 2 1 | 1 2 3 4
```

Left laterotrusion

```
                  3 4 5 6 7
  7 6   4 3 2 1 | 1 2 3 4
```

Protrusion

```
              3 4 5 6 7
  7 6   4 3 2 1 | 1 2 3 4
```

Tooth surface loss

General tooth surface loss (caries)

```
              3 4 5 6 7
  7 6   4 3 2 1 | 1 2 3 4
```

Bruxofacets – mild

```
              3 4 5 6 7
  7 6   4 3 2 1 | 1 2 3 4
```

Erosion – not apparent

```
              3 4 5 6 7
  7 6   4 3 2 1 | 1 2 3 4
```

Attrition – mild

```
              3 4 5 6 7
  7 6   4 3 2 1 | 1 2 3 4
```

Toothbrush abrasion – minimal

```
              3 4 5 6 7
  7 6   4 3 2 1 | 1 2 3 4
```

Dental charting

Tooth no.	Clinical findings	Prognosis	Comments
18	Missing		Nil
17	Missing		Nil
16	Missing		Nil
15	Missing		Nil
14	Missing		Nil
13	Missing		Nil
12	Missing		Nil
11	Missing		Nil
21	Missing		Nil
22	Missing		Nil
23	MPD composite	Good	Nil
24	MODL composite	Good	Nil
25	MOD amalgam	Good	Nil
26	MOD amalgam	Good	Nil
27	MOD amalgam	Good	Nil
28	Missing		Nil
38	Missing		Nil
37	Missing		Nil
36	Missing		Nil
35	Missing		Nil
34	L amalgam, deep root caries	Poor	Tooth is not restorable
33	Unrestored	Good	Nil
32	Unrestored	Good	Nil
31	MOL composite	Good	Nil
41	MOL composite	Good	Nil
42	Unrestored	Good	Nil
43	L amalgam	Good	Nil
44	L amalgam	Good	Nil
45	Missing		Nil
46	FGC	Good	Nil
47	Amalgam crown + pins	Questionable	Difficult to clean, very large amalgam, but there is no opposing dentition
48	Missing		Nil

Visualised dental charting

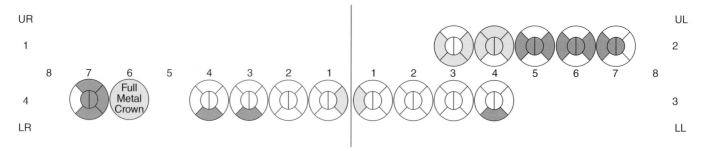

Previous prosthesis – N/A

   Teeth replaced

       3 4 5 6 7

7 6 5 4 3 2 1   1 2 3 4 5 6 7 8

	Mandible	Maxilla
Age	12 years	
Type	Metal base	
	Distal extension base	
Kennedy classification	Class II	
Appearance	Acceptable	
VDO	Metal stop in 36, would need relining	
Stability	Abutment tooth 34 will be extracted compromising stability that is now fair	
Support	Wear in acrylic teeth	
Retention	Good	
Hygiene	Acceptable	
Patient opinion	No complaints	

Special tests

Test	Performed	Additional information
Percussion	√	No teeth sensitive to percussion
Palpation	√	No tenderness
Vitality	√	Teeth 34, 46, 47 not responsive
Cusp loading	√	Normal
Other	√	Saliva test reported above

Radiographs

- Panoramic radiographs (Figures 15.1.3, 15.1.4 & 15.1.5).
- Periapical/full mouth series radiographs (Figure 15.1.6).

Information obtained from clinical and radiographic examinations and prognostic ratings for 10 years of remaining teeth.

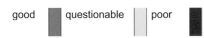

good ▮ questionable ▯ poor ▮

FDI	Finding	Prognosis	FDI	Finding	Prognosis
18	Missing		38	Missing	
17	Missing		37	Missing	
16	Missing		36	Missing	
15	Missing		35	Missing	
14	Missing		34	L amalgam, deep root caries	
13	Missing		33	Unrestored	
12	Missing		32	Unrestored	
11	Missing		31	MOL composite	
21	Missing		41	MOL composite	
22	Missing		42	Unrestored	
23	MPD composite		43	L amalgam	
24	MODL composite		44	L amalgam	
25	MOD amalgam		45	Missing	
26	MOD amalgam		46	FGC, asymptomatic periapical radiolucency	
27	MOD amalgam		47	Amalgam crown + pins, asymptomatic periapical radiolucency	
28	Missing		48	Missing	

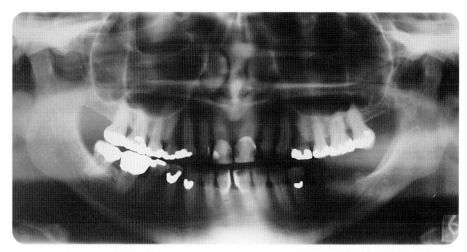

Figure 15.1.3 Panoramic radiograph in 2001.

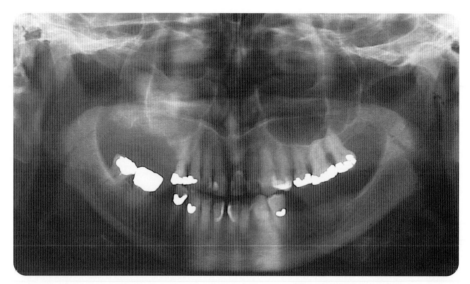

Figure 15.1.4 Panoramic radiograph in 2005 after diagnosis of carcinoma and extraction of several maxillary teeth.

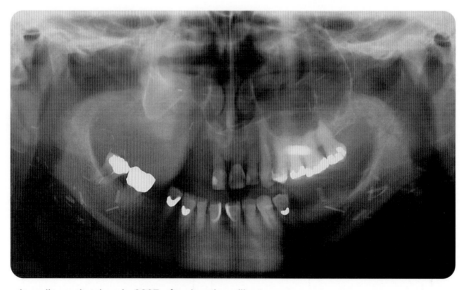

Figure 15.1.5 Panoramic radiograph taken in 2007 after hemimaxillectomy.

Study casts (Figure 15.1.7)

Articulation	Position	ICP
	Face bow	Yes
Diagnostic wax-up	OVD change	+1 mm
	Occlusal adjustment	Nil
	Crown lengthening	Nil

Provisional diagnosis

Category	Diagnosis/problem list
Medical conditions	Surgically removed SCC with removal of right parotid gland and regional lymph nodes Cardiovascular disease Medications with possible side-effects such as bleeding and xerostomia Osteoarthritis
TMD	Nil
Orofacial pain	Nil
Aesthetics	Lip collapse due to the lack of teeth and maxillary bone
Phonetics	Unable to speak properly due to the lack of anterior maxillary teeth
Soft tissues	Collapse of the upper lip
Oral hygiene	Nil
Occlusion	Occlusal contact only between 23 and 24, and 33 and 34. Tooth 34 must be extracted
Saliva	Xerostomia
Tooth surface loss	Unremarkable
Edentulism	Maxillary and mandibular partially edentulous
Restorative	Heavily restored dentition
Prosthodontics	Maxilla: lack of hard and soft tissue support for the restoration of anterior teeth; lack of maxillary bone in the right side; poor bone quantity and quality in the region of 11–22; heavily restored remaining maxillary teeth Mandible: class II Kennedy with the distal extension base as the only region with opposing dentition suitable for chewing
Periodontics	History of mild periodontitis
Endodontics	Asymptomatic periapical radiolucency 37 and 36

Treatment goals
Short-term
- Control of disease (periodontitis and dental caries).
- Control dry mouth.
- Minimise dental treatment.
- Issue of a provisional vacuum form denture for 11, 21, 22.
- Diet and oral hygiene advice.

Long-term
- Restore anterior maxillary teeth for aesthetics and phonetics with a prosthesis that does not interfere with the skin graft.
- Restore mandibular missing/extracted teeth to allow for acceptable function.
- Restore occlusal stability.
- Minimise maintenance.
- Replace missing or extracted teeth.
- Protect remaining tooth structure.
- Preservation existing tooth structure.
- Preservation periodontal tissues.

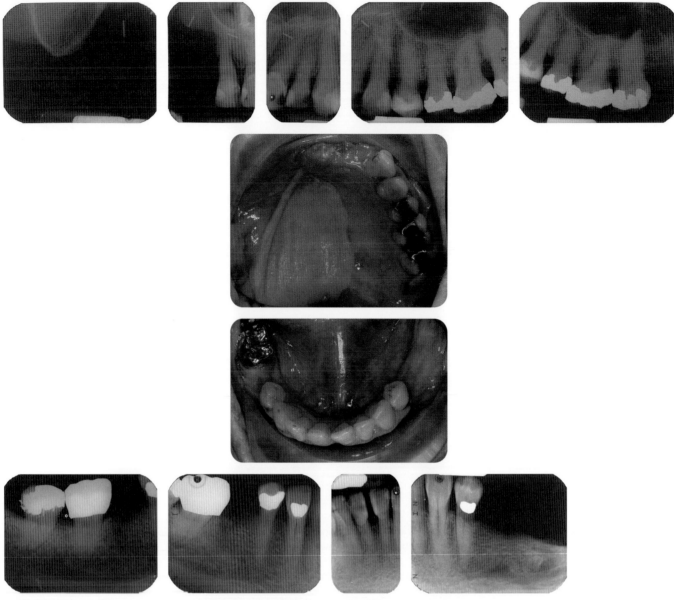

Figure 15.1.6 Periapical radiographs and corresponding intraoral views.

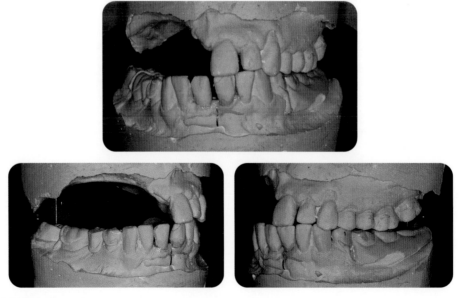

Figure 15.1.7 Articulated study casts.

Treatment options

All treatment options include:

- preliminary OHI;
- supportive periodontal treatment;
- palliative treatment for xerostomia.

Maxilla

Treatment option 1: Conventional metal-base partial RDP limited up to tooth 13
- Advantages:
  - minimal intervention;
  - inexpensive.
- Disadvantages:
  - the effort arm would be too long compared with the resistance arm, creating a lever action;
  - poor tissue support in the edentulous area.

Treatment option 2: Telescopic crowns of 24, 25, 26, tooth-supported metal-base partial RDP limited up to tooth 13
- Advantages: greater support and rigidity than option 1.
- Disadvantages:
  - the effort arm would be too long compared with the resistance arm;
  - poor tissue support in the edentulous area;
  - it requires more interarch space;
  - understanding, communication and ability of the dental technician is crucial;
  - it requires tooth preparation.

Treatment option 3: Milled metal-ceramic splinted crowns on 24, 25, 26, tooth-supported metal-base partial RDP limited up to tooth 13
- Advantages:
  - greater support and rigidity than option 1;
  - simpler procedure than option 2.
- Disadvantages:
  - the effort arm would be too long compared with the resistance arm, creating a lever action;
  - poor tissue support in the edentulous area;
  - requires tooth preparation.

Treatment option 4: Milled metal-ceramic splinted crowns of 24, 25, 26, insertion of one or two implants in the region of 11 and 22; tooth and implant-supported metal-base partial RDP limited up to tooth 13
- Advantages:
  - best support, retention and resistance;
  - rigidity better than in option 1;
  - level action minimised;
  - fully tooth- and implant-supported denture;
  - best protection for the skin graft.
- Disadvantages:
  - involves a surgical procedure;
  - the effort arm would be too long compared with the resistance arm, creating a lever action;

- poor tissue support in the edentulous area;
- requires teeth preparation;
- expensive treatment, although the fees are partially supported by dental companies.

Mandible

Treatment option 1: extraction of tooth 34; conventional metal-base partial removable dental prosthesis
- Advantages:
  - minimal intervention;
  - inexpensive.
- Disadvantages:
  - the denture would have a distal extension base opposing the natural dentition;
  - the distal extension base is where the patient is actually chewing;
  - lever effect on tooth 33.

Treatment option 2: extraction of tooth 34; insertion of one implant in the edentulous saddle; metal-base implant–tooth retained overdenture
- Advantages: greater support and rigidity than option 1.
- Disadvantages:
  - involves a surgical procedure;
  - relatively expensive.

Treatment option 3: extraction of tooth 34; insertion of two implants in the edentulous saddle; fixed partial dental prosthesis to replace missing teeth quadrant 3
- Advantages:
  - best support;
  - chewing efficiency.
- Disadvantages:
  - involves a surgical procedure;
  - expensive treatment.

Treatment plan accepted

- Preliminary OHI.
- Supportive periodontal treatment.
- Palliative treatment for xerostomia.

Maxilla (option 4)
- Partial vacuum form denture.
- Periodontal flap quadrant 2.
- Insertion of two implants in the region of teeth 11 and 22.
- Bone grafting.
- Milled metal-ceramic splinted crowns 24, 25, 26.
- Tooth- and implant-supported metal base partial overdenture.

Mandible (option 1)
- Extraction tooth 34.
- Distal extension base metal base RDP.

Treatment sequence

Treatment phase	Detail
Diagnostic phase	Data collection Examination Radiographs Study casts Articulation Wax-up CT scan Presentation of treatment options Informed consent
Control phase	Preliminary OHI Supportive periodontal treatment Palliative treatment for xerostomia
Surgical phase I (2 weeks after the previous phase)	Periodontal flap quadrant 2 Extraction tooth 34 Repair existing denture
Surgical phase II (after 2 months) (Figure 15.1.8)	Insertion of the implants Bone grafting
Prosthetic phase I (within phases) (Figure 15.1.9)	Preparation of 24, 25, 26 Impression Copper plating MMR articulation Master casts
Surgical phase III (3 months after stage 1)	Uncovering of the implants
Prosthetic phase II (after 4 weeks) (Figure 15.1.10)	Altered cast technique New articulation Issue distal extension base partial metal-base denture
Prosthetic phase III (within 1 month) (Fig 15.1.11)	Implant assessment Abutments and attachments selection Issue milled MCC and new provisional Abutment level impression MMR – articulation Fabrication of bar Issue bar and tooth-implant-supported partial overdenture
Maintenance (Figure 15.1.12)	Review at 2 weeks, 1 month, 6 months Review every 4 months Supportive periodontal treatment Cancer screening Radiographs Reinforcement of oral hygiene Examination / occlusion Periodontal probing

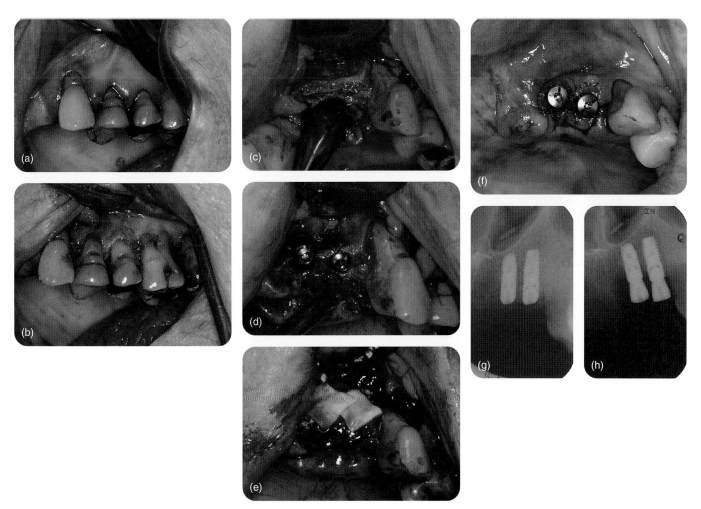

Figure 15.1.8 Surgical phases Periodontal flap and implant insertion. Subgingival calculus was removed with a periodontal flap and bone architecture was re-established (a, b). Two short (8 mm) implants were inserted in the anterior maxilla and allograft material with a collagen membrane was positioned to cover some of exposed labial wall implant threads (c–e). After 4 months, the implants were uncovered (f) and bone levels verified with periapical radiographs (g, h).

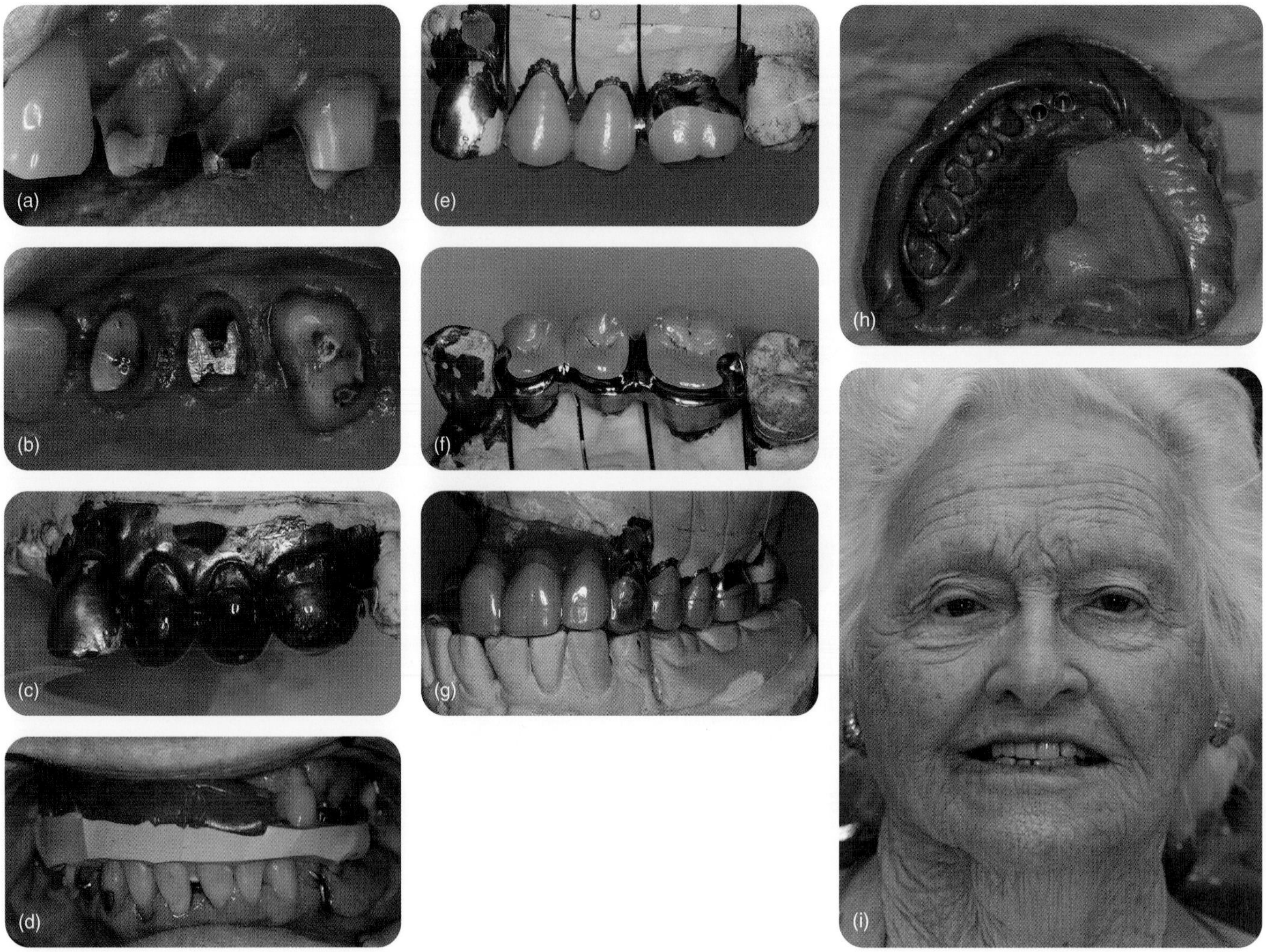

Figure 15.1.9 Prosthetic phase I Maxilla. The maxillary teeth which had a good prognosis were prepared to retain a temporary removable dental prosthesis. Preparation of teeth 24, 25, 26 (a, b). An acrylic resin base and silicon material were use to record the maxillomandibular relationship (c, d,). Milled-metal ceramic crowns were issued with a vacuum-pressed provisional prosthesis to provide lip support (e g). Impression with polyether material of the cemented crowns and implants (h). A metal base removable dental prosthesis was prepared and tried-in (i).

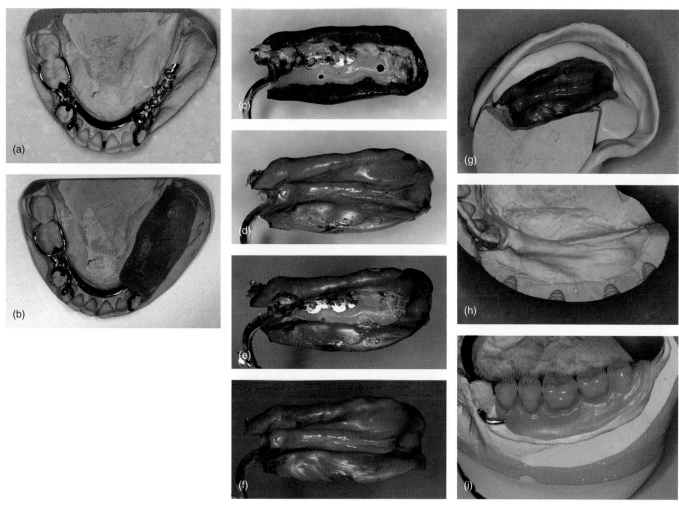

Figure 15.1.10 Prosthetic phase II Mandible. A mandibular partial removable dental prosthesis with a metal base was fabricated following the altered-cast technique. The base on the first master cast (a) with the customised tray (b). The secondary impression with thermoplastic material for denture border moulding followed by layers of polyether impression material (c–f). The final master cast with the edentulous saddle and the wax try-in (g–i).

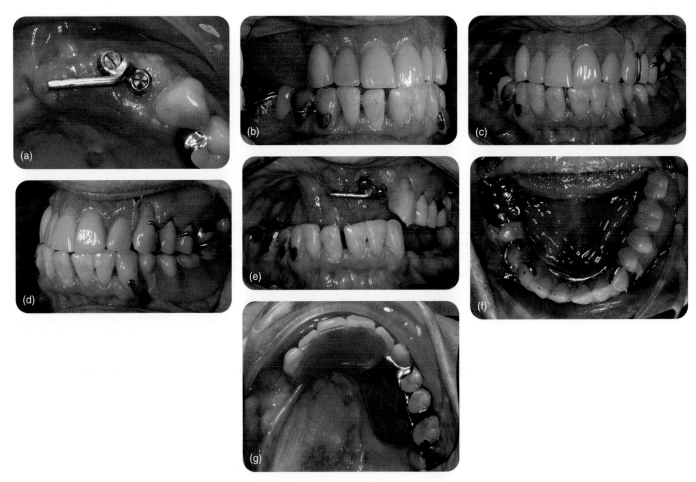

Figure 15.1.11 Prosthetic phase III Issue of definitive prosthesis. Milled metal-ceramic crowns and bar with distal cantilevered extensions supported by implants were used to retain the mandibular partial removable dental prosthesis (a–e). Intraoral view with the new removable prosthesis (f).

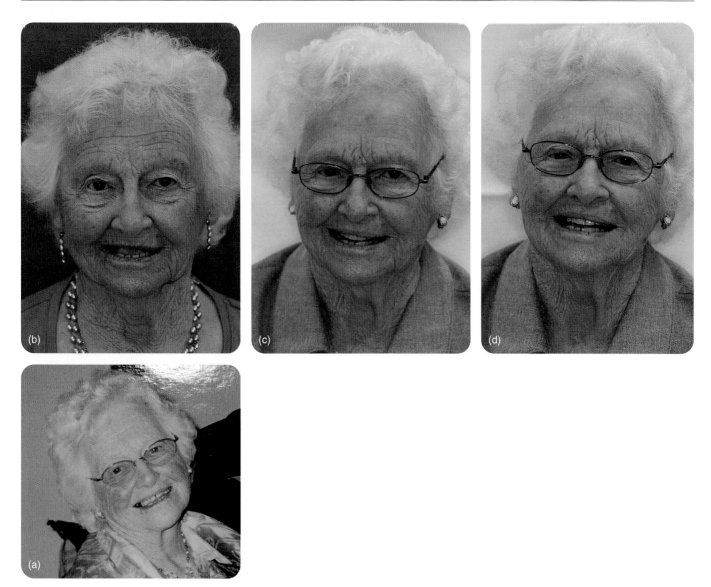

Figure 15.1.12 Extraoral views. Prior to the hemimaxillectomy (a). Prior to prosthodontics (b). After completion of oral rehabilitation (c, d).

Treatment discussion
Selected treatment for the maxilla

Ms K underwent surgical treatment for SCC consisting of removal of the teeth in the vicinity and partial removal of the maxilla corresponding to quadrant 1. This surgical procedure often results in communication between oral and nasal cavities. This opening is often repaired with an acrylic obturator prosthesis. In this case, the maxillary defect was sealed with a skin graft. Loading of the area of the skin graft is not possible as there is no maxillary bone underneath to grant support.

The main objective of the treatment was to restore some missing maxillary anterior teeth to allow lip support and to re-establish acceptable appearance and proper speech. Ideally, teeth 13, 12, 11, 21 and 22 should be restored. The restoration of the maxillary anterior teeth will result in a significant cantilever, which is exacerbated by the inability of the soft tissue to provide support. The following treatment options have been considered and discussed with the patient:

- conventional metal-base partial RDP;
- conical CMCs of 24, 25, 26; tooth-supported metal-base partial RDP;
- milled CMCs of 24, 25,26; tooth-supported metal-base partial RDP;
- milled metal ceramic splinted crowns of 24, 25, 26, insertion of one or two implants in the region of 11 and 22; tooth and implant-supported metal-base partial RDP limited up to tooth 13.

During discussion of possible treatment options, the following matters were considered before a decision was made on the most suitable treatment for Ms K:

- bone quality/quantity;
- cost/aesthetics/function;
- risk;
- patient expectations;
- stability;
- support facial tissues;
- clinical outcome;
- cleanliness;
- maintenance;
- complications.

Conventional metal-connector RDP

The use of a conventional metal-connector RDP would have the advantages of limited cost as well as minimal intervention. On the other hand, it is unlikely that this option provides retention and resistance to dislodgment for a sufficient period of time without causing damage to abutment teeth. In particular, in this case the effort arm would be too long compared with the resistance arm, creating a lever action which would not be sufficiently counteracted by tissue support in the edentulous area.

There are no studies that investigate the patient satisfaction and the longevity of conventional RDPs used in comparable clinical scenarios. In general, patient's satisfaction and longevity of conventional RDPs is influenced by patient's age, general health, previous experiences with RDPs and opposing dentition (Frank et al. 1998). According to Waliszewski (2005), the satisfaction of patients wearing an RDP seems to be more related to denture aesthetics than functional outcome. The patient was given a provisional denture with acrylic teeth embedded into a plastic vacuum form retained by the remaining teeth. Assessment of denture appearance and function was negative. However, the patient considered the provisional appliance a significant improvement for her condition, showing a positive attitude towards the treatment and ability to adapt. Ms K agreed to explore other options that may offer better stability and longevity.

Conical metal-ceramic crowns of 24, 25, 26; tooth-supported metal-connector removable partial dental prosthesis

The use of conical telescopic crown-retained dentures was first advocated by Korber (Igarashi & Goto 1997) and has been commonly used in Germany, Japan and north Europe. Wostmann et al. (2007) reported the long-term outcome of 554 telescopic crown-retained RDPs after an average follow-up period of 2.5 years. They found that the rigid connection between the tooth and the denture through the telescopic system reduced mobility and favoured axial loading and stress distribution. Survival rate at 5 years was 95% and decreased with the decrease of the number of abutments available. The main disadvantages are the unsupported cantilever; the need for greater tooth preparation; cost; and lack of experienced technical support.

Milled metal-ceramic crowns of 24, 25, 26; tooth-supported metal-connector removable partial dental prosthesis

An alternative to the concept of telescopic crowns with similar retention can be achieved with milled metal-ceramic crowns. Guide planes, occlusal rests and ideal undercuts can be created in the crowns to facilitate a conventional clasp-designed RDP. Crowns splinted together optimised retention and stability of the denture and stabilised periodontally compromised teeth. This technique is described by Chaiyabutr and Brudvik (2008). The option of conical crowns does not address the lack of support of the cantilever area of the denture, the cost is significant and the teeth require preparation.

Milled metal ceramic splinted crowns for 24, 25, 26, one or two implants in the region of 11 and 22; tooth and implant-supported metal-base RDPs (selected treatment option)

The use of dental implants to improve support for RDPs with large edentulous areas and unfavourable distribution of remaining teeth is now common practice. For example, Chikunov et al. (2008) proposed the use of implants in the contralateral quadrant (the edentulous quadrant) in unfavourable maxillary Kennedy class II patients (transformed into class IV) to improve stability and retention. Mijiritsky et al. (2005) demonstrated the effectiveness of dental implants used to increase support in Kennedy class II patients with few remaining teeth. They reported that a limited number of implants in conjunction with remaining natural teeth improves denture design by significantly reducing the effort arm and improving the fulcrum line position. This prevents rotation towards the tissue during function. These authors also investigated the clinical outcome of tooth-implant-supported dentures in 15 patients followed for 2–7 years and reported a survival rate for implants and prostheses of 100% with only minor complications.

A denture design as proposed by Mijiritsky et al. (2005) may be used for Ms K. A CT scan indicated that two implants may be placed in 11 and 22 positions. Selection of abutments, given the implant position in the CT reconstruction, excludes magnets, locator and ball attachments. A bar would allow the use of implants with unfavourable angles and the matrix would be placed as close to the implants as possible to minimise cantilever action. This design would result in a tooth-implant-supported RDP and optimise function and comfort.

Bone assessment
Bone showed that two short implants could have been used and that bone grafting was required.

This option also presented disadvantages: it required surgical procedures and preparation of teeth; and the cost was greater.

Risk analysis for the maxillary prosthesis
- The risk analysis of restoration of the mandibular arch.
- Risk factors linked to the patient's medical conditions, parafunctions and habits; the surgical procedure; and the selected prosthetic option.

Risk factors linked to the patient's local and systemic factors
Age, cardiovascular disease and hormone replacement therapy are weak contraindications for dental implant treatment (Goodacre et al. 2003, Moy et al. 2005). It is also widely accepted that the quality and quantity of the bone are the major risk factors for dental implant treatment (Moy et al. 2005).

Risk factors linked to the surgical procedure
Infections (3%), implant loss, poor healing, bleeding and increased bone loss have been reported in most studies on clinical outcomes of dental implants (Adell et al. 1990). In the case of Ms K, bleeding may be significant due to prescription aspirin; however, presurgical screening confirmed that the international normalised ratio (INR) was suitable to undergo surgical procedures.

Risk factors linked to the prosthetic procedure
Possible complications must be considered for metalceramic FDPs, conventional dentures as well as implant-retained overdentures.

Walton (2009) reported the outcome of 997 metal ceramic single crowns and 331 FDPs in a study on the impact of implant dentistry on outcomes of metal-ceramic tooth-supported single crowns and FDPs in specialist practice. Complications were classified as minor (could be undertaken in no more than 30 minutes), major (treatment required more than 30 minutes or referral to another specialty) or failure (involving modification of the tooth/restoration margin). The modes of failure were classified as biological (tooth–coronal fracture, tooth–root fracture periodontal breakdown, endodontic failure, dental caries), mechanical (lost retention, porcelain fracture, metal fracture) and aesthetic factors. The most common complications were loss of vitality, corono-radicular fracture and loss of retention. The most common failures were tooth–root fracture (especially in FDPs), periodontal breakdown, endodontic failure and dental caries.

De Backer et al. (2007) reported the outcome of 165 three-unit FDPs over 20 years by undergraduate students. Of the 134 FDPs available for analysis, 21 failed (15%). The main reasons for failure were dental caries (38%), loss of retention (10%), metal fracture (10%), and periodontal breakdown (5%). Complications of implant-retained overdentures may be summarised from Naert et al. (2004) and Trakas et al. (2006):

- Mechanical complications:
  - wear of resilient retention elements was the most frequent complication, which may be considered as maintenance when it arises infrequently;
  - fracture of the abutment;
  - loosening of the abutment screw;
  - overdenture fracture;
  - acrylic tooth fracture or de-bonding;
  - food impaction.
- Biological complications:
  - decubitus ulcers;
  - mucosal hyperplasia;
  - pain;
  - mucositis;
  - fungal infections.

Mijiritsky et al. (2005) investigated clinical outcomes of tooth-implant-supported dentures in 15 patients followed 2–7 years; this procedure and clinical situation is comparable to the treatment for Ms K. The authors reported high survival rate and only minor complications (such as one rest rupture occurring within the follow-up period).

The complications of RDPs are related to design and the consistency of the professional and home oral and denture hygiene. Infrequent professional cleaning and maintenance may lead to biological complications, including dental caries and periodontal breakdown (Bergman et al. 1995). The failure rate of abutment teeth is, in general, higher as a result of oral hygiene difficulty and the influence of mechanical stress (Saito et al. 2002). On the other hand, mechanical complications, such as acrylic resin fracture and metal components, are rare.

With Ms K, three teeth were prepared and restored with milled crowns, which should optimise stress distribution and minimise loading on abutments.

Treatment options for the mandible

Clinical and radiographical examination showed that tooth 34 has deep, unrestorable root caries and is currently providing retention for a distal extension RDP; tooth 33 is sound and immobile but with limited labial undercut. The restoration of the quadrant 3 is important because this quadrant is the only region that can be used for chewing. The following treatment options have been considered:

- conventional metal-base partial RDP;
- placement of one implant in the edentulous area with an implant- and tooth-retained overdenture;
- insertion of two implants in the edentulous area and a partial FDP.

Comfort and function of conventional RDPs for restoration of a Kennedy class II situation are affected by lack of a distal abutment and the need for soft tissue support. The lack of rigidity of the distal extension creates rotation around the fulcrum between the direct retainers, generating horizontal forces that may damage the abutments.

This deleterious mechanism may be minimised with appropriate denture design and impression technique. The periphery of the denture is fully extended and a wide base (concept of the snowshoe as described by Carr et al. 2005) allows better distribution of the masticatory load.

The master cast was constructed with a two-impression altered cast technique. With the first impression, a material that provides maximum accuracy for tooth reproduction (such as polyvinyl siloxane) is used and the metal connector is constructed on this cast. The edentulous section of the case is then removed and a second impression with thermoplastic and polyether materials is taken. This technique provides the best accuracy and therefore minimises potential vertical displacement of the distal extension of the denture. The accuracy of these techniques has been compared with conventional single-phase techniques (Leupold et al. 1992, Frank et al. 2004) and both studies concluded that with the altered cast technique there was less space (0.15 and 0.19 mm) between the ridge and denture base. Optimal performance was obtained with the altered cast technique, but the authors questioned the clinical relevance of the minimal space with the increased complexity and cost of the procedure.

The use of dental implants has been proposed to change a Kennedy class I or II into a class III by adding a distal abutment. Ohkubo et al. (2008) showed that this option significantly improved the comfort, chewing, retention and stability.

Finally, the use of two or more implants would allow an FDP. The implant option offered significant advantages; however, these options were not selected because of:

- minimal thickness of the alveolar ridge;
- age and patient's medical conditions;
- cost of the procedure;
- time (the patient was keen to complete the treatment as soon as possible so she could visit her daughter interstate).

Risk analysis for the selected treatment plan

With the maxillary complete RDP, the anatomy of the maxilla is unfavourable to provide stability and retention of the prosthesis. The new denture was based on the 'neutral zone' concept: combination of muco-compressive and mucostatic impression and a balanced occlusal scheme, to achieve optimum stability. However, in the long term the patient may be disappointed with loss of stability due to a flabby ridge and progressive bone resorption. Regular relining and adjustments of the occlusion would be required.

Maintenance and definition of clinical success

After completion of treatment, the patient is reviewed at 6 months and then on a yearly basis. At reviews the following will be assessed:

- plaque control;
- mucosal condition;
- presence of soft tissue inflammation;
- peri-implant probing depth;
- width of keratinised mucosa;
- implant mobility/discomfort;
- bone loss;
- retention of the denture;
- integrity of the denture;
- occlusion;
- wear of the retentive elements.

Such parameters were updated in the 2004 ITI consensus (Salvi & Lang 2004).

Clinical success for the implants has been defined by Testori et al. (2003) as:

- no clinically detectable mobility;
- no evidence of peri-implant radiolucency;
- no peri-implant infection;
- no pain;
- no paraesthesia;
- no crestal bone loss exceeding 1.5 mm by the end of the first year and 0.2 mm/year in the subsequent years.

Most authors agree that the majority of complications and need for maintenance occur within the first year. It appears that the patient and the denture need time to adapt (Sadowsky 2001, Trakas *et al.* 2006). The complete maxillary prosthesis and the overdenture will require:

- occlusal adjustments (review every 6 months);
- relining (variable may be needed after 1–4 years of service);
- change-resilient components (variable).

Rationale for the treatment plan

The rationale for the treatment is supported by the data indicated; the most important points are summarised as follows:

- the primary objective of the treatment for the maxillary arch was to provide a denture to support the lip and improve aesthetics and speech;
- the construction of a tooth-supported RDP would result in a significant cantilever that can only be reduced by the use of implants;
- the extension of the denture was limited to tooth 13 to minimise the cantilever;
- the insertion of the implants is surgically driven due to the limited quantity of bone and the need to minimise treatment;
- a bar-shaped attachment is indicated for retention of the denture on the implants;
- milled crowns have been selected to create denture support;
- milled crowns are preferred as it is more conservative of tooth structure;
- occlusally approaching clasps will be used for retention and to facilitate the removal of the denture;
- a conventional RDP was preferred for the mandibular arch to minimise treatment intervention;
- altered cast technique was used to achieve maximum accuracy for the edentulous areas and minimise prosthesis movements.

References

Adell, R., Erickson, B., Lekholm, U. *et al.* (1990) A long-term follow-up study of osseointegrated implants in the treatment of totally edentulous jaws. *International Journal of Oral & Maxillofacial Implants*, 5 (4), 347–359.

Bergman, B., Hugoson, A. & Olsson, C.O. (1995) A 25 year longitudinal study of patients treated with removable partial dentures. *Journal of Oral Rehabilitation*, 22 (8), 595–599.

Carr, A.B., McGivney, G.P. & Brown, D.T. (2005) *McCracken's removable partial prosthodontics*, 11th edn. Elsevier Mosby, St Louis.

Chaiyabutr, Y. & Brudvik, J.S. (2008) Removable partial denture design using milled abutment surfaces and minimal soft tissue coverage for periodontally compromised teeth: a clinical report. *Journal of Prosthetic Dentistry*, 99 (4), 263–266.

Chikunov, I., Doan, P. & Vahidi, F. (2008) Implant-retained partial overdenture with resilient attachments. *Journal of Prosthodontics*, 17 (2), 141–148.

De Backer, H., Van Maele, G., Decock, V. *et al.* (2007) Long-term survival of complete crowns, fixed dental prostheses and cantilever fixed dental prostheses with posts and cores on root canal-treated teeth. *International Journal of Prosthodontics*, 20 (3), 229–234.

Frank, R.P., Milgrom, P., Leroux, B.G. *et al.* (1998) Treatment outcomes with mandibular removable partial dentures: a population-based study of patient satisfaction. *Journal of Prosthetic Dentistry*, 80 (1), 36–45.

Frank, R.P., Brudvik, J.S. & Noonan, C.J. (2004) Clinical outcome of the altered cast impression procedure compared with use of one-piece cast. *Journal of Prosthetic Dentistry*, 91 (5), 468–476.

Goodacre, C.J., Bernal, G., Rungcharassaeng, K. *et al.* (2003) Clinical complications with implants and implant prostheses. *Journal of Prosthetic Dentistry*, 90 (2), 121–132.

Igarashi, Y. & Goto, T. (1997) Ten-year follow-up study of conical crown-retained dentures. *International Journal of Prosthodontics*, 10 (2), 149–155.

Leupold, R.J., Flinton, R.J. & Pfeifer, D.L. (1992) Comparison of vertical movement occurring during loading of distal-extension removable partial dentures made by three impression techniques. *Journal of Prosthetic Dentistry*, 68 (2), 290–293.

Mijiritsky, E., Ormianer, Z., Klinger, A. *et al.* (2005) Use of dental implants to improve unfavourable removable partial denture design. *Compendium of Continuing Education in Dentistry*, 26 (10), 744–752.

Moy, P.K., Medina, D., Shetty, V. *et al.* (2005) Dental implant failure rates and associated rick factors. *International Journal of Oral & Maxillofacial Implants*, 20 (4), 569–577.

Naert, I., Alsaadi, G. & Quirynen, M. (2004) Prosthetic aspects and patient satisfaction with two-implant retained mandibular overdentures: a 10-year randomized clinical study. *International Journal of Prosthodontics*, 17 (4), 401–410.

Ohkubo, C., Kobayashi, M., Suzuki, Y. *et al.* (2008) Effect of implant support on distal-extension removable partial dentures: in vivo assessment. *International Journal of Oral & Maxillofacial Implants*, 23 (6), 1095–1101.

Sadowsky, S.J. (2001) Mandibular implant-retained overdentures: a literature review. *Journal of Prosthetic Dentistry*, 86 (5), 468–473.

Saito, M., Notani, K., Miura, Y. *et al.* (2002) Complications and failures in removable partial dentures: a clinical evaluation. *Journal of Oral Rehabilitation*, 29 (7), 627–633.

Salvi, G.E. & Lang, N.P. (2004). Diagnostic parameters for monitoring peri-implant conditions. *International Journal of Oral & Maxillofacial Implants*, 19 (Suppl.), 116–127.

Testori, T., Del Fabbro, M., Szmukler-Moncler, S. *et al.* (2003) Immediate occlusal loading of Osseotite implants in the completely edentulous mandible. *International Journal of Oral & Maxillofacial Implants*, 18 (4), 544–551.

Trakas, T., Michalakis, K., Kang, K. *et al.* (2006) Attachment systems for implant retained overdentures: a literature review. *Implant Dentistry*, 15 (1), 24–34.

Waliszewski, M. (2005) Restoring dentate appearance: a literature review for modern complete denture esthetics. *Journal of Prosthetic Dentistry*, 93 (4), 386–394.

Walton, T.R. (2009) Changes in the outcome of metal-ceramics tooth-supported single crowns and FDPs following the introduction of osseointegrated implant dentistry into a prosthodontic practice. *International Journal of Prosthodontics*, 22 (3), 260–267.

Wostmann, B., Balkenhol, M., Weber, A. *et al.* (2007) Long-term analysis of telescopic crown retained removable partial dentures: survival and need for maintenance. *Journal of Dentistry*, 35 (12), 939–945.

Conclusion

Iven Klineberg

A defined commitment for prosthodontics and prosthodontists has been the basis of the specialty programme at the University of Sydney, and was the encouragement to prepare this material. The focus is on (i) evidence-based clinical decisions; and (ii) interdisciplinary treatment planning and delivery to optimise treatment and ensure patient-centred outcomes, and in the process to engage patients to enhance their oral awareness and oral health.

The concept of oral health management

Prosthodontics or oral rehabilitation is a key element of oral health management and has a beneficial impact on general health, both of which are important in defining its roles. The introduction of oral implant treatment in oral rehabilitation has been a catalyst for interdisciplinary collaboration in treatment planning and case management. These developments have helped mould contemporary prosthodontics.

It is acknowledged that other disciplines are engaged in oral implant management and traditionally periodontics and OMFS have provided a collaborative role in interdisciplinary treatment. This was encouraged by the Branemark protocol, which initially defined the need for specialists to plan and deliver care to optimise outcomes. Endodontics is developing an extended role, which includes placing implants in selected cases as well as providing temporary FDPs, while orthodontics applies implants for intraoral anchorage. Contemporary management of the clinical environment presents ongoing challenges for oral rehabilitation and it is apparent that implant treatment has been embraced by several dental disciplines and is not the exclusive domain of a particular discipline. The corollary is that implant dentistry is not a specialty but a component of the disciplines contributing to oral rehabilitation and oral health care.

Breadth of clinical responsibility

The prosthodontics discipline and clinical and academic community of necessity need to recognise the breadth of commitment of prosthodontics to oral and general health, including psychological health. The academic and clinical responsibilities of co-ordinating case assessment, treatment planning and delivery of oral rehabilitation are significant and a comprehensive training curriculum needs to incorporate this breadth of discipline content in undergraduate, postgraduate and continuing professional education programmes.

Clinical responsibilities of oral rehabilitation are often transformational for individuals whose needs may arise from developmental, occupational and environmental causes as well as the inevitable impact of trauma. In addition, the need for rehabilitation is often derived from iatrogenic causes of 'limited-vision dentistry', which follows a piecemeal approach to individual tooth restoration, without consideration of functional occlusion with intra- and interarch tooth relationships.

Oral health

Oral rehabilitation has a focus on form and function and an initial commitment to ensuring that disease processes are addressed – in particular dental caries and periodontal disease – and that oral health home care is optimised to allow rehabilitation planning to be set within a disease-free and well-managed oral environment. Optimal preparation of the mouth needs to be recognised as an essential prelude to oral rehabilitation. Form is integral to patient-centred treatment and aesthetic enhancement with concern for facial and particularly lip form and proportions, and rehabilitation of lower face height correlated with restoration of occlusal vertical dimension. These

Oral Rehabilitation: A Case-Based Approach, First Edition. Edited by Iven Klineberg, Diana Kingston.
© 2012 Blackwell Publishing Ltd. Published 2012 by Blackwell Publishing Ltd.

tasks require comprehensive assessment and planning, often with interdisciplinary involvement in an integrated and staged process, co-ordinated by the prosthodontic requirements. Obtaining informed consent is an essential requirement in oral health care and ensures patient engagement with the process as a key element of successful outcome.

Form and function

- *Form and aesthetic enhancement.* The concept of aesthetics includes facial form, facial profile, lip form and smile, which are integrated with tooth position, shape, orientation and colour. These features have a profound significance for patients' psychosocial well-being, social confidence and social interaction, and are directly related to the informed consent that drove the decision to proceed with a particular treatment plan.
- *Function.* The functions of mastication and swallowing influence diet and nutrition, which impacts on long-term health of oral soft and hard tissues. The influence of mastication on general health is of special significance. The impact of mastication on cognition has been comprehensively reviewed by Weijenberg *et al.* (2010) and Ono *et al.* (2010), which are the first definitive reviews on the topic. Data from animal and human studies confirm a causal relationship between mastication and executive cognition, with particular concerns for the elderly. However, the evidence is also reported from animal and human data for young subjects and clearly indicates that optimising mastication enhances cognitive functions. Studies confirm that mastication develops enhanced concentration and memory, with more rapid information processing and spatial and numeric recall, which enhance learning. The possible

mechanisms underlying these direct neuroplastic changes include many areas of the brain involved with cognition as well as sensorimotor functions. Executive function representation is linked to the prefrontal cortex and the striatum (Salat *et al.* 2004), while memory and recall are linked to the hippocampus (Viard *et al.* 2009), which when impaired affects memory recall. In addition, the ascending activating system appears to drive general arousal, which may also be reduced with impaired mastication.

These remarkable correlates with mastication, and their implications for nutrition as well as cognition and executive cerebral function, place the very significant responsibility of oral rehabilitation in the hands of clinicians with appropriate training to optimise mastication and swallowing. These data add to the evidence base to emphasise the importance of oral rehabilitation for general health and well-being across young and older adult populations.

References

Ono, Y., Yamamoto, T., Kubo, K.Y. *et al.* (2010) Occlusion and brain function: mastication as a prevention of cognitive dysfunction. *Journal of Oral Rehabilitation*, 37 (8), 624–640.

Salat, D.H., Buckner, R.L., Snyder, A.Z. *et al.* (2004) Thinning of the cerebral cortex in aging. *Cerebral Cortex*, 14 (7), 721–730.

Viard, A, Lebreton, K., Chetelat, G. *et al.* (2009) Patterns of hippocampal–neocortical interactions in the retrieval of episodic autobiographical memories across entire life-span of aged adults. *Hippocampus*, 20 (1), 153–165.

Weijenberg, R.A. Scherder,E.J. & Lobbezoo, F. (2010) Mastication for the mind – the relationship between mastication and cognition in ageing and dementia. *Neuroscience and Biobehavioral Reviews*, 6, 1–15.

Section 5

Appendices

Appendix 1

Programme Overview

Iven Klineberg

Prosthodontics Specialty Programme, Faculty of Dentistry, the University of Sydney: Doctor of Clinical Dentistry (Prosthodontics)

1. Historical background

The Doctor of Clinical Dentistry (Prosthodontics) programme commenced in 1980 and was the first of the contemporary postgraduate programmes in prosthodontics in Australia. It was previously the Master of Dental Science (Prosthodontics) programme and originally the Master of Dental Surgery programme.

The programme was developed following the return to Sydney of the course co-ordinator from the University of Michigan. While at the University of Michigan, the prosthodontics specialty programmes in the USA were studied and this background provided the opportunity to develop a programme in Sydney that followed the format developed in US dental schools. The programme was designed for international equivalence.

The programme commenced as a 2-year programme in 1980, and changed to 3 years full-time in 1988. It includes all components of prosthodontics – removable, fixed and maxillofacial – with the application of dental implants as an integral part of oral rehabilitation. In addition the programme includes management of TMD and orofacial pain as an essential aspect of clinical case management. The programme has been the benchmark programme in Australia. It is accredited by the Australian Dental Council and is peer reviewed by the Academy of Australian and New Zealand Prosthodontists, which is the senior prosthodontic organisation in Australasia.

The programme is strongly supported by Faculty and prosthodontic specialists from practice who assist in presentation of seminars, journal club sessions, clinical mentoring and assessment. The oral rehabilitation philosophy is a contemporary one, where decision-making is evidence based and student centred, encouraging student maturity in clinical assessment, decision making and treatment planning, with a focus on patient-centred decisions.

The programme follows the University of Sydney philosophy of inclusion of local and international graduates, which has provided a breadth of backgrounds of students who work together as a team in each year. With an intake each year (since 1998) and an average of four new students each year, the senior students effectively support the junior students.

The introduction of an annual intake commenced in 2000. This was delayed until there were sufficient graduates from the programme in practice to assist with both undergraduate and postgraduate prosthodontics supervision, and followed the programme's relocation to the Westmead Centre for Oral Health. This relocation was to support interdisciplinary (with other specialty programmes in dentistry) and interprofessional (with medicine primarily) case management.

In 2005, a submission to the University of Sydney was approved for a restructure of the first year into the first semester Graduate Certificate in Clinical Dentistry (Restorative), and the first and second semesters as a Graduate Diploma in Clinical Dentistry (Restorative). These qualifications may be separate exit qualifications or allow continuity, if assessment permits, to complete the second and third years of the Doctor of Clinical Dentistry (Prosthodontics). This structure in the first year was pioneered by Prosthodontics to provide the opportunity for candidates to complete a one- or a two- semester programme and to gain a graduate qualification in restorative dentistry, or to continue for 3 years to complete the prosthodontic specialty programme.

In addition in 2005, following broad discussion with, and with the support of, the Academy of Australian and New Zealand Prosthodontists (NSW Branch), a proposal

Oral Rehabilitation: A Case-Based Approach, First Edition. Edited by Iven Klineberg, Diana Kingston.
© 2012 Blackwell Publishing Ltd. Published 2012 by Blackwell Publishing Ltd.

was accepted by the University of Sydney to allow a select intake of mature dental practitioners who wished to study prosthodontics, to complete the programme by allowing an agreed proportion of clinical treatment to be undertaken in practice with specialist mentor supervision. This required a restructuring of the academic and practical coursework, which was formerly delivered progressively throughout each year, to be delivered in a series of coursework blocks. This structure provided the opportunity for external candidates to complete coursework blocks, and for selected clinical components to be completed in practice. The clinical components that are to be completed in practice with clinical mentor guidance vary with each external candidate and depend on a candidate's clinical background and availability of appropriate specialist mentors. This was an innovative additional admission possibility and this programme was the only one nationally to have offered this. The development has proven to be successful and student interactions in the years where there are external candidates have been advantaged by the varied input provided by their clinical maturity and experience.

The programme has allowed specialist description by the Dental Boards of each of the Australian states and territory and is recognised by the Australian Dental Board which centralised dental and specialist registrations nationally from 2010.

2. Course information
2.1 General information

The course is a clinical coursework programme in prosthodontics, leading to specialisation in the discipline. Biological science subjects are integrated with clinical subjects horizontally and vertically over 3 years. The 3-year programme includes the major clinical components of fixed prosthodontics, removable prosthodontics and maxillofacial prosthodontics, orofacial pain and TMDs and occlusion, and candidates are expected to become competent in each area.

Graduate students in the programme may be appointed as Registrars in Prosthodontics in the Department of Oral Restorative Sciences, Westmead Centre for Oral Health and the Sydney Dental Hospital, and an average of six clinical sessions each week are devoted to patient care; in a particular semester, this may vary with coursework requirements, research and teaching commitments. Clinical sessions are supervised by visiting clinical teaching staff, full-time Faculty staff or hospital specialist staff.

The completion of a research project is an essential Faculty and University requirement, and completing a research project in a Faculty Research Unit is encouraged.

The degree, DClin Dent (Prosthodontics), is recognised by the Australian Dental Council, the Australian Dental Boards, and the Australian and New Zealand Academy of Prosthodontists, as fulfilling coursework requirements for registration and specialist description in Prosthodontics.

The Royal Australasian College of Dental Surgeons (RACDS) accepts the programme as fulfilling coursework requirements for entry into the Membership in the Special Field of Prosthodontics. The final DClin Dent (Prosthodontics) examination may be taken in conjunction with the RACDS Membership Special Field examination.

Location
The clinical and seminar programmes take place primarily in the Department of Oral Restorative Sciences (ORS), Westmead Centre for Oral Health, Westmead Hospital.

In first year, clinic sessions are scheduled from Monday to Thursday and clinic hours are 8.00 am to 12.30 pm and 1.30 pm to 5.00 pm. In the first semester candidates may be rostered to am/pm clinic sessions (Monday to Thursday) and alternate Fridays.

Rotations to the Department of Restorative Dentistry, Sydney Dental Hospital, may take place in second and third years.

In general, seminars are arranged with the blocks; additional seminars may be arranged before or after clinics on some days, and additional seminars and clinical activities may take place in other locations. In first semester, a core seminar programme is also scheduled as a block of coursework shared across DClin Dent programmes.

Eligibility
Dental graduates with acceptable qualifications and special interests in Prosthodontics may apply.

Applicants are assessed over 4 days in Sydney. They may be required to satisfactorily complete a skills test and a written examination, and will be required to present a case report and an interview. They must also have an acceptable level of general practice experience.

The Planning Committee prefers applicants to have completed a minimum of 4 years after graduation working in general dental practice. In some instances, candidates may be accepted with a shorter time in general practice, if it is clear that their experience focused on a broad range of prosthodontic and restorative treatments.

The assessment panel includes the Course Coordinator, a representative from Westmead Centre for Oral Health, up to two representatives from the Faculty and possibly up to two specialist Prosthodontists from practice.

Applicants are advised within a month after applications if they are short-listed for the programme. The University date for receipt of applications is 31st March each year. The short-list, interviews and follow-up referee reports usually allows offers to be made by June.

Selection
- Local students: places are offered based on skills assessment, interviews/viva, case presentation and referee reports.

- International students: places are offered based on a written paper, skills assessment, interview/viva, case presentation and referee reports.

External candidature

There are specific requirements, which are considered on an individual basis, concerning the possibility of external candidature:

- the number of years in practice: 8–10 years is in general required;
- the type of experience gained in practice; in particular the breadth of general practice experience in restorative and prosthodontics treatments, and interaction with other disciplines such as periodontics, endodontics and oral surgery;
- clinical maturity in decision-making and discussion of the case presentation;
- access to suitable mentors and specialised clinics;
- an additional qualification, either university or college-based.

Orientation

A structured orientation is offered in the November/December preceding commencement of the programme as an introduction to ensure that candidates are prepared for the start of the programme in February the following year.

The orientation includes:

- discussion on clinical procedures, log books and clinical requirements;
- clinical transfer records;
- handling articulators;
- photographic records.

Candidates may be required to complete a diagnostic wax-up of selected procedures by the beginning of first semester.

Further information is available in the *Faculty of Dentistry Graduate Student Handbook*.

2.2 Research

A *minor project* is required during September of the first year. Topics will be selected in consultation with the Course Coordinator. These projects will be based on a critical appraisal of a prosthodontic topic and, where possible, may include experimental data recording and analysis.

The *major project* is required to be completed as a thesis and submitted to the Course Coordinator by the end of August of third year. This will allow time for thesis examination and completion of corrections where possible for graduation the following March. If the thesis is submitted later in third year, graduation may not be possible in March of the following year.

The major project of relevance to prosthodontics is completed under supervision of a member of staff.

Projects of a clinical or laboratory nature are possible, but depend on the availability of resources and funding. The time for preparation and completion of the research project is limited and all details must be carefully planned in conjunction with the supervisor, to ensure completion by the appropriate time. The overall time for research in the programme varies from 30% to 40% over the 3 years of the programme, with most time being spent in second and third years.

Note:

- Unless otherwise approved by the Faculty Postgraduate Committee on the recommendation of the course coordinator, candidates will be required to complete and submit a manuscript for publication derived from their research work before completing final examinations.
- Faculty requires that the research project and outcomes are written in a form that is suitable for publication in a refereed journal.
- The thesis submitted is to contain a critical review of the literature and the research paper.
- An internal and an external examiner are appointed (separate from the clinical examiners) for assessment of the research project.

2.3 Assessment

Candidates are required to satisfactorily complete summative assessment at the end of the first semester of first year, and at the end of the first, second and third years. Continuation in the prosthodontics programme is dependent on satisfactorily completing all aspects of the first- and second-semester coursework of first year. Formative assessment will be conducted throughout the course.

Assessment will take the following forms.

Written examinations

Written examinations may include

- Short-answer questions: cover a broad range of topics, require integration of clinical and basic sciences information and formulation of thoughts in an organised way.
- Long-answer questions: cover limited topics but allow assessment of creative writing skills, scientific knowledge and current literature. At least one long-answer question will be included for end-of-year papers in first, second and third years.
- Scenario questions: request broadly based answers that assess clinical reasoning, knowledge of current literature, and ability to synthesise and prioritise facts.

Clinical assessment

A full-time commitment to patient care is expected by the Planning Committee and the Executive of WCOH. This is essential to maximise clinical experience and service.

Clinical assessment is continuous during all clinical activities and contributes to the semester and annual clinical assessment:

- Case presentation seminars for prosthodontic treatment are conducted fortnightly and feedback is provided.
- Treatment planning seminars for orofacial pain and oral implant treatments are conducted weekly and feedback provided.
- A log book, indicating progress of cases, breadth of cases and clinical proficiency is assessed for each end-of-year exam. Unseen clinical cases may be included:
  - short cases – 5/10 minutes (with 5 minutes reporting) show ability to take a quick history and examination, and rapidly synthesise information;
  - long cases – 30 minutes (with 20 minutes reporting) require a full history, examination, diagnosis and treatment plans.
- Completed clinical cases: require a summary and discussion of treatment planning decisions and outcomes of treatment. A report or questionnaire on treatment outcomes, including patient satisfaction, as a before and after comparison (use of a questionnaire/visual analogue scale, etc.).

Seminars
Seminar contribution is monitored and formative feedback is provided. A summary of each seminar topic is usually required.

Self-reflection portfolio (year 1)
A portfolio on self-evaluation of progress as a component of assessment is to be submitted in October of the first year as a formative assessment. This is submitted as a written reflection of the year as a component of personal and professional development.

Case presentations
In years 2 and 3, case presentations will assess ability to progressively develop confidence in:

- patient assessment and treatment planning, with reference to the current literature;
- oral presentation among peers, allowing feedback;
- developing presentation skills.

Case presentations are formative and continue through the programme.

Oral examinations (viva voce) (years 1, 2 and 3)
- Viva voce is a structured separate assessment to further consider a candidate's breadth of knowledge and maturity, clinical reasoning and judgement (such as in diagnosis), and knowledge of current literature.
- There may be an additional and optional oral examination to allow examiners to further assess aspects of a candidate's written answers.

Year 3 final
The final examination will be held at the end of the third year (September–October) or if required, early the following year (January–February).

This examination will consist of:

- presentation of at least five fully documented completed cases, demonstrating a range of clinical prosthodontics;
- a detailed log book;
- written and viva voce examinations.

It is possible for arrangements to be made to allow the final DClin Dent examination to be taken in association with the Membership in the Special Field of Prosthodontics of the Royal Australasian College of Dental Surgeons. Candidates wishing to sit both examinations are required to advise the Course Coordinator in writing during the first semester of third year.

The research is examined separately. To allow adequate time as prescribed by the University (i.e. 2–3 months for research assessment and for corrections to be completed), the thesis should be submitted in its final form by the end of August of the final year.

2.4 Treatment philosophy
Clinical management and treatment planning with an emphasis on biology is a paradigm for best practice.

Simple, conservative and minimally invasive procedures are preferred, with acknowledgement of patient preferences and maintaining where possible natural teeth and tissues.

Complex treatment may be indicated but needs to be carefully considered within the context of long-term oral health, psychosocial well-being and the likely evidence-based long-term outcome.

General
Current best practice requires a patient-centred approach to patient care, where the patient's concerns, expectations and social circumstances are a key component of informed consent, case planning, treatment agreement and treatment delivery.

Central neuroplasticity allows adaptation to small and large modifications to the intraoral environment. This may vary from tooth adjustment and restoration, tooth loss, the provision of fixed and removable prostheses, and the rehabilitation of the edentulous state.

The occlusal scheme requirements include determining optimal OVD, stable tooth contact arrangement across the arch, appropriate tooth guidance to encourage fluent function, and an anterior tooth arrangement that meets each patient's aesthetic expectations.

Assessment
Patient assessment at the commencement of treatment provides the opportunity to evaluate expectations and to acknowledge matters that may impact on outcomes.

Assessment should include:

- General medical history, medications and their implications for oral function.
- Psychometric assessment such as the SCL-90-R inventory, which considers nine behavioural domains, the details of which may bear directly on patient acceptance of treatment and its outcomes in the short and long term.
- Patient outcome assessment is valuable at the conclusion of treatment to ensure that there is an opportunity for patient feedback on their management and treatment experience, as distinct from the clinician's opinion. The outcome assessment is directly influenced by the patient's psychosocial status at the commencement of treatment and their experiences during treatment.

Treatment planning
- Avoid options as a way of demonstrating what you know, but focus on optimising outcomes and offer the most rational (i.e. not the 'ideal') option and consider the cost–benefit analysis to define effectiveness in the long term.
- Use provisional restorations to confirm your rational and evidence-based proposals:
  - if appropriate build on existing prostheses (e.g. increase OVD or splints);
  - 28 teeth, all ideally aligned, with a perfect curve of Spee, symmetry and minimal interproximal spaces is not a realistic goal – this is 'textbook mechanics'.
- Consider the whole mouth: soft tissues, hard tissues, facial form, OVD, TMD, etc.:
  - add medical background and implications especially of medications;
  - recognise age-specific requirements;
  - do not be influenced by the patient's views or media hype about aesthetics, but focus on an optimum blend of form with function;
  - patient preference needs to be tempered by: the evidence-base for optimising outcomes, the cost–benefit analysis, and realistic expectations.
- Change (e.g. attritional wear, increase in OVD) needs to acknowledge that compensatory tooth eruption occurs with attritional wear, and muscle adaptation (lengthening by additional sarcomere in series) also occurs as a biological response to increase in OVD.
- Partial denture design should expose the maximum and cover the minimum of soft tissue.

In summary:

- think biologically in the context of best evidence for decision-making;
- acknowledge normative values, rather than a theoretical or textbook ideal;
- consider simple approaches, and what is likely to work best – do not focus on complexity!

Further Information

For information on DClin Dent (Prosthodontics) access http://sydney.edu.au/handbooks/dentistry/postgraduate/coursework/dr_clinical_dentistry/prosthodontics.shtml

For University of Sydney Faculty of Dentistry general course information, access http://sydney.edu.au/dentistry

For Faculty of Dentistry handbooks access http://sydney.edu.au/handbooks/handbooks_admin/dentistry.shtml or http://sydney.edu.au/handbooks/dentistry/

Appendix 2

Evidence Base for Case 10.2 (Mr Graeme S)

1. Outcome of direct composite restorations

Direct composite restorations can be used effectively to restore the worn dentition of the anterior mandible. The need for re-intervention is acceptable and is offset by the cost and simplicity compared with complications and loss of tooth structure that alternative options, such as indirect veneers and crowns, may present (Poyser et al. 2007).

The outcome is different when direct and indirect restorations of posterior teeth are compared. Generally, there is a preference for amalgam and direct composite restorations because of less time and cost compared with indirect restorations. However, longevity of direct restorations is questioned, especially with large posterior restorations.

A randomised trial by Bernardo et al. (2007) on 472 young patients who received 1748 restorations reported data for up to 7 years. Half were treated with posterior amalgam restoration and half with composite resin restorations. The survival rate of amalgam restorations was 94%, and that of composite restorations was 85%. The annual failure ranged from 0.1% to 3% for amalgam and from 0.9% to 9.5% for composite. This study was conducted on young patients and a range of cavity designs were included. From this study, the clinical indication that may apply to Mr S is that greater longevity is expected from amalgam compared with composite restorations and, in particular, in large multisurface posterior restorations.

Opdam et al. (2007) compared longevity of 2867 composite and amalgam class I and II restorations with a follow-up of 10 years. The survival rate for small posterior restorations was similar for composite materials (82% at 10 years) compared with amalgam (79% at 10 years). These two studies indicate that composite restorations perform as well as amalgam for small cavities. The longevity of direct composite restorations decreases significantly (compared with amalgam), as the size of the cavity increases and the available enamel for bonding decreases. In addition, the quality of the remaining tooth structure may affect the bonding and longevity of the restoration. An in vitro study by Kwong et al. (2000) reported that the lack of resin tags and hybrid layer in worn and sclerotic dentine significantly weakened the strength of the bond between composite material and tooth structure.

The performance of composite materials may be disappointing when used in worn posterior dentitions (Bartlett & Sundaram 2006), where direct and indirect composite restorations were used to restore 32 teeth in 16 patients with worn dentitions and 26 teeth in 13 patients with normal dentitions. After a follow-up of 3 years, 50% of the restorations in the worn dentition group were lost, compared with a failure of 20% in the normal dentition. The authors advise that composite resin restorations are not indicated for the posterior worn dentition.

The longevity and need for re-intervention and maintenance of teeth restored with large amalgam restorations or crowns were investigated by Kolker et al. (2005). They followed 518 teeth (equally divided in two groups, amalgam or crown) over 10 years and recorded type and frequency of intervention, patient characteristics, failure mode and facture rate. At 10 years, amalgam failure was 22% versus 12% for crowns, with the odds of teeth with large amalgam restorations needing major treatment being 2:1 teeth with crowns. A total of 64% of the amalgam restorations required subsequent treatment versus 32% of crowns over the 10 years.

Data indicate that anterior mandibular teeth and posterior teeth that require small restorations can be effectively restored with direct composite resin. This technique is acceptable even when the restorations are used to increase the OVD. However, tooth-supported and implant-supported indirect restorations should be considered for the posterior heavily restored or missing dentition respectively.

2. Outcome of single crowns and fixed dental prostheses

Tooth-supported single crowns may be fabricated with gold alloys, ceramo-metal or all-ceramic materials. Gold alloys are ideal for posterior teeth, especially when there is insufficient interarch space for veneering porcelain. The mechanical properties of this material are optimal; however, not all patients accept its appearance (Wataha 2002).

Walton (2009) analysed the impact of the introduction of implant dentistry on the outcome of metal-ceramic tooth-supported single FDPs in a specialist practice. Patients were divided into two groups: group 1 was patients treated from 1989 to 1993 (when few implants were used) and data were analysed in 1998; group 2 was patients treated from 1997 to 2001 (when the use of implants increased significantly) and the outcome was determined in 2006. There was no significant difference in the cumulative survival rate at 10 years of tooth-supported single crowns (approximately 94%) and tooth-supported FDPs (approximately 90%). Comparison of data regarding vital and non-vital abutment teeth showed that in group 1 the cumulative survival rate of non-vital teeth was significantly lower than that of vital teeth. Statistical significance is not apparent for group 2. The difference was explained by the fact that in group 2, implants were used more frequently instead of teeth when the prognosis of the tooth was poor. This study showed that the long-term survival rate of CMCs and FDPs is excellent, and that the integrity of the remaining tooth structure is more important than its vitality in determining the prognosis of the tooth and prosthesis.

A similar conclusion was described by De Backer et al. (2006, 2007, 2008a,b) in their long-term survival of single crowns (1037), three-unit FDPs (134), multi-unit FDPs (322) and cantilevered FDPs. The data included vital and non-vital teeth with post cores. In contrast to the study by Walton, all prostheses were made by undergraduate students under supervision. The estimated survival rate for single crowns was: vital teeth single crowns: 94% (year 6), 86% (year 12) and 75% (year 18); non-vital teeth single crowns: 95% (year 6), 85% (year 12) and 75% (year 18). The estimated survival rate for three-unit FDPs was: vital teeth FDPs 95% (year 5), 90% (year 10) and 83% (year 15); non-vital teeth FDPs 95% (year 5), 85% (year 10) and 76% (year 15).

There was no statistical difference among the groups, although with the three-unit FDPs some divergence is evident after 10 years. As in the study by Walton, the investigation by De Backer et al. supports acceptable long-term survival of metal-ceramic single crowns and three-unit FDPs, and that endodontically treated teeth

perform as well as vital teeth provided there is sufficient tooth structure.

All-ceramic materials have become more popular because of enhanced aesthetic possibilities. Pjetursson et al. (2007) described survival rates of all-ceramic single crowns at 5 years from 87% (glass-ceramic) to 96% (fully sintered alumina); clinical outcome of anterior ACCs is similar to that of CMCs. It appears that the mechanical properties of the ceramic relate directly to the clinical outcomes and longevity of these materials. In general, crowns made with stronger and tougher core materials have longer survival than lower strength and fracture toughness materials (Odman & Andersson 2001, Fradeani & Redemagni 2002, Segal 2001). In vitro studies reported that yttria partially stabilised zirconia ceramics have the highest flexural strength and fracture toughness and therefore restorations made from these materials should have the lowest incidence of in-service fractures (Guazzato et al. 2004a,b,c,d, 2005). Since in-service all-ceramic restorations fail mechanically, the interest of clinicians and research has focused on the fracture resistance of three- and multi-unit zirconia-based FDPs and, to date, no studies on single crowns have been published. Of particular interest are studies on zirconia-based FDPs by Raigrodski et al. (2006) Sailer et al. (2007) and Tinschert et al. (2008).

The prospective clinical cohort study by Sailer et al. (2007) determined success rate of three- to five-unit yttria-stabilised tetragonal zirconia polycrystal (Y-TZP) FDPs over 5 years. A total of 45 patients and 57 FDPs were included; however, only data on 33 FDPs were analysed. The success and survival rates of this study are invalid because of questionable interpretation of success and survival. For example, seven patients with seven FDPs were excluded from statistical analysis as unacceptable (owing to biological and technical complications) before the 5-year follow-up. These FDPs should have been included in the analysis as 'failure'. At the 5-year follow-up, an additional 12 FDPs were replaced due to biological (caries) and mechanical complications (chipping of the porcelain). Of the 45 patients included initially, 11 patients with 17 FDPs withdrew from the study (lost to follow-up). The authors reported a survival rate of 74%, when in reality only 21 FDPs of the initial 57 FDPs were in service and examined at 5 years. Despite these shortcomings, the data were interesting when the failure of the remaining FDPs was analysed. Of the 33 FDPs examined, one fractured as a result of trauma, and chipping of the veneering porcelain was reported in 15%.

A prospective study by Raigrodski et al. (2006) assessed the outcome of 20 three-unit FDPs over 36 months. None of the frameworks fractured; however, cohesive fracture of the veneering porcelain was seen in 25%. The authors suggested that since no adhesive fracture was seen, the bond strength between the Y-TZP core and the veneering porcelain was adequate. They considered the chipping of the porcelain to be related to the design of the Y-TZP frameworks, to the mechanical properties of the veneering porcelain, or to a mismatch of the coefficient of thermal expansion.

Tinschert et al. (2008) investigated clinical outcome of 65 FDPs over a mean period of 38 months. Although some prostheses had up to four pontics, no framework fractures were recorded. However, as consistently reported in previous studies, porcelain chipping was seen in four FDPs. In this study, the authors considered the loss of veneering material to be related to the lack of sufficient support of the porcelain by the Y-TZP core and recommended optimising support of the veneering porcelain by designing the frame with an anatomical contour.

Marchack et al. (2008) also supported the concept of optimising the design of Y-TZP restorations by increasing framework thickness and described the customisation of milled zirconia copings to provide an even porcelain thickness. They claimed, without evidence, that this design would decrease cohesive porcelain fracture and other failures.

Although more studies with larger sample sizes and longer follow-up periods are required, these investigations indicate that mechanical properties of Y-TZP are sufficient for dental applications. However, the cohesive fracture of the veneering porcelain has been consistently reported and its incidence is greater than that recorded in ceramo-metal prostheses.

The longevity data of all-ceramic materials and zirconia in particular does not support their use in this case; however, the material was selected as an alternative to option 2 of acrylic provisional crowns on implants and direct composite restorations for the existing teeth (a favourable arrangement with the laboratory allowed it be provided without cost).

References

Bartlett, D. & Sundaram, G. (2006) An up to 3-year randomized clinical study comparing indirect and direct resin composites used to restore worn posterior teeth. *International Journal of Prosthodontics*, 19 (6), 613–617.

Bernardo, M., Lius, H., Martin, M.D. et al. (2007) Survival and reasons for failure of amalgam versus composite posterior restorations placed in a randomized clinical trial. *Journal of the American Dental Association*, 138 (6), 775–783.

De Backer, H., Van Maele, G, De Moor, N. et al. (2006) Single-tooth replacement: is a 3-unit fixed partial denture still an option? A 20-year retrospective study. *International Journal of Prosthodontics*, 19 (6), 567–573.

De Backer, H., Van Maele, G., Decock, V. et al. (2007) Long-term survival of complete crowns, fixed dental prostheses and cantilever fixed dental prostheses with posts and cores on root canal-treated teeth. *International Journal of Prosthodontics*, 20 (3), 229–334.

De Backer, H., Van Maele, G, De Moor, N. et al. (2008a) Long-term results of short-span versus long-span fixed dental prostheses: an up to 20-year retrospective study. *International Journal of Prosthodontics*, 21 (1), 75–85.

De Backer, H., Van Maele, G, De Moor, N. et al. (2008b) An up to 20-year retrospective study of 4-unit fixed dental prostheses for the replacement of 2 missing adjacent teeth. *International Journal of Prosthodontics*, 21 (3), 259–266.

Fradeani, M. & Redemagni, M. (2002) An 11-year clinical evaluation of leucite-reinforced glass-ceramic crowns: a retrospective study. *Quintessence International*, 33 (7), 503–510.

Guazzato, M., Albakry, M., Ringer, S.P. et al. (2004a) Strength, fracture toughness and microstructure of a selection of all-ceramic materials. Part I: pressable and alumina glass-infiltrated ceramics. *Dental Materials*, 20 (5), 441–448.

Guazzato, M., Albakry, M., Ringer, S.P. et al. (2004b) Strength, fracture toughness and microstructure of a selection of all-ceramic materials. Part II: Zirconia-based dental ceramics. *Dental Materials*, 20 (5), 449–456.

Guazzato, M, Albakry, M., Quach, L. et al. (2004c) Influence of grinding, sandblasting, polishing and heat treatment on the flexural strength of a glass-infiltrated alumina-reinforced dental ceramic. *Biomaterials*, 25 (11), 2153–2160.

Guazzato, M., Proos, K., Quach, L. et al. (2004d) Strength, reliability and mode of fracture of bilayered porcelain/zirconia (Y-TZP) dental ceramics. *Biomaterials*, 25 (20), 5045–5052.

Guazzato, M., Quach, L., Albakry, M. et al. (2005) Influence of surface and heat treatments on the flexural strength of Y-TZP dental ceramics. *Journal of Dentistry*, 33 (1), 9–18.

Kolker, J.L., Damiano, P.C., Caplan, D.J. et al. (2005) Teeth with large amalgam restorations and crowns: factors affecting the receipt of subsequent treatment after 10 years. *Journal of the American Dental Association*, 136, 738–748.

Kwong, S.M., Tay, F.R., Yip, H.K. et al. (2000) An ultrastructural study of the application of dentine adhesive to acid-conditioned sclerotic dentine. *Journal of Dentistry*, 28 (7), 515–528.

Marchack, B.W., Futatsuki, Y., Marchack, C.B. et al. (2008) Customization of milled zirconia copings for all-ceramic crowns: a clinical report. *Journal of Prosthetic Dentistry*, 99 (3), 169–173.

Odman, P. & Andersson, B. (2001). Procera AllCeram crowns followed for 5 to 10.5 years: a prospective clinical study. *International Journal of Prosthodontics*, 14 (6), 504–509.

Opdam, N.J., Bronkhorst, E.M., Roeters, J.M. et al. (2007) A retrospective clinical study on longevity of posterior composite and amalgam restorations. *Dental Materials*, 23 (1), 2–8.

Pjetursson, B.E., Sailer, I., Zwahlen, M. et al. (2007) A systematic review of the survival and complication rates of all-ceramic and metal–ceramic reconstructions after an observation period of at least 3 years. Part I: Single crowns. *Clinical Oral Implants Research*, 18 (Suppl. 3), 73–85.

Poyser, N.J., Briggs, P.F., Chana, H.S. et al. (2007) The evaluation of direct composite restorations for the worn mandibular anterior dentition – clinical performance and patient satisfaction. *Journal of Oral Rehabilitation*, 34 (5), 361–376.

Raigrodski, A.J., Chiche, G.J., Potiket, N. et al. (2006) The efficacy of posterior three-unit zirconium-oxide-based ceramic fixed partial dental prostheses: A prospective clinical pilot study. *Journal of Prosthetic Dentistry*, 96 (4), 237–244.

Sailer, I., Feher, A., Filser, F. et al. (2007) Five-year clinical results of zirconia frameworks for posterior fixed partial dentures. *International Journal of Prosthodontics*, 20 (4), 383–388.

Segal, B.S. (2001) Retrospective assessment of 546 all-ceramic anterior and posterior crowns in a general practice. *Journal of Prosthetic Dentistry*, 85 (6), 544–550.

Tinschert, J., Schulze, K.A, Natt, G. *et al.* (2008) Clinical behaviour of zirconia based fixed-partial dentures made of DC–Zirkon: 3 year results. *International Journal of Prosthodontics*, 21 (3), 217–222.

Walton, T.R. (2009) Changes in the outcome of metal-ceramics tooth-supported single crowns and FDPs following the introduction of osseointegrated implant dentistry into a prosthodontic practice. *International Journal of Prosthodontics*, 22 (3), 260–267.

Wataha, J.C. (2002) Alloys for prosthodontic restorations. *Journal of Prosthetic Dentistry*, 87 (4), 351–363.

Appendix 3

Evidence Base for Case 11.1 (Mr Divo C)

1. Clinical outcomes of implant-retained overdentures

Mericske-Stern (1990) reported the clinical outcome of 62 edentulous patients (124 implants) restored with mandibular overdentures retained by bars or ball attachments on two implants. Patients were followed for up to 66 months; two implants failed. The conclusion was that overdentures are a simple and effective treatment.

Attard and Zarb (2004) reported the long-term outcome (10–19 years) of 42 mandibular overdentures retained by a bar on implants. After follow-up of at least 10 years, 30 patients were reviewed. Six implants failed, giving a prosthetic and implant cumulative survival in excess of 90%. Gender, bicortical stabilisation, bone quality and healing time were predictors of bone loss, but only in the first year. On average, the longevity of the prostheses was 12 years, and laboratory relining was required every 4 years.

Cooper et al. (1999) reported clinical outcomes of mandibular overdentures retained by ball attachments. Fifty-eight patients (116 implants) were restored with mandibular overdentures and followed for 5 years in a prospective study. Five implants failed immediately after loading, resulting in a survival rate of approximately 96%. The main prosthetic complications were: one fractured abutment, three loose abutments and one fractured overdenture.

2. Patient satisfaction with implant-retained fixed prostheses, implant-retained overdentures or conventional prostheses

Fenlon and Sherriff (2008) studied 723 patients with new complete dentures to investigate patient satisfaction. Relevant history, anatomical factors and denture performance were recorded. The study indicated that quality of the mandibular alveolar ridges, retention and stability, accuracy of recording of jaw relationships and patient adaptability strongly correlated with satisfaction. In this case, a complete removable denture was successful on the basis of the quality and quantity of the edentulous ridges, but there were doubts about the patient's ability to adapt to the new dentures.

Studies by Feine and colleagues (1994) investigated the performance and outcomes of implant-retained overdentures. An early study demonstrated, via a within-subject cross-over clinical trial, that masticatory efficacy of a long-bar overdenture was comparable to an implant-retained FDP. The study was repeated (Heydecke et al. 2003), where 16 patients were given overdentures and fixed prostheses. Comfort, speech, stability, aesthetics, ease of cleaning and occlusion details were recorded after 2 months of use.

Patients preferred overdentures to FDPs, especially where aesthetics, ability to speak and ease of cleaning were concerned. Nine patients chose to keep the overdenture and four preferred an FDP. Fontijn-Tekamp et al. (2000) showed that biting and chewing efficacy of patients wearing a mandibular implant-retained overdenture was greater than patients wearing a conventional complete denture, but was significantly less than that of patients with natural dentition.

Emami et al. (2009) conducted a meta-analysis of randomised controlled trials and concluded that despite almost 20 years of studies showing that implant-retained overdentures may be more satisfying for edentulous patients than new conventional dentures, the magnitude of the effect was uncertain. This study indicated the need for more evidence on cost effectiveness.

Sadowsky (2001) drew attention to the following considerations with treatment planning for patients with edentulous mandibles:

Oral Rehabilitation: A Case-Based Approach, First Edition. Edited by Iven Klineberg, Diana Kingston.
© 2012 Blackwell Publishing Ltd. Published 2012 by Blackwell Publishing Ltd.

- compared with a complete removable denture, an implant-retained mandibular denture appears to maintain the bone in the anterior mandible;
- in younger patients and those edentulous for less than 10 years, a fixed implant denture may preserve bone better than an overdenture;
- patients who consider stability to be more important than hygiene prefer an FDP.

In addition, Chee and Jivraj (2006) reported that patients who have worn a removable denture are often content with an implant-retained overdenture, while patients with some remaining teeth or who have experienced pain with complete dentures prefer an FDP.

Divo C's priority was the stability of the mandibular denture and improved function. He accepted the cost and the difficulty in cleaning an FDP. Treatment options and indications of implant-supported FDPs are discussed on the basis of loading and outcomes.

3. Clinical outcomes of mandibular fixed prostheses with differing techniques and loading protocols

There is a current view that new implant surfaces and protocols developed by manufacturers indicate that an undisturbed load-free healing of 3–6 months, as suggested by Branemark and coworkers, is no longer required and that the new implant surfaces allow implants to integrate successfully, even when loaded immediately on placement. The period of time from implant insertion to their loading was classified by Ostman (2008) as conventional or delayed (when implants are loaded after at least 3 months), early (when implants are loaded within days or few weeks) and immediate loading (when implants are loaded within 48 hours). The first step in the treatment plan was to compare the long-term clinical outcome of each of the loading options. Research articles and reviews provide a picture of the data. Ostman (2008) and Del Fabbro et al. (2006) have shown that, in general, implant survival of the three options appears to be similar, ranging from 87% to 100%. However, the differences in protocols, period of follow-up and implant designs and surfaces make it difficult to interpret the data accurately. It is more relevant to select articles for each technique and protocol and compare outcomes, advantages and disadvantages.

4. Clinical outcomes of implant-supported mandibular fixed prostheses: conventional loading (delayed) protocol

A prospective study by Lindquist et al. (1996) reported data on 47 edentulous patients treated with 273 machined implants, restored with FDPs and followed for 12–15 years. Three implants (1%) were lost, two before denture issue. The cumulative success rate was 98.9% and all dentures were functioning at follow-up. Marginal bone loss was 0.5mm the first year and then 0.05mm per year

following. Anterior implants lost more bone than the posterior implants. Smoking and poor oral hygiene had a significant influence on bone loss, whereas occlusal loading, maximal bite force, tooth clenching and length of the cantilever were considered to be of minor importance.

Branemark et al. (1995) reported on the 10-year survival rate of FDPs on four or six implants in 156 fully edentulous patients. The survival rate for the mandible FDPs (72 patients) at 10 years was 88% and 93%. Considering that 7mm and 10mm turned implants were used (shorter implants have poorer prognosis) and that four implants were used when the bone condition did not allow more implants (poorer quantity and quality), the data indicated that four implants may be used instead of six in the mandible.

5. Clinical outcomes of implant-supported mandibular fixed prostheses: early loading protocol

Engquist et al. (2005), Friberg et al. (2005) and De Bruyn et al. (2001) were selected on the basis of the level of evidence on early loading of implants in the edentulous mandible.

Engquist et al. (2005) compared outcomes of one-stage surgery (group A), delayed loading two-stage surgery (group B, control group), one-piece implants (group C) and an early loading (group D). A total of 108 patients were treated with 432 implants and followed up for 3 years. The survival rate was 93% in three tested groups (groups A, C and D) versus 97.5% for the two-stage and delayed loading protocols as the control group. Although the number of failures was slightly greater in the early loading group, there was no statistical difference. Failures in the early loading group that occurred after loading indicate that the loading protocol affected outcomes.

Friberg et al. (2005) compared short-term outcomes of the one-stage surgical procedure and early loading of FDPs with the conventional loading protocol. A total of 750 implants were inserted in 152 edentulous patients (average five implants) and restored with FDPs within 42 days. The control group had 68 subjects. The cumulative survival rate at 1 year was 97.5%, compared with 99.7% for the conventional protocol. There was a significant difference; however, the data were influenced by the inclusion of three patients with cluster failure related to cancer, bruxism and smoking habits. A further seven implants failed after insertion into fresh extraction sockets, and this condition does not compare with the conventional protocol, as it introduces an additional risk factor. The study suggests that this protocol is reliable and successful although not to the level of the conventional protocol.

De Bruyn et al. (2001) attempted to reduce the financial burden by reducing the number of implants and the number of surgical procedures. In a multicentre prospective study, success rates of 10- to 12-unit fixed prostheses restored on implants were reported. Twenty patients were treated and 19 received five implants (two left buried) of which three were functionally loaded with an FDP within 30 days. A total of 10% of the implants and 15% of the FDPs failed within the first year, suggesting that early loading, especially on only three implants, does not provide an equivalent outcome obtained with four or six implants.

6. Clinical outcomes of implant-supported mandibular fixed prostheses: immediate loading protocol

A number of studies on immediate loading were noted but only three protocols had long-term data and included the Branemark Novum Concept, the All-on-Four and the DIEM protocol.

The Branemark Novum Concept is described by Engstrand et al. (2003), where 95 patients with edentulous mandibles were treated with three implants specifically designed for this protocol. Implants were immediately splinted with a prefabricated substructure and an FDP and follow-up was for up to 5 years. The Kaplan-Meier estimated survival was 95% at 1 year and 93% at 5 years, and mean bone loss was similar to other studies. The cumulative prosthesis survival rate was 99%, although 6.3% of the implants failed. Further data on whether the prostheses survived on the two remaining implants, or whether another implant was subsequently inserted, were not provided. The authors concluded that prosthesis stability rates are similar to that of the conventional procedure, although the failure rate of the implants was greater. The authors also analysed factors that may have been linked with implant failure. Bone quality was the only statistically significant factor but it is important to note that:

- the influence of smoking and bruxism was not significant;
- the type of opposing dentition was not significant, although more failures were recorded when the opposing dentition was an implant-supported prosthesis;
- more failures were reported with wider diameter implants.

The All-on-Four immediate function concept is documented by Malo et al. (2003) in a retrospective study on 44 patients with mandibles restored with acrylic on metal FDPs. In this study, immediate loading of four implants for each patient (total of 176 implants) was followed for 2 years. The cumulative survival rate was 97% for the development group and 98% for the routine group. The prostheses survival was 100%, despite the failure of five implants in five patients. With this technique the most posterior implants are tilted distally in order to increase the AP spread and minimise the cantilever. A total of 30% of the acrylic prostheses fractured in the development group, whereas no facture was recorded in the routine group.

The DIEM protocol is documented in two studies from Testori et al. (2003) with 103 implants in 15 patients (five to six implants in each patient) loaded with a provisional hybrid prosthesis within a few hours. The provisional prosthesis was replaced within 6 months with a titanium–acrylic denture. The cumulative success rate up to 48 months was 98.9%; one implant failed immediately after the surgical procedure, but none of the prostheses failed. The authors suggested that the use of five to six implants was sufficient to minimise micromotion and improve survival rate. This is also supported by a histological study carried out on a selected patient showing bone to implant contact greater on immediate loaded implants, at 85% at 4 months of loading. This is consistent with the lower bone loss recorded in this study compared with the bone loss expected in a conventional protocol. In the second study (a prospective multicentre study), 62 patients were treated with 325 implants. The prosthesis was issued and fabricated with the same protocol. Two implants failed within 2 months, giving a cumulative implant success rate of 99.4% in a period of 12–60 months; bone loss was comparable with the delayed protocol. The implant surface was rough and not machined as in previous studies.

The advantages and disadvantages of the loading protocol in this case were as follows:

- The delayed loading protocol is well documented and the success rate is high and consistent; however, there is need for a provisional RDP.
- With immediate loading, success rate is less consistent, is affected by the technique and is less well documented. However, it overcomes the need for a provisional prosthesis and a second surgical procedure, and data indicate that bone and soft tissue healing is improved.

7. Criteria for immediate loading with DIEM protocol

The DIEM protocol was selected on the basis of the evidence. In addition, the use of more than four implants for immediate loading of the edentulous mandible is supported in the ITI Consensus Statement in 2004 (Cochran et al. 2004). Provided there are no contraindications for surgical procedures the criteria that need to be fulfilled to minimise the risk of failure for immediate loading in the edentulous mandible, according to the DIEM protocol are:

- adequate bone quality (types I, II or III),
- sufficient bone height (12 mm) for a minimum length of the implants of 10 mm;
- sufficient bone width (approximately 6 mm);
- sufficient primary stability ($>30 \, N/cm^2$);
- ability to achieve adequate AP spread.

8. Material options for the implant-supported fixed prostheses

Fixed prostheses may be fabricated with the following materials: titanium and acrylic; gold alloy and acrylic; gold alloy and porcelain; and zirconia and porcelain.

A titanium framework veneered with acrylic for the reproduction of the teeth and soft tissues has become a commonly used option. Milling of titanium results in a passive frame that is not subject to distortion when veneered with acrylic. The cost is less than that of the alternative options. It is believed that the elasticity of the frame and the acrylic contribute to absorbing part of the stresses that otherwise would be borne by the implants. On the other hand, fracture and staining of the acrylic have been reported in several studies as a frequent complication (Malo et al. 2003, Jemt & Johansson 2006, Bryant et al. 2007).

Gold alloy frameworks veneered with acrylic were widely used when Branemark introduced the first protocols for the restoration of the edentulous mandible (Branemark et al. 1995, Lindquist et al. 1996). The high cost of gold alloy frameworks, which are cast, introduces the possibility of distortion and therefore a non-passive fit. As a result, titanium has progressively replaced the use of gold alloys for frameworks.

More recently, zirconia has been introduced in combination with porcelain as a viable alternative. The advantages of zirconia/porcelain prostheses are: biocompatibility, accuracy, passive fit, colour stability, wear resistance and aesthetics (Holst et al. 2006, Van Dooren 2007, Wohrle & Cornell 2008). However, chipping of the veneering porcelain has been reported. It is also believed that contrary to what happens in the case of titanium/acrylic prostheses, the high elastic modulus of zirconia may increase and concentrate the stresses borne by the implants. In addition, there are no long-term studies documenting the clinical outcomes of zirconia/porcelain prostheses used to restore the edentulous mandible.

References

Attard, N.J. & Zarb, A. (2004) Long-term treatment outcomes in edentulous patients with implant overdentures: the Toronto study. *International Journal of Prosthodontics*, 17 (4), 425–433.

Branemark, P.-I., Svensson, B. & van Steenberghe, D. (1995) Ten-year survival rates of fixed prostheses on four or six implants ad modum Branemark in full edentulism. *Clinical Oral Implants Research*, 6 (4), 227–231.

Bryant, S.R., MacDonald-Jankowski, D. & Kim, K. (2007) Does the type of implant prosthetic affect outcomes for the completely edentulous arch? *International Journal of Oral & Maxillofacial Implants*, 22 (Suppl.), 117–139.

Chee, W. & Jivraj, S. (2006) Treatment planning of the edentulous mandible. *British Dental Journal*, 201 (6), 337–347.

Cochran, D.L., Morton, D. & Weber, H.P. (2004) Consensus statement and recommended clinical procedures regarding loading protocols for endosseous dental implants. *International Journal of Oral & Maxillofacial Implants*, 19 (Suppl.), 109–113.

Cooper, L.F., Scurria, M.S., Lang, L.A. et al. (1999) Treatment of edentulism using Astra Tech implants and ball abutments to retain mandibular overdentures. *International Journal of Oral & Maxillofacial Implants*, 14 (5), 646–653.

De Bruyn, H., Kish, J., Collaert, B. et al. (2001) Fixed mandibular restorations on three early-loaded regular platform Branemark implants. *Clinical Implant Dentistry and Related Research*, 3 (4), 176–184.

Del Fabbro, M., Testori, T., Francetti, L. et al. (2006) Systematic review of survival rates for immediately loaded dental implants. *International Journal of Periodontics & Restorative Dentistry*, 26 (3), 249–263.

Emami, E., Heydecke, G., Rompre, P.H. et al. (2009) Impact of implant support for mandibular dentures on satisfaction, oral and general health-related quality of life: a meta-analysis of randomized-controlled trials. *Clinical Oral Implants Research*, 20 (6), 533–544.

Engquist, B., Astrand, P., Anzen, B. et al. (2005) Simplified methods of implant treatment in the edentulous lower jaw: a 3-year follow-up report of a controlled prospective study of one-stage versus two-stage surgery and early loading. *Clinical Implant Dentistry and Related Research*, 7 (2), 95–103.

Engstrand, P., Grondahl, K., Ohrnell, L.-O. et al. (2003) Prospective follow-up study of 95 patients with edentulous mandibles treated according to the Branemark novum concept. *Clinical Implant Dentistry and Related Research*, 5 (1), 3–10.

Feine, J., Maskawi, K., de Grandmont, P. et al. (1994) Within-subject comparisons of implant supported mandibular prostheses: evaluation of masticatory function. *Journal of Dental Research*, 73 (10), 1646–1656.

Fenlon, M.R. & Sherriff, M. (2008) An investigation of factors influencing patients' satisfaction with new complete dentures using structural equation modelling. *Journal of Dentistry*, 36 (6), 427–434.

Fontijn-Tekamp, F.A., Slagter, A.P., Van Der Bilt, A. et al. (2000) Biting and chewing in overdentures, full dentures, and natural dentitions. *Journal of Dental Research*, 79 (7), 1519–1524.

Friberg, B., Henningsson, C. & Jemt, T. (2005) Rehabilitation of edentulous mandibles by means of turned Branemark system implants after one-stage surgery: a 1-year retrospective study of 152 patients. *Clinical Implant Dentistry and Related Research*, 1 (1), 7–9.

Heydecke, G., Boudrias, P., Awad, M.A. et al. (2003) Within-subject comparisons of maxillary fixed and removable implant prostheses. Patient satisfaction and choice of prosthesis. *Clinical Oral Implants Research*, 14 (1), 125–130.

Holst, S., Bergler, M., Steger, E. et al. (2006) The application of zirconium oxide frameworks for implant superstructures. *Quintessence of Dental Technology*, 29, 103–112.

Jemt, T. & Johansson, J. (2006) Implant treatment in the edentulous maxillae: a 15-year follow-up study on 76 consecutive patients provided with fixed prostheses. *Clinical Implant Dentistry and Related Research*, 8 (2), 61–69.

Lindquist, L.W., Carlsson, G.E. & Jemt, T. (1996) A prospective 15-years follow-up study of mandibular fixed prostheses supported by osseointegrated implants. Clinical results and marginal bone loss. *Clinical Oral Implants Research*, 7 (4), 329–336.

Malo, P., Rangert, B. & Nobre, M. (2003) 'All-on-Four' immediate-function concept with Branemark System implants for completely edentulous mandibles: a retrospective clinical study. *Clinical Implant Dentistry and Related Research*, 5 (Suppl. 1), 2–9.

Mericske-Stern, R. (1990) Clinical evaluation of overdenture restorations supported by osseointegrated titanium implants: a retrospective study. *International Journal of Oral & Maxillofacial Implants*, 5 (4), 375–383.

Ostman, P.O. (2008) Immediate /early loading of dental implants. Clinical documentation and presentation of a treatment concept. *Periodontology* 2000, 47, 90–112.

Sadowsky, S.J. (2001) Mandibular implant-retained overdentures: a literature review. *Journal of Prosthetic Dentistry*, 86 (5), 468–473.

Testori, T., Del Fabbro, M., Szmukler-Moncler, S. *et al.* (2003) Immediate occlusal loading of Osseotite implants in the completely edentulous mandible. *International Journal of Oral & Maxillofacial Implants*, 18 (4), 544–551.

Van Dooren, E. (2007) Using zirconia in esthetic implant restorations. *Quintessence of Dental Technology* 30, 119–128.

Wohrle, P.S. & Cornell, D.F. (2008) Contemporary maxillary implant-supported full-arch restorations combining esthetics and passive fit. *Quintessence of Dental Technology*, 31, 1–47.

Appendix 4

Case Summary Template

Patient (Name and Date of birth):

Presenting complaints

Chief complaint
Subsidiary complaints
History of complaints
Patient's expectations

History
Medical history

Medical Practitioner

Respiratory

Cardiovascular

Gastrointestinal

Neurological

Endocrine

Developmental

Musculoskeletal

Genitourinary

Haematological

Other

Allergies
Smoking
Infectious diseases
Pregnancy
Hospitalisation
Medications

Social history

Marital status

Children

Occupation

Smoking   Type
                   Frequency
                   Period

Recreational drugs

Diet   ☐   Soft drinks
                   ☐   Sports drinks
                   ☐   Lemons
                   ☐   Acidic foods
                   ☐   Sweet foods
                   ☐   Water
                   ☐   Tea
                   ☐   Coffee
                   ☐   Alcohol
                   ☐   Hard/brittle foods
                   ☐   Ice crunching

Habits/hobbies   ☐   Musical instrument
                   ☐   Exercise
                   ☐   Oral habits

Oral Rehabilitation: A Case-Based Approach, First Edition. Edited by Iven Klineberg, Diana Kingston.
© 2012 Blackwell Publishing Ltd. Published 2012 by Blackwell Publishing Ltd.

Dental history

	Additional information
Date of last examination	
Oral hygiene ☐ Brushing	
☐ Flossing	
☐ Mouthwash	
☐ Toothpaste	
Treatment ☐ Restorations	
☐ Endodontics	
☐ Periodontics	
☐ Orthodontics	
☐ RDP	
☐ FDP	
☐ TMD	
☐ OMFS	

Extraoral examination
Aesthetics

Facial symmetry	
Profile	
Nasolabial angle	
Facial folds	
Midlines	Face/maxillary centrals
	Maxillary central alignment
	Maxillary/mandibular centrals
Lip posture	Symmetry
	Upper lip
	Lower lip
	Competence
	Tooth display
Occlusal plane	Parallel to ala tragus line
	Parallel to interpupillary line
	Over-eruption
Vertical	FWS
	OVD assessment
Smile assessment	Symmetry
	Lip line
	Gingival display
	Tooth display
	Buccal corridor

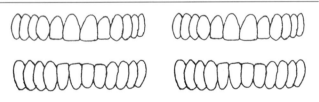

At rest   Broad smile

Phonetics

	Normal	Abnormal
Labial (m)	☐	☐
Labiodental (f/v)	☐	☐
Linguodental (th)	☐	☐
Interdental (s)	☐	☐
Linguopalatal (k/ng)	☐	☐

Temporomandibular assessment

TMJ	Additional information
Click ☐	
Crepitus ☐	
Tenderness ☐	

Muscle tenderness	Right	Left
Temporalis	☐	☐
Masseter	☐	☐
Posterior mandible	☐	☐
Anterior mandible	☐	☐

Glands
Nodes

Jaw movement	Measurement (mm)	Reference points
Maximal opening		
Right laterotrusion		
Left laterotrusion		
Midline deviation		
Maximal protrusion		
Opening pathway		
Overjet		
Overbite		

Further investigation required

Intraoral examination
Soft tissues

Tissue	Healthy	Abnormal	Additional information
Lips	☐	☐	
Labial vestibule	☐	☐	
Cheeks	☐	☐	
Palate	☐	☐	
Oropharynx	☐	☐	
Tongue	☐	☐	
Floor	☐	☐	
Frenal attachments	☐	☐	

Ridges	Maxilla	Mandible
Arch shape		
Resorption		
Palatal vault		
Tori		
Frenal attachments		
Mucosa		
Pathology		

Oral cleanliness

Condition	Yes	No
Plaque	☐	☐
Calculus	☐	☐
Food impaction	☐	☐
Stains	☐	☐
Halitosis	☐	☐

Saliva

Water intake
Quality
Quantity
Pathology
Medications affecting

Further investigation required

Periodontium

CPITN

Gingiva — Biotype, Colour, Contour, Consistency

Papillae — Colour, Contour

Periodontal charting

Maxillary buccal

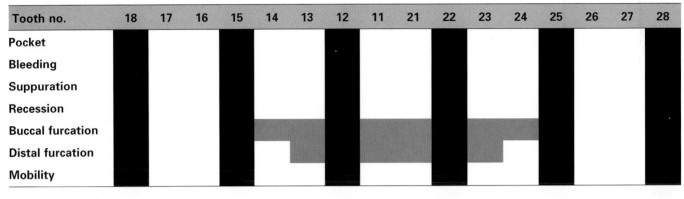

Maxillary palatal

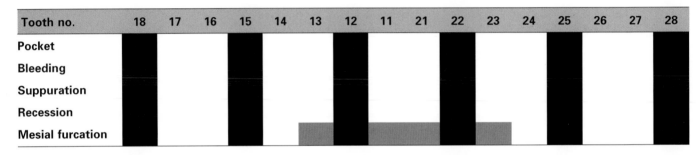

Mandibular lingual

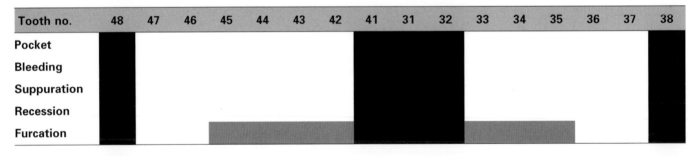

Mandibular buccal

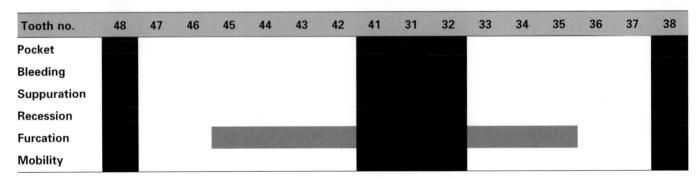

Occlusion

Skeletal classification
Dental occlusion
Angle right
Angle left
Anterior overbite
Anterior overjet
Cross-bites
Open-bites
Curve of Spee
Curve of Wilson
RP to IP slide
FWS

Tooth guidance

Right laterotrusion

<u>8 7 6 5 4 3 2 1 | 1 2 3 4 5 6 7 8</u>

8 7 6 5 4 3 2 1   1 2 3 4 5 6 7 8

Left laterotrusion

<u>8 7 6 5 4 3 2 1 | 1 2 3 4 5 6 7 8</u>

8 7 6 5 4 3 2 1   1 2 3 4 5 6 7 8

Protrusion

<u>8 7 6 5 4 3 2 1 | 1 2 3 4 5 6 7 8</u>

8 7 6 5 4 3 2 1   1 2 3 4 5 6 7 8

Tooth surface loss

Caries

<u>8 7 6 5 4 3 2 1 | 1 2 3 4 5 6 7 8</u>

8 7 6 5 4 3 2 1   1 2 3 4 5 6 7 8

Attrition

<u>8 7 6 5 4 3 2 1 | 1 2 3 4 5 6 7 8</u>

8 7 6 5 4 3 2 1   1 2 3 4 5 6 7 8

Erosion (specify surface)

<u>8 7 6 5 4 3 2 1 | 1 2 3 4 5 6 7 8</u>

8 7 6 5 4 3 2 1   1 2 3 4 5 6 7 8

Abrasion (specify surface)

<u>8 7 6 5 4 3 2 1 | 1 2 3 4 5 6 7 8</u>

8 7 6 5 4 3 2 1   1 2 3 4 5 6 7 8

Abfraction (specify surface)

<u>8 7 6 5 4 3 2 1 | 1 2 3 4 5 6 7 8</u>

8 7 6 5 4 3 2 1   1 2 3 4 5 6 7 8

Dental charting

Tooth no.	Clinical findings	Comments
18		
17		
16		
15		
14		
13		
12		
11		
21		
22		
23		
24		
25		
26		
27		
28		
38		
37		
36		
35		
34		
33		
32		
31		
41		
42		
43		
44		
45		
46		
47		
48		

Previous dentures

Teeth replaced   <u>8 7 6 5 4 3 2 1 | 1 2 3 4 5 6 7 8</u>

8 7 6 5 4 3 2 1 1 2 3 4 5 6 7 8

	Maxilla	Mandible
Age/number		
Type		
Kennedy classification		
Appearance		
LFH		
Stability		
Support		
Retention		
Hygiene		
Patient opinion		

Special tests

	Performed	Additional information
Percussion	☐	
Palpation	☐	
Vitality	☐	
Cusp loading	☐	
Transillumination	☐	
Selective anaesthesia	☐	
Other	☐	

Radiographs
Orthopantomogram (date)

Features	Radiographic data
TMJ	
Bone loss	
Sinuses	
Mandibular foramen and canal	
Mental foramen	
Retained roots	
Pathology	

Periapical films

Information		Information
18		38
17		37
16		36
15		35
14		34
13		33
12		32
11		31
21		41
22		42
23		43
24		44
25		45
26		46
27		47
28		48

Other radiographs

	Date	Radiographic data
OPG		
Lat ceph		
OPG		
Lat ceph		

Study casts

Articulation	Position
	Face bow
Diagnostic wax-up	OVD change
	Occlusal adjustment
	Crown lengthening

Problem list

Problem list	Details
Medical condition	
Aesthetics	
Speech	
TMD	
Soft tissue	
Oral hygiene	
Saliva	
Periodontal	
Edentulism	
Occlusion	
Tooth surface loss	
Restorative	
Prosthetic	
Endodontic	

Treatment options
Maxilla

Treatment option 1	Treatment time	Cost
	Total	$

Treatment option 2	Treatment time	Cost
	Total	$

Treatment option 3	Treatment time	Cost
	Total	$

Treatment option 4	Treatment time	Cost
	Total	$

Mandible

Treatment option 1	Treatment time	Cost
	Total	$

Treatment option 2	Treatment time	Cost
	Total	$

Treatment option 3	Treatment time	Cost
	Total	$

Treatment plan
• Maxilla: Treatment option
• Mandible: Treatment option

Treatment phase	Detail	Timeline	Cost
Hygiene phase			
Pre-prosthetic pretreatment phase I			
Pre-prosthetic pretreatment phase II			
Prosthetic phase			
Maintenance			
		Total	$

18	**17**	**16**	**15**	**14**	**13**	**12**	**11**	**21**	**22**	**23**	**24**	**25**	**26**	**27**	**28**
48	**47**	**46**	**45**	**44**	**43**	**42**	**41**	**31**	**32**	**33**	**34**	**35**	**36**	**37**	**38**

ACC, all-ceramic crown; MCC, metal-ceramic crown; P, pontic; I, implant.

Treatment sequence

Appointment	Procedure	Time (minutes)	Cost
1			
2			
3			
4			
5			
6			
7			
8			
9			
10			
11			
12			
13			
14			
15			
16			
17			
18			
Total			$0

Treatment discussion

References

Index

Oral Rehabilitation: A Case-Based Approach, First Edition. Edited by Iven Klineberg, Diana Kingston.
© 2012 Blackwell Publishing Ltd. Published 2012 by Blackwell Publishing Ltd.